河南省中医药文化著作出版资助专项
（编号：TCMCB2023015）

河南省高等学校青年骨干教师培养项目
（编号：2020GGJS112）

河南省高等教育教学改革研究与实践（研究生教育类）项目
（编号：2023SJGLX223Y）

2023 年教育部产学研协同育人项目：
基于虚拟现实技术的河南中医药大学翻译硕士（MTI）实践基地建设研究
（编号：230805701080157）

2024 年河南省哲学社会科学规划青年项目：
数字人文视域下中医药国际传播的话语形象建构与提升路径研究

U0194952

Bilingual (English) Communication in
Traditional Chinese Medicine Application

中医应用双语(英语)交流

何 阳 李 蕊 宋文刚 王琳琳 主编

河南大学出版社
HENAN UNIVERSITY PRESS
·郑州·

图书在版编目(CIP)数据

中医应用双语(英语)交流 / 何阳等主编. -- 郑州：
河南大学出版社,2024.6. -- ISBN 978-7-5649-5970-8

Ⅰ. R2

中国国家版本馆 CIP 数据核字第 20246HB893 号

中医应用双英(英语)交流

ZHONGYI YINGYONG SHUANGYU (YINGYU) JIAOLIU

责任编辑 　马　博　　时二凤
责任校对 　王　珂
封面设计 　马　龙

出版发行 　河南大学出版社
　　　　　　地址:郑州市郑东新区商务外环中华大厦 2401 号　　　邮编:450046
　　　　　　电话:0371-22860116(南方出版中心)
　　　　　　　　 0371-86059701(营销发行中心)　网址:hupress.henu.edu.cn
排　版 　郑州市今日文教印制有限公司
印　刷 　广东虎彩云印刷有限公司
版　次 　2024 年 6 月第 1 版　　　　　**印　次** 　2024 年 6 月第 1 次印刷
开　本 　787 mm×1092 mm　1/16　　**印　张** 　33.5
字　数 　767 千字　　　　　　　　　**定　价** 　89.00 元

(本书如有印装质量问题,请与河南大学出版社营销发行中心联系调换。)

Preface

前 言

习近平新时代中国特色社会主义思想关于推动中医药健康养生文化创造性转化、创新性发展的指示精神,特别是习近平"一带一路"倡议为中西医文化交流、中医药走向世界指明了方向。机遇来临的同时,势必对中医、西医诊疗从业人员专业提升、对外学术沟通交流能力提出更高的要求:(1)如何让从事西医临床的国内外同行了解中医、认识中医,同时又能借助于地道的语言媒介"助我中医,走向世界"?(2)多元文化格局下如何实现中西医文化平等交流,优势互补?(3)如何向世界推介我们的中医国粹,为喜爱中医、中国传统文化的外国朋友搭建一个学习交流、沟通的平台?本书旨在满足以上需求,消除沟通障碍。

全书中英文对照,按照医院真实中西医诊疗流程分为六个章节,涵盖导医、中西医问诊、检查诊断、处方与指导用药、住院与出院等各个环节,附有真实情景对话案例以及全方位的多种替换情景,"点"(词汇)、"线"(替换情景)、"面"(对话案例)结合,重在突出其实际交流应用价值。同时,本书以中医文化和中医问诊部分为重要章节内容,立足祖国传统医学,凸显中医辨证治则、经络脉诊、方剂用药、养生保健等文化特色,尊重多元文化格局下的中西医文化平等原则,有利于重构中医文化主体话语意识,既可满足河南中西医学临床人员病案融合交流,拓展专业视野、走向国际的语言交流需求,又顺应了关注中医治未病、药食同源、绿色大健康等天人合一中医哲学思维治则新趋势。本书最后还将国际知名医学期刊、机构的中英文名称作为附录部分,希望助力国内的医疗科研人员论文、论著的检索、发表、出版与世界接轨,并为中国援非医疗队国内专业英语培训借鉴和使用。

本书理论依据具有以下三个方面的显著特点:

文化性:语言是文化的载体,"The bridge of understanding and friendship cannot be built without language.——Yang Jiechi"(没有语言,就无法搭建起

理解与友谊的桥梁。——杨洁篪),传承文化离不开鲜活的语言交流。致中致和、生生不息的中医传统文化蕴含着天人合一的中国哲学独特审美与治疗原则,理应与西医文化体系平分秋色,和谐共生;英语作为全球通用的语言,是实现"一带一路"所倡导的与沿线各国文化交流、坚持"中医药走出去"的工具,符合推动中医药走向世界的指示精神。

科学性:树立文化自信,重构中医文化的主体话语意识;尊重多元文化差异,构建平等多元文化交流语境意识;打造复合型英语交际人才,强化中医文化知识储备意识;立足西医系统临床体系,建立中西医学经典病案融合交流意识。

普及性:繁荣中医药文化,推动中医药强省战略实施,服务健康中原建设,消除中西医学交流障碍,"助我中医,走向世界"已摆在每一个从事中医药文化传承及关系国民健康医疗人员的面前。

衷心感谢在本书的编写过程中,给予大力鼓励、专业指导与支持的河南中医药大学副校长田力博士/主任医师,河南省医药科学研究院何伟博士/研究员,郑州大学第一附属医院主任医师王晓娟,河南省中医药研究院副主任医师张爱华,中国援厄立特里亚第 14 批医疗队队长、焦作市中医院赵延兵院长/主任医师,以及心血管内科外籍专家 Mikias Legesse Gebrenedhin(米基亚斯·莱格塞·格布雷内丁)。

同时,还要把最真诚的感谢送给为完成这部书稿精诚合作、付出努力的援非医疗队的战友和同事:漯河医学高等专科学校病理学宋文刚副教授(负责第一、三章,合计 16 万字),河南中医药大学外语学院李蕊副教授(负责第二、六章,合计 20 万字)、王琳琳副教授(负责第四、五章及附录,合计 16 万字)。

由于水平有限,加之医疗范围涉及甚广,挂一漏万,在所难免,书中不当之处,恳请读者朋友批评指正。

编 者

2023 年 1 月 6 日于郑州

Contents

目 录

Chapter 1   Registration at the Entrance

第 1 章   导医问诊

Section 1   Registration

第 1 节   挂号

Ⅰ. Dialogues 情景对话

1. Registration 挂号

Doctor：Do you want to see a doctor?

请问，你是要看病吗？

Patient：Yes, where can I register?

是的，在哪儿挂号？

Doctor：Here, have you ever been here before?

这儿，你以前来过吗？

Patient：Yes, half a year ago. / No, this is my first visit.

是的，半年前来过。/ 没有，我这是第一次来。

Doctor：Have you a registration card?

你有挂号证吗？

Patient：Yes, here it is. / No, I forgot to bring it.

有，在这儿呢。/ 没有，我忘带了。

Doctor：Do you remember your card number?

那你还记得挂号证号码吗？

Patient：Yes, it is W dash six, six, eight, five, eight. / No, I can't remember it.

记得,是 W-66858. / 不,不记得了。

Doctor：When did you come last?

你上次是什么时候来的呢?

Patient：About a week ago.

一个星期以前吧。

Doctor：Then I will find out for you. Oh, yes. Mr. Smith, you are working in the Japanese Embassy. Please pay for the registration.

那好,我帮你查查。你是在日本大使馆工作的史密斯先生吧。请交挂号费。

Patient：Oh, yes, thank you. How much?

哦,是的,谢谢。多少钱?

Doctor：Five yuan.

五块钱。

2. Appointment 预约

Receptionist：Good morning, madame.

早上好,夫人。

Mrs. Ford：Good morning, Miss Receptionist. I'm Mrs. Ford. Can I make an appointment to come and see Dr. Barber some time today?

早上好,接线员小姐。我是福特夫人,请问我今天能预约个时间来看巴伯医生吗?

Receptionist：Certainly. I'm Miss White. Wait, let me see, while, can you come at half past ten, Mrs. Ford?

当然可以啦。你叫我怀特小姐好了。请稍等,让我看看,噢,你能十点半来吗,福特夫人?

Mrs. Ford：Fine. Thank you, Miss White.

好的,可以。谢谢你,怀特小姐。

II. Sentences 替换句型

(1) May I help you?

我能帮你什么忙?

(2) Take care, please. Nurses are used to dealing with sick people gently and patiently.

放心,护士习惯于温和、耐心地接待病人。

(3) Grip my hand. Please come this way.

握紧我的手,请这边走。

(4) I shan't hurt you. Just lie still and relax.

我不会弄疼你,躺着别动,请放松。

(5) If doctor is examining the patient, wait outside the door.

如果医生正在给病人做检查,请在门外等候。

(6) Can you speak Chinese?

你会说汉语吗?

(7) Remember to bring your hospital appointment card with you every time.

每次来医院就医请记着带上你的预约卡。

(8) Is registration for initial visit at counter No. 1?

请问初诊挂号是在1号窗口吗?

(9) Registration for second visit is at counter No. 2.

复诊挂号请到2号窗口。

(10) Please show me your ID card (diplomatic certificate, passport, experts card…).

请出示你的身份证(外交官证、护照、专家证……)。

(11) What is your position in the ambassy?

请问你在大使馆是做什么工作的?

(12) I'm the ambassador (minister, commercial/administrative/political counsellor, first/second/third secretary, consul…).

我是大使(公使、商务/行政/政务参赞、一/二/三等秘书、领事……)。

(13) What is your work here?

你在这儿做什么工作?

(14) I'm a delegate (a businessman, a pilot, an engineer, a teacher, a musician, a taxi-driver, a retired worker, a housewife…).

我是一名代表团成员(商人、飞行员、工程师、教师、音乐人、出租车司机、退休工人、家庭主妇……)。

(15) How long do you intend to stay here?

你准备在这儿待多久?

(16) I am a tourist. I am leaving tomorrow morning (About a week/ Till the end of this year…).

我是一名游客,明天早上就走(在这儿待一周/ 在这儿待到今年年底……)。

(17) I'll make a file for you, please write down your full name in block letters.

我给你填一份病历,请用印刷体写上你的全名。

(18) Are you married or single, and your address, please?

你结婚了还是单身? 你的住址在哪儿?

(19) I'm divorced. And I live in Huayuan Hotel (… Embassy, … road… building… block… number).

我离婚了。我住在花园酒店(……使馆,……路……号楼……单元……号)。

(20) Have you any small change?

你有零钱吗?

(21) Here is your receipt and change. And this is you registration card. Please don't lose it and carry it with you whenever you come.

这是你的收据和找回的零钱。另外,还有你的挂号证,请收好,记得每次就诊时带上。

(22) What's wrong with you today? And which department do you want to register with?

你今天哪儿不舒服? 要挂哪科的号?

(23) I don't know which clinic. I have a rash all over my body, and it itches badly.

我也不知道挂哪科。我浑身起红疹,而且痒得厉害。

(24) You should see a dermatologist first, I think. If necessary I'll transfer you to the physician.

那你先看看皮肤科吧,需要的话再转内科。

(25) My baby has had diarrhea since yesterday and kept on vomiting. I'd like him to see a pediatrician.

我孩子从昨天开始腹泻,一直呕吐,我想让他看看儿科。

(26) I want to see a physician (an internist, a surgeon, a gynaecologist,

an obstetrician, a pediatrician, a neurologist, a dermatologist, an oculist, an ENT. specialist, a TCM doctor, an allergist, a urologist, an orthopedist, a dentist, an endocrinologist…).

我要看病，挂（内科，外科，妇科，产科，儿科，神经科，皮肤科，眼科，耳鼻喉科，中医科，过敏反应科，泌尿科，骨科，牙科，内分泌科……）的号。

（27）I want to have a denture fitted/my teeth cleaned, could you please make an appointment for me?

我想镶牙/洗牙，请给我约个时间好吗？

（28）Sorry, the department of orthopedics is closed today. Please observe the clinical hours.

对不起，今天整形外科不开诊。请你按门诊时间来就诊。

（29）Under the National Health Service poor people go to their doctors more than they used to.

在国家医疗保健服务体系下，穷人比过去更看得起医生了。

（30）Ophthalmology is only open till noon every day.

眼科每天只有上午半天的门诊。

（31）Your turn is next. (It's your turn now. / There are only two more patients before you. The patient before you is a rather complicated case, I'm so sorry that you have to wait at least half an hour.)

下一个就轮到你了。（该你看病了。/你前面还有两个病人。抱歉，你前面的那个病人病况较为复杂，你至少还得再等半个小时。）

（32）Nurse, I feel uncomfortable now. Could you please fetch me a glass of water?

护士，我现在很不舒服，请你给我拿杯水，好吗？

Ⅲ. Words and Expressions 单词和短语

1. At the Entrance 在候诊大厅

clinic /ˈklɪnɪk/ n. 门诊室
corridor /ˈkɒrɪdɔː/ n. 走廊
counter /ˈkaʊntə/ n. 窗口
dispensary /dɪˈspensəri/ n. 药房
elevator /ˈelɪveɪtə/; lift /lɪft/ n. 电梯

emergency room 急救室
examination room 诊室
initial visit 初诊
inpatient department 住院部
outpatient clinic; outpatient department 门诊部

privy /'prɪvi/; necessary /'nesəsəri/ n. 厕所

reception /rɪ'sepʃn/ n. 问讯处；服务台

register /'redʒɪstə/ v. 挂号

register's office 挂号处

second visit 复诊

waiting room/waiting hall 候诊室/厅

water closet; toilet /'tɔɪlət/; lavatory /'lævətri/ n. 厕所；洗手间

2. External Parts of the Body
身体外部名称

adam's apple 喉结

ankle /'æŋkl/ n. 踝；脚腕

arm /a:m/ n. 臂

armpit /'a:mpɪt/ n. 腋下

back /bæk/ n. 背

back of head 后脑勺

back of the hand 手背

belly /'beli/; abdomen /'æbdəmən/ n. 腹

bend of the arm 胳臂弯

big toe 大脚趾

breast /brest/ n. 胸

buttock /'bʌtək/ n. 臀部

calf /ka:f/ n. 小腿肚

cheek /tʃi:k/ n. 面颊

chest /tʃest/; thorax /'θɔ:ræks/ n. 胸腔

chin /tʃɪn/ n. 下巴(颏)

crown /kraʊn/ n. 头顶

elbow /'elbəʊ/ n. 肘

finger /'fɪŋgə/ n. 手指

fist /fɪst/ n. 拳

foot /fʊt/ n. 足

forearm /'fɔ:ra:m/ n. 前臂

forehead /'fɒrɪd/ /'fɔ:hed/ n. 额

groin /grɔɪn/ n. 鼠蹊(大腿根儿)

hand /hænd/ n. 手

head /hed/ n. 头

heel /hi:l/ n. 踵；脚跟

hip /hɪp/ n. 胯

index finger 食指

instep /'ɪnstep/ n. 脚背

jaw /dʒɔ:/ n. 颚

kneecap /'ni:ˌkæp/ n. 膝盖

knee-hollow; ham /hæm/ n. 腘；腿弯子

knee /ni:/; genu /'dʒenju:/ n. 膝

knuckle /'nʌkl/ n. 指节

leg /leg/ n. 腿

little finger 小指

loin /lɔɪn/ n. 腰眼

lower leg; shank /ʃæŋk/ n. 小腿

lower limbs 下肢

middle finger; long finger 中指

moon /mu:n/ n. 月牙儿

nail bed; nail matrix 甲床

nail /neɪl/ n. 指甲

nape /neɪp/ n. 脖梗子；颈背

navel /'neɪvl/ n. 脐

neck /nek/ n. 颈

palm /pa:m/ n. 手掌

ring finger 无名指

shoulder /'ʃəʊldə/ n. 肩

sole /səʊl/ n. 脚底

temple /'templ/ n. 太阳穴

thigh /θaɪ/ n. 股；大腿

thumb /θʌm/ n. 拇指

toe /təʊ/ n. 脚趾

trunk /trʌŋk/ n. 躯干

upper arm 上臂

upper limbs 上肢

waist /weɪst/ *n.* 腰

wrist /rɪst/ *n.* 手腕

Section 2　Emergency
第 2 节　急诊

I. Dialogues 情景对话

1. Appendicitis 阑尾炎

Patient：Doctor，I've got an awful pain in my stomach. I feel like vomiting.

医生，我肚子疼，恶心想吐。

Doctor：How long have you had it?

疼了有多久了？

Patient：Since last night，it was in the middle at first around my belly. But this morning it moved to the right.

昨天晚上开始的，先是肚子当中疼，可今天早晨就转移到右边了。

Doctor：Has it moved again?

疼又向别处窜了吗？

Patient：No. It's been steady for four hours.

没有，固定在这儿已经四个小时了。

Doctor：Is it there all the time?

一直持续不断这样疼吗？

Patient：No, it just comes and goes.

不是，好一阵，坏一阵。

Doctor：Have you had any diarrhea?

有腹泻吗？

Patient：No, I haven't had a bowel movement for two days.

没有，我已经两天没有大便了。

Doctor：Have you had any nausea and vomiting?

你恶心、呕吐吗?

Patient：Well，now it's a bit better. But last night I vomited every two hours, soon after the pain began.

现在好些了。可是昨天晚上我差不多每两小时吐一次,一疼就吐。

Doctor：Have you had a temperature?

你发烧吗?

Patient：Last night I took my temperature. It was 38℃.

昨晚我量的体温是38℃。

Doctor：Show me where it hurts most right now.

给我指一指你现在最疼的部位。

Patient：Just here.

就这儿。

Doctor：Please lie down. Let me examine your abdomen. Do you feel any pain when I press here? Does it hurt you when I withdraw my hand suddenly? … you have appendicitis. You must have an operation.

躺下,我检查一下你的肚子。我按的这个地方疼吗? 我突然抬手时疼得是否更重了呢? ……你得阑尾炎了,需要手术治疗。

Patient：Is it serious?

危险吗?

Doctor：It could be if we don't operate.

如果不手术,可能会有危险的。

Patient：All right, doctor. I agree.

好吧,医生,我同意。

Doctor：While, we must have your consent. Please sign this paper consenting to have the operation.

可是我们必须征得你的同意才行。那就请在这单子上签上你同意做手术吧。

Patient：All right.

好的。

Doctor：Don't worry, everything will be OK.

不用担心,一切都会好起来的。

Patient：I really hope so, doctor, thank you very much.

但愿如此吧。谢谢你啊,医生。

2. Inquiry 问询

Doctor：Did you have any childhood diseases?

你童年患过什么疾病吗?

Patient：As far as I remember I had whooping cough, chicken-pox and measles, but most of the times I had a healthy childhood.

我记得我得过百日咳、水痘和麻疹,但大多数时候还是很健康的。

Doctor：Is any member of your family suffering from any special diseases, such as tuberculosis, hypertension, diabetes or cancers, etc.?

你家族成员中有无患肺结核、高血压、糖尿病或者什么癌症的呢?

Patient：No, never.

不,从没有。

Doctor：And are you allergic to any medicine?

那你对什么药物过敏吗?

Patient：Sorry, I don't know.

抱歉,我不知道。

Ⅱ. Sentences 替换句型

(1) You'd better ring 120 for an ambulance at once.

你最好马上打 120 叫一辆救护车。

(2) They promise they will come right away.

他们说了马上就来。

(3) Dad, can you tolerate this pain? / Is this pain bearable?

爸爸,你能忍受住疼痛吗?

(4) Foreign bodies may still lodge in the trachea.

异物可能还滞留在气管内。

(5) Open your mouth as wide as you can, and put tongue out (stick out

your tongue) as far as you can, please.

请尽量张大嘴,并尽力伸出舌头。

(6) Come, please help him lie on his back(stomach, right side, left side).

来,请帮一下忙,让他仰卧(俯卧、右侧卧、左侧卧)。

(7) Let me take your body temperature, and please put the thermometer under your arm.

来,把体温计放在腋下,我给你量一下体温。

(8) Be quick. Take his blood pressure, and then feel his pulse.

快点,量一下他的血压,再测一下他的脉搏。

(9) OK, please bend your knees, relax, and breathe deeply (normally).

好的,请屈膝,放松,深呼吸(正常呼吸)。

(10) The most common cause of facial injury is the road traffic accident.

脸部外伤最常见的原因是公路交通事故。

(11) Acute anaphylaxis is one of the most urgent and alarming emergencies.

急性过敏是最紧急和令人担忧的急诊之一。

(12) Can you tell me what bothered you most? / And what do you find is the most uncomfortable?

告诉我,你哪儿最难受?

(13) The patient complained of epigastric pain accompanied by distension, belching and nausea.

病人感到胃脘(即上腹部)疼痛,并伴有腹胀、打嗝和恶心现象。

(14) Please do let me know if you become more sick.

你感觉再有不舒服时,告诉我一声。

(15) When did you have your last dizzy spell?

你最近的一次眩晕发作是什么时候?

(16) Do you drink or smoke? We have evidence that cigarette smoking exerts a harmful effect on the heart.

你喝酒或抽烟吗? 研究证实,吸烟的确对心脏有害。

(17) Every day (Sometimes), a lot (a little).

天天(有时)喝,喝很多(很少)。

(18) —How many cigarettes do you smoke every day? —A pack.

——你一天抽多少支烟呢? ———一包吧。

(19) My neighbor was giving artificial mouth-to-mouth respiration while her husband was rushing to get a doctor.

我邻居正在进行口对口人工呼吸,这时她的丈夫正忙着找医生。

(20) He might collapse.

他可能会虚脱。

(21) The patient underwent closed mitral valvotomy last year.

病人去年做了闭式二尖瓣切开术。

(22) What is his eating habit? And does he eat regularly?

他吃饭习惯怎样? 进餐是否规律呢?

(23) Does she have regular movement (tend to have constipation, tend to have diarrhea)?

她大便每天是否正常(是否便秘、腹泻)?

(24) Do you sleep well? And how many hours can you sleep?

你睡眠好吗? 你一天你能睡几个小时呢?

(25) Did you use to get cramp?

你过去经常抽筋吗?

(26) The patient went to bed to relieve the pain of lumbar strain and a few hours later found he could not void.

病人上床睡觉来缓解腰肌劳损疼痛,而几小时后他发现自己不能排泄了。

(27) Early diagnosis makes all the difference in tuberculous meningitis.

早期诊断在结核性脑膜炎的治疗中关系重大。

(28) One reason for keeping beds empty in a ward is to prepare emergent admissions.

在病房内保留空床位的一个原因是保证急诊病人的住院需要。

(29) The casualty officer said: "The X-ray shows a Colles fracture. We'll have to make a plaster for your wrist. I'll ask the plaster technician to do this for you."

外伤急救官说:"X光片显示科勒斯氏(桡骨下端)骨折,我们不得不在你的腕上打石膏,我让石膏技师给你打上。"

(30) The surgeon will be ready to operate by ten o'clock.

外科医生将在十点准备好手术。

Ⅲ. Words and Expressions 单词和短语

1. Departments in the Hospitals 医院大部门

children's ward 儿科病房
disinfectious room 消毒室
dressing room 换药室
emergency unit/department 急救科
general office of hospital 医院办公室
general ward 普通病房
inquiry room 医务咨询室
intensive care unit (ICU) 重症监护室
isolation ward 隔离病房
laboratory /ləˈbɒrətri/ /lbrətəːri/ n. 化验室
lying-in room; delivery room 产房
male ward 男科病房
observation room 观察室
operation room 手术室
pharmacy /ˈfaːməsi/ n. 药房
private ward 头等/特护病房
recovery room 复苏室
treatment room 治疗室

2. Various Emergencies 各种急症

asphyxia /æsˈfɪksiə/;
　asphyxiation /əsˌfɪksiˈeɪʃn/ n. 窒息
drowning /ˈdraʊnɪŋ/ n. 溺死, 淹死
emergency /iˈmɜːdʒənsi/;
　accident /ˈæksɪdənt/ n. 急诊; 紧急
gas poisoning 煤气中毒
hanging /ˈhæŋɪŋ/ n. 绞死
homicide /ˈhɒmɪsaɪd/ n. 他杀
poisoning /ˈpɔɪzənɪŋ/ n. 中毒
strangulation /ˌstræŋɡjʊˈleɪʃn/ n. 勒死

suicide /ˈsuːɪˌsaɪd/; self-murder; self-slaughter n. 自杀
sunstroke /ˈsʌnstrəʊk/ n. 中暑
thermoplegia /ˌθɜːməʊˈpliːdʒiə/ n. 热射病
to take poison 服毒

3. Symptoms 症状

ache /eɪk/ n. 酸痛
asphyxiate /əsˈfɪksieɪt/ v. 使窒息
blocked (stuffed-up) nose 鼻塞
body temperature 体温
centigrade temperature 摄氏温度
choke /tʃəʊk/ v. 憋气
cold fits 阵冷
cold /kəʊld/ n. 发冷
cold sweat 冷汗
colic /ˈkɒlɪk/ n. 绞痛
cough /kɒf/ n. 咳嗽
difficult breathing; dyspnea /dɪsˈpniːə/ n. 呼吸困难
drowsy /ˈdraʊzi/; sleepy /ˈsliːpi/ adj. 思睡的; 嗜睡的
fahrenheit temperature 华氏温度
fever /ˈfiːvə/ n. 发烧
feverish /ˈfiːvərɪʃ/ adj. 发烧的
flatulence /ˈflætjʊləns/;
　flatus /ˈfleɪtəs/ n. 胃肠气胀
hacking cough 不停干咳
hawking /ˈhɔːkɪŋ/ n. 咳痰
hurt /hɜːt/ v. 发痛
inertia /iˈnɜːʃə/ n. 无力
insomnia /ɪnˈsɒmniə/ n. 失眠

loss of appetite 食欲不振

nausea /'nɔːsiə/ *n.* 恶心

night sweat 盗汗

nose bleeding; epistaxis /ˌepɪˈstæksɪs/
　　n. 鼻出血

other discomforts 其他不适

pain /peɪn/ *n.* 疼痛

paroxysmal cough 阵咳

running nose 流鼻涕

shaking /'ʃeɪkɪŋ/; shivering /'ʃɪvərɪŋ/;
　　trembling /'tremblɪŋ/ *n.* 战栗

sharp pain 剧痛

sleepless /'sliːpləs/ *adj.* 失眠的

sneeze /sniːz/ *n.* 打喷嚏

sore /sɔː/ *n.* 伤痛处

sputum /'spjuːtəm/; phlegm /flem/;
　　expectoration /ɪkˌspektəˈreɪʃn/ *n.* 痰

stabbing pain; pricking /'prɪkɪŋ/ *n.*;
　　prickling /'prɪklɪŋ/ *n.* 刺痛

stomach-ache /'stʌməkˌeɪk/ *n.* 胃痛

suffocation /ˌsʌfəˈkeɪʃn/ *n.* 堵闷

superacidity /sjuːpərəˈsɪdɪti/;
　　hyperacidity /ˌhaɪpərəˈsɪdɪti/ *n.*
　　胃酸过多

sweating /'swetɪŋ/;
　　perspiration /ˌpɜːspəˈreɪʃn/ *n.* 出汗

tenderness /'tendənəs/ *n.* 压痛

tender /'tendə/ *adj.* 疼痛的

vomit /'vɒmɪt/ *v.* 呕吐

yawn /jɔːn/ *v.* 打哈欠

Chapter 2　The Chinese Medicine

第 2 章　中医问诊

Section 1　Key Concepts of Chinese Medicine: Yin and Yang Theory

第 1 节　中医文化关键概念：阴阳理论

I. Key Concepts 核心概念

1. Yin and Yang 阴阳

Yin and yang are a philosophical concept in ancient China, containing the plain view of dialectics. Yin-yang theory of Chinese medicine is a theoretical system which combines ancient philosophical thoughts and medical practices. It includes two major aspects. First, yin and yang are the fundamental laws of nature, the principles of everything in creation, and the sources for all creatures to grow, develop, and change. Second, yin and yang are opposite, interdependent, mutually waxing and waning, as well as transforming. The theory runs through the entire medical field, aiming to expound the human structure, physiology, pathology, diagnosis, prevention, and treatment.

阴阳是中国古代哲学术语，含有朴素的辩证观。中医阴阳学说是古代哲学思想与医学实践相结合而形成的理论体系。其主要内容包括两个方面：首先，阴阳是自然界的根本规律，万物的纲纪，一切生物生长、发展和变化的根源。其次，阴阳是相对、互根的，是互相消长且互相转化的。这一理论贯穿于解释人体的结构、生理、病理、诊断和防治等整个医学领域中。

All phenomena in the universe may be ascribed to yin and yang. Each individual phenomenon depend upon and counterbalance each other. Further, they are mutually convertible, since either may change into the other.

宇宙中的一切现象都可以归因于阴阳。每个个别的现象都相互依存和平衡。而且它们是相互转化的,因为其中一个可以变成另一个。

The following principles may be observed in the application of the yin-yang theory to yin and yang as the fundamental categories of all phenomena：In medicine，the concepts of yin and yang are generally used to categorize both anatomic parts and physiological functions. For example，the back is yang and the abdomen is yin；the six fu-organs are yang and the five zang-organs are yin；qi is yang and blood is yin；agitation is yang and depression is yin.

在将阴阳理论应用于作为所有现象基本范畴的阴阳的过程中,可以观察到以下原则:在医学中,阴阳的概念通常用于分类解剖部位和生理功能。例如,背部是阳,腹部是阴;六腑是阳,五脏是阴;气是阳,血是阴;烦躁是阳,沉郁是阴。

2. Yin and Yang Are Divisible 阴阳可分

Every phenomenon may be classified as yin or yang in contrast to the other. Each yin or yang phenomenon itself possesses both yin and yang aspects that may be further divided in the same way.

每个现象都可以对比为阴或阳。每个阴或阳现象本身都具有阴阳两个方面,可以以同样的方式进一步划分。

3. Yin and Yang Are Rooted in Each Other 阴阳互根

The notion that yin and yang are rooted in each other means that they are mutually indispensable and engendering. Yin and yang are interdependent. Blood and qi，two fundamental elements of the human body，provide an example：blood is yin and qi is yang. It is said that "qi engenders blood"，i. e.，blood formation relies on the power of qi to move and transform food；"qi moves blood"，meaning that blood circulation relies on the warmth and driving power of qi.

阴阳互根意味着它们相互不可或缺且相互生成。阴阳是相互依存的。人体的两个基本要素——血和气,就提供了一个例子:血是阴,气是阳。有一种说法是"气生血",即血液的形成依赖于气的力量来移动和转化食物;"气行血",意味着血液循环依赖于气的温暖和推动力。

4. Yin and Yang Counterbalance Each Other 阴阳平衡

The yin and yang aspects of the body counterbalance each other. A deficiency of one naturally leads to an excess of the other, while an excess of one weakens the other. In both cases, yin and yang no longer counterbalance each other, and disease arises as a result. In medicine, the notion of counterbalancing is widely applied in physiology, pathology, therapeutics, etc.

身体的阴阳方面相互平衡。一方面的不足自然导致另一方面的过剩,而一方面的过剩会削弱另一方面。在这两种情况下,阴阳不再相互平衡,疾病就会产生。在医学中,平衡的概念在生理学、病理学、治疗学等方面有着广泛的应用。

Ⅱ. Key Words 核心词语

1. The Yang Qi (The Yang Principle) 阳气

It is the opposite of the yin qi (the yin principle) and a generalized term for one aspect of the two opposites. It usually refers to the functional activities of the viscera.

与阴气相对而言,泛指它们所代表的事物的两个对立面之一。一般多指脏腑的机能活动。

2. The Yin Qi (The Yin Principle) 阴气

It is the opposite of the yang qi (the yang principle) and a generalized term for one aspect of the two opposites. It usually refers to the refined materials in the viscera.

与阴气相对而言,泛指它们所代表的事物的两个对立面之一。一般多指脏腑所藏的精微物质。

3. The Yang Aspect of Yang and the Yin Aspect of Yang 阳中之阳,阳中之阴

An object belonging to the category of yang may, in turn, be subdivided into two parts: its yin and its yang. Its yang part is called "the yang aspect of yang" and its yin part, "the yin aspect of yang".

指属阳的事物中又可分为阴阳两个方面,其中分属于阳的一面,称为"阳中之阳";分属于阴的一面,称为"阳中之阴"。

4. The Yin Aspect of Yin and the Yang Aspect of Yin 阴中之阴,阴中之阳

An object belonging to the category of yin may, in turn, be subdivided into two opposites: its yin and its yang. The former is called "the yin aspect of yin" and the latter, "the yang aspect of yin".

指属阴的事物又可分为阴阳两个方面,其中分属于阴的一面,称为"阴中之阴";分属于阳的一面,称为"阴中之阳"。

5．The Flourishing Yin Based on the Vivified Yang 阳生阴长

Yang must be vivified normally in order that yin may flourish. This explains the aspect of the flourishing state of matters.

阳气生化正常,阴气才能不断滋长,以此说明事物生发的一面。

6．Yang Restrained and Yin Concealed 阳杀阴藏

When yang is restrained, yin becomes dormant or concealed. This explains the aspect of the restraining state of matters.

阳气收束时,则阴气也潜藏,以此说明事物敛藏的一面。

7．The Interdependence of Yin and Yang 阴阳互根

The existence of one of the two opposites, yin and yang, depends on the very existence of the other. Neither of them can exist and flourish independently. At the same time, yin or yang may transform itself into the opposite under certain defined circumstances. For example, such interdependent relationship exists between matter and its function.

阴阳双方均以对方的存在为前提,任何一方均不能单独存在和运动。同时,阴阳双方又可在一定的条件下互相转化。如物质与机能之间就存在着这种互根关系。

8．Yin Generated from Yang 阴生于阳

The existence of yin must depend on the prior existence of yang. For example, the essence of yin in the human body must invoke the activities of the yang principle in order to develop.

指阴以阳的存在为自己存在的前提。如人体中的阴精是通过阳气的活动而化生的。

9．Yang Generated from Yin 阳生于阴

The existence of yang must depend on the prior existence of yin. For example, the yang principle in the human body must invoke the essence of yin in order to develop.

指阳以阴的存在为自己存在的前提。如人体中的阳气是通过阴精而化生的。

10．Ebb and Flow of Yin and Yang 阴阳消长

Yin and yang coexist in a dynamic state in which one rises while the other declines. An excess of one will lead to the decline of the other and vice versa.

指阴阳双方此盛彼衰、此消彼长的动态变化。若一方太过,就会引起另一方不足;反之,一方不足,也会导致另一方太过。

11. Mutual Metamorphoses of Yin and Yang 阴阳转化

Under certain defined circumstances, yin and yang may be mutually transmutable. Yin may be transmuted into yang, and yang into yin. For example, cold reaching its extreme may produce heat and heat reaching its extreme may generate cold. A yin syndrome may metamorphose into a yang one and vice versa.

阴阳双方在一定条件下可以互相转化,阴可以转化为阳,阳也可以转化为阴。如寒极生热,热极生寒;阴证可以转化为阳证,阳证也可以转化为阴证。

12. Yin Flourishing Smoothly and Yang Vivified Steadily 阴平阳秘

The yin principle flourishes smoothly while the yang principle is vivified steadily. They regulate themselves so as to maintain their relative kinetic equilibrium. This is the basic principle to promote the normal activities of life and keep healthy.

阴气平顺,阳气固守,两者相互调节而保持其相对的动态平衡,这是机体生命活动与健康的基本条件。

13. Imbalance of Yin and Yang 阴阳失调

It is the disharmony of yin and yang, and leads to pathologic changes with excesses of one and deficiencies of the other, disturbances of qi (vital energy) and blood, malfunctioning of the viscera, etc.

即阴阳不和,它可导致阴阳双方偏盛偏衰、气血紊乱、脏腑机能失常等病理变化。

14. Failure of Yin to Sustain Yang 阴不抱阳

This is due to abnormal changes of yin. When it cannot maintain the normal stance of the yang principle, pathologic changes would appear, such as "deficiency of yin with excess of yang", and "excess of yin with exclusion of yang", etc.

由于阴的病变,不能维系阳气的正常固守而出现的病理现象,如"阴虚阳亢""阴盛格阳"皆是。

15. Dissociation of Yin and Yang 阴阳离决

It denotes a disintegration of the relationship between yin and yang, and is used to express the end of life.

指阴阳双方互根关系的毁灭,表示生命停止。

16. Yang Representing Qi and Yin the Matter 阳化气,阴成形

Yin and yang are used to explain the interdependence and mutual transmutation between the material (the form) and the function (qi). When appearing as functional activities, the matter belongs to "yang"; and when appearing as formed materials, it belongs to "yin".

是以阴阳说明物质(形)和机能(气)之间相互依存、相互转化的关系。当事物表现为机能活动时属"阳",而成为有形物质时便属"阴"。

17. Excess of Yin Causing Disorder of Yang 阴盛则阳病

When the principle of yin-cold is intensified, the yang principle would be affected, resulting in disease (with dissipation of the yang principle or restriction of its activities).

当阴寒之气偏盛时,就要影响阳气而得病(如阳气虚弱或阳气活动受到限制)。

18. Excess of Yang Causing Disorder of Yin 阳盛则阴病

When the principle of yang-heat is intensified or the debilitating heat is impetuous, the yin-liquid would be dissipated, and disease would result.

当阳热之气亢奋或虚火妄动时,就要耗损阴液而得病。

19. Deficiency of Yin Affecting Yang 阴损及阳

A deficiency of the yin-essence would cause a shortage of the yang principle. For example, if the kidney yin is damaged for long, it will lead to a deficiency of the kidney yang.

阴精亏损会导致阳虚弱。如肾阴亏损日久,就可出现肾阳不足。

20. Deficiency of Yang Affecting Yin 阳损及阴

An impairment of the yang principle would lead to the dissipation of the yin-essence. For example, if the kidney yang is impaired for long, it will result in a shortage of the kidney yin.

阳气虚弱会导致阴精亏乏。如肾阳虚衰日久,就可出现肾阴亏乏。

21. The Superposed Yang 重阳

It refers to the simultaneous presence of two forms of the yang property in a single entity. For example, day belongs to the category of yang and noon, the yang aspect of yang. Thus, noon is called "the superposed yang".

两种属于阳的性质同时出现在同一事物上。如白昼为阳,中午为阳中之阳,故称中午为"重阳"。

22. The Superposed Yin 重阴

It refers to the simultaneous presence of two forms of the yin property in a single entity. For example, night belongs to the category of yin and midnight, the yin aspect of yin. Thus, midnight is called "the superposed yin".

两种属于阴的性质同时出现在同一事物上。如夜晚为阴,夜半为阴中之阴,故称夜半为"重阴"。

23. Inevitable Transmutation of the Superposed Yin into Yang 重阴必阳

A disease may be characterized by an excess of the yin principle. When this excess of its yin principle reaches a certain limit, it may exhibit yang characters or metamorphose toward yang. For example, when a syndrome of chills develops to its climax, fever manifestations may appear.

疾病的性质源属阴气偏盛,但当阴气偏盛到一定限度时,就会出现阳的现象或向着阳的方向转化。如寒证发展到极点,就可能出现热象。

24. Inevitable Transmutation of the Superposed Yang into Yin 重阳必阴

A disease may be characterized by an excess of the yang principle. When this excess of its yang principle reaches a certain limit, it may exhibit yin characters or metamorphose toward yin. For example, when a fever syndrome reaches its climax, manifestations of chills may appear.

疾病的性质源属阳气偏盛,但当阳气亢盛到一定限度时,就会出现阴的现象或向着阴的方向转化。如热证发展到极点,就可能出现寒象。

25. While Yang Often in Excess, Yin Often in Shortage 阳常有余,阴常不足

This is a theory formulated through clinical practice and advocated by the famous physician, Zhu Danxi (A. D. 1281-1358) of the Yuan Dynasty. He held that the essence and blood (yin) of the human body were the material foundation of activities of life. They were continuously consumed, easily dissipated, and difficult to restore. Thus, yin tended to be deficient. The yang principle was liable to be stimulated, and the debilitating heat would become impetuous, resulting frequently in a surplus of the yang principle. When yin was deficient and yang excessive, many diseases might occur. Zhu advocated that essence and blood must be preserved and enriched in order to maintain the dynamic equilibrium of yin and yang of the body. This was the theoretical basis of his emphasis on nourishing yin clinically.

这是元朝著名医家朱丹溪(1281－1358)通过临床实践提出的一种学说。他认为人身精血(阴)是生命活动的物质基础,不断消耗,易损难复,故阴常不足。阳气易亢,虚火妄动,故阳常有余。阴虚阳亢,则百病丛生。因此,朱氏主张保重精血以维持身体阴阳相对平衡,这是临床上侧重滋阴法的理论根据。

26. Inability for the Excessive Yang to Congeal, Leading to an Exhaustion of the Yin Principle 阳强不能密,阴气乃绝

When the yang principle is excessive, it can hardly maintain the integrity of the body surface and protect muscles against trauma, but also may cause the yin-liquid of yin to be dissipated and evaporated from the body. Hence, the yin principle becomes deficient and exhausted.

当阳气过于亢盛时,既不能固护肌表、抵御外伤,又可使在内的阴液受损耗而蒸逼外泄,以致阴气亏损/耗竭。

27. Alternate Excesses of Yin and Yang 阴阳胜复

It refers to the conditions in which excesses of yin and yang occur alternately. Sometimes, such a situation may be utilized to prognosticate diseases clinically.

即阴阳双方交替出现偏盛偏衰的局面。临床上有时可根据这种局面判断疾病的预后。

28. Re-Establishment of Equilibrium Between Yin and Yang 阴阳自和

Pathological disharmony of yin and yang may progress to a relative equilibrium between the two. It is shown as an improvement or a recovery of the disease.

病理上的阴阳失调趋向相对平衡的建立,表示疾病好转或痊愈。

29. The Internal Yin as the Source of Yang 阴在内,阳之守也

Materials (yin) inside the body are (is) the foundation for producing vital functions (yang).

物质(阴)居于体内,是产生功能(阳)的基础。

30. The External Yang as the Representaion of Yin 阳在外,阴之使也

Vital functions (yang) as manifested externally reflect(s) the changes of the materials (yin) inside the body.

功能(阳)表现于外,是内在物质(阴)运动的体现。

31. The Complexity of the Human Anatomy Representable Exclusively by Yin and Yang 人生有形,不离阴阳

The formation, growth and development of the human body may be generally expressed in terms of yin and yang in spite of their complexity.

人体的成形、生长、发育尽管复杂,但总体上可以用阴阳来概括。

32. Mutual Conversion of Yin and Yang 阴阳转化

The term means either yin or yang can be converted to its opposite under certain circumstances, which is the basic form of movement between yin and yang. Under certain conditions, one becomes the other, i. e., yin can be converted to yang and yang can be converted to yin. This conversion could be manifested in either a gradual process or in a sudden manner. In physiology, it is manifested in the conversion between function and substance as well as in the mutual rooting of yin and yang, i. e., yin engenders yang and yang engenders yin. In pathology, mutual conversion of yin and yang is manifested in the fact that extreme cold will engender heat and extreme heat will engender cold.

指的是阴阳双方在一定条件下向其各自相反的方向转变,这是阴阳运动的基本形式。在一定的条件下,阴阳双方可以相互转化,即阴可以转化为阳,阳也可以转化为阴。阴阳的相互转化,既可以表现为渐变形式,又可以表现为突变形式。在生理上,阴阳转化的表现形式为功能与物质的转换,以及阳生于阴、阴生于阳的互根。在病理上,阴阳转化的表现为寒极生热和热极生寒。

33. Waxing and Waning of Yin and Yang 阴阳消长

The term describes the ebb and flow of yin and yang within a certain limit in terms of motion. Because of the relationship of mutual opposing and rooting, yin and yang within any phenomenon are not fixed but in a state of continuous mutual growth and diminishment, maintaining dynamic balance in the process of waxing and waning. Yin and yang aspects in nature are opposite, and are in constant rise-and-fall changes. It is the mutual opposition and constraint as well as the mutual rooting and promotion of yin and yang that causes the waxing and waning of yin and yang, in which the former is primarily involved.

指的是阴阳之间互为增减盛衰的运动变化。对立互根的阴阳双方不是一成不变的,而是处于不断的增长和消减的变化之中,并在彼此消长的运动过程中保持着动态平衡。自然事物中的阴阳双方是对立的,总是此盛彼衰、此消彼长地变化。导致阴阳出现消长变化的根本原因是阴阳之间存在着的相互对立、相互制约及互根互用的关系,其中阴阳之间的相互对立与制约尤为重要。

Ⅲ. Dialogues 情景对话

1. Dialogue 1 对话 1

Student：Yin-yang theory is a very fascinating concept，and something I've really wrapped my head around in the last few days.

阴阳理论是一个非常吸引人的概念，在过去的几天里我真的很着迷。

Professor：Good for you.

太好了。

Student：But something doesn't add up. When you said "the opposition of yin and yang"，I was thinking immediately "OK, I got this, it is just like the desk is round and the desk is not round." And then you lost me when you said，"Yin and yang can be converted into each other." How can the desk be round and not round at the same time?

但有些事情我有些迷惑。当你说"阴阳对立"时，我立刻在想"好吧，我明白了，这就像桌子是圆的和桌子不是圆的"。然后你说"阴阳可以相互转换"时，我又迷惑了。桌子怎么可能同时是圆的和不圆的？

Professor：That's a very interesting question. The problem，I believe，might lie in the fundamental difference between western logic and its Chinese counterpart. The latter places the opposition of yin and yang in a constantly changing mode，just as the alternations between day and night. Day，with the characteristics of yang，is the opposite of night，yin. However，time does not stop at any point. Day will turn into night when it has reached its point of exhaustion. Does it make sense to you?

这是一个非常有趣的问题。我认为，问题可能在于西方逻辑与中国逻辑的根本区别。后者将阴阳对立置于一种不断变化的模式中，就像昼夜交替一样。白天具有阳的特征，与夜晚的阴相反。然而,时间不会在任何时候停止。当白天到了精疲力竭的地步时,就会变成夜晚。你能明白吗?

Student：Yes, it does. Just as it is said，"Change is at the root of everything."

是的。正如人们所说的:"改变是一切的根源。"

Professor：What's more, it's believed classically that yin-yang has a name but not a form. As a result，the term is designated for a universally observed phenomenon rather than an object such as a desk.

更重要的是,传统上认为阴阳有名无形。因此,这个词是指一种普遍观察到的现象,而不是桌子之类的物体。

Student：I see. Your explanation is very helpful. How I wish you could be around when other questions pop up!

我明白了。你的解释很有帮助。当其他问题突然出现时,我多么希望你能在身边!

2. Dialogue 2 对话 2

Student A：Could you spare me a couple of minutes before class?

上课前你能抽出几分钟时间吗?

Student B：My pleasure. It was pretty interesting，what you asked in class. I didn't even know that angle existed.

当然可以,我的荣幸。你在课堂上问的问题很有趣。我甚至不知道那个角度的存在。

Student A：Speaking of which，another thing just popped into my mind. You guys keep calling the yin-yang concept a theory，right? For me，it sounds like a perspective，an alternative perspective.

说到这里,我突然想到了另一件事。你们一直把阴阳概念称为理论,对吧? 对我来说,这听起来像是一种视角,一种对立的视角。

Student B：We call it a theory since it serves as a basic guideline in almost every aspect of traditional Chinese medicine，physiology for instance，do you remember what we've learned?

我们称之为理论,是因为它几乎在中医的各个方面都是一个基本的指导方针,比如生理学,你还记得我们学过什么吗?

Student A：Yes. It says that all substances with form such as the organs, tissues and body fluids are yin, while their physiological functions are yang. Life depends on both. Based on this concept, signs like insomnia, emotional disorders or epilepsy are interpreted as kidney yin in deficiency, and thus the sea of marrow fails to be nourished. That's a perspective. Another one is that the damage of brain cells may also lead to these symptoms. Here's where I become confused. You see, a scientific theory can only earn its name after being proven methodically. The cells are substantiated to be in existence, but how about kidney yin?

是的。所有有形体的物质,如器官、组织和体液都是阴的,而它们的生理功能是阳的。生命取决于两者。基于这一概念,失眠、情绪障碍或癫痫等症状被解释为肾阴不足,因此骨髓无法得到滋养。这是一种观点。另一种观点是脑细胞的损伤也可能导致这些症状。这就是我感到困惑的地方。你看,一个科学理论只有经过有条不紊的证明才能获得名字。这些细胞被证实是存在的,但肾阴呢?

Student B：I see your point. I think this might just be another difference between China and the West. For us, the inductive mindset dominates. We tend to spend generations observing and trying to accumulate wisdom through observation. Yin-yang is a law, not an entity. It started to become a perspective after viewing things in the universe, but it's certainly been verified by years of TCM clinical practice in diagnosis and treatment.

我明白你的意思。我认为这可能只是中国和西方的另一个区别。对我们来说,归纳思维占主导地位。我们倾向于花几代人的时间观察,并试图通过观察积累智慧。阴阳是一种规律,而不是一个实体。在观察宇宙万物后,它开始成为一种视角,但多年的中医临床诊疗实践无疑证实了这一点。

Student A：You mean treatments based on pattern identification?

你的意思是基于模式识别的治疗？

Student B：Yes. First we need to identity signs like cold body and limbs, pale and dark complexion, unwillingness to speak up, long voiding of clear urine, watery stools, etc. as yin patterns. Then diagnosis can be made that yang qi is in decline, while yin cold is on the rise. In order to regain a healthy state, or equilibrium within the human body, treatment should involve warming yang. In this practice, the concept of yin and yang plays a theoretical role in putting the puzzles together. With so many successful case histories supporting its validity, the word "theory" sounds reasonably in order.

是的。首先，我们将身体和四肢发冷、面色苍白、不愿意说话、长时间排尿清便和水样便等症状识别为阴型。诊断为阳气下降，阴寒上升。为了在人体内恢复健康状态或平衡，治疗方式主要为温阳。在这一实践中，阴阳概念对解谜起到了理论作用。有这么多成功的案例支持它的有效性，"理论"这个词听起来很合理。

Student A：I think I'm starting to understand more about the Chinese mentality as my study of traditional Chinese medicine advances.

随着我对中医的学习逐渐深入，我想我开始对中国人的心态有了更多的了解。

Section 2　Key Concepts of Chinese Medicine：Five Elements
第2节　中医文化关键概念：五行

Ⅰ. Key Concepts 核心概念

The Theory of the Five Elements (Five Activities of Five Principles in Action) 五行学说

It is one of the philosophical theories in ancient China adapted in the medical practice, becoming an important part of the theory of traditional Chinese medicine. It relates the properties of the five elements(metal, wood, water, fire and earth) to universally interdependent and mutually restraining relationships of matters. It played a definitive role in the development of traditional Chinese medicine.

是中国古代哲学理论与医学实践相结合的学说之一，为中医理论的一个重要组成部分。它用五种物质(金、木、水、火、土)的属性，说明事物间相互依存又相互制约的关系，对中医的发展起到了一定的作用。

The concept refers to the five basic substances including metal, wood, water, fire, and earth, as well as their motions and changes. The application of five elements in traditional Chinese medicine is mainly concentrated on the corresponding relationship between five elements and five zang-organs, which has been developed into one of the basic theories of traditional Chinese medicine. On the basis of five elements corresponding to five zang-organs, meridians help connect the whole body, which demonstrates the wholism. It also explains the unity of man and nature when combined with the concepts of five directions and four seasons based on the observation in nature and development of clinical practice. In addition, the generation, restriction, over-restriction, and counter-restriction among the five elements illustrate the interdependence and inter-restriction relationships of five zang-organs, which reflects the principle of prevention and treatment of diseases in combination with the theory of yin and yang.

五行指金、木、水、火、土五类要素及其运动变化。五行在中医上的应用主要以五行配五脏为中心,逐步发展为中医的基本理论之一。在五行配五脏为中心的基础上,通过经络联系全身,说明了人体的整体性;通过自然现象的观察和临床实践的发展与五方、四时联系在一起,说明了人与自然的统一性。另外,以五行的生、克、乘、侮阐述五脏之间相互依存和相互制约的关系,并与阴阳学说贯通一起,可以体现防病治病的道理。

Two major relationships between the elements exist under normal physiological conditions in the body:

在身体正常的生理条件下,这些元素之间存在两种主要关系:

The generation cycle: The promoting relationship that describes the generation, nourishment and support given by the "mother" in the sequence to its "son". For example, fire is the son of wood and another of earth, and so on.

世代循环:指顺序中"母亲"给予"儿子"的生成、滋养和支持的促进关系。例如,火由木生,并与土相生相连,等等。

The restraining cycle: The relationship that describes how elements interact and constrain each other, forming a dynamic equilibrium within the system. For example, earth controls water and is itself controlled by wood.

约束循环:描述元素之间相互影响,相互制约,形成一种系统内部的动力平衡。例如,土控制着水,而它本身又由木控制。

Several disharmonious relationships can occur when there is an imbalance between the elements, usually as a result of an excess or deficiency of one or more of the elements. Such imbalances can lead to disease. Disharmonious relationships in the restraining cycle are:

当元素之间不平衡时,可能会发生几种不和谐的关系,通常源于一种或多种元素的过量或缺乏。这种不平衡可能导致疾病。约束循环中的不和谐关系为:

Overacting: This can occur more readily if the element that is normally controlled becomes weakened or deficient. The lung is associated with metal, and the liver with wood, metal can overcome wood.

过度作用:如果正常控制的元素变弱或不足,这种情况可能会更容易发生。肺属金,肝属木,金可以克木。

Counter-acting: The element that is normally controlled in the restraining sequence become the controller and attacks the element that would normally control it. The abnormal relationships in the generation cycle may manifest as disorders of "the mother affecting the son", and disorders of "the son affecting the mother".

反作用：约束序列中正常受控制的元素变成控制者，并攻击本应正常控制它的元素。世代循环中的异常关系可能表现为"母亲影响儿子"的障碍，以及"儿子影响母亲"的障碍。

The five-element theory is used as a model to explain the functions of the body's internal organs and tissues in terms of the characteristics of the five elements and analyze the dynamic relationship between the organs. For example, the kidney corresponds to the element of water since it regulates water metabolism.

以五行学说为模型，根据五行的特点来解释人体内部器官和组织的功能，并分析器官之间的动态关系。例如，肾脏对应于水元素，因为它调节水代谢。

The theory may be applied during the analysis of signs and symptoms in order to make a diagnosis. For example, a person with red, swollen eyes and a bitter taste in the mouth is likely to have a problem in the liver, since a bitter taste is associated with the element of wood and the eyes are sense organs related to the liver.

该理论可以应用于体征和症状的分析，以便进行诊断。例如，眼睛红肿、口腔有苦味的人很可能会有肝脏问题，因为苦味与木元素有关，而眼睛是与肝脏有关的感觉器官。

The theory may also be used in clinical treatment. For example, if the liver is overacting on the spleen, herbs may be given to calm the liver and strengthen the weakened spleen. Acupuncture points may also be chosen according to five-element theory. For example, specific acupuncture points are selected according to the theory to "reinforce the mother" in the case where the "son" element is weak. In medicine, the concept of counterbalancing is widely applied in physiology, pathology, and therapy.

该理论也可用于临床治疗。例如，如果肝脏对脾脏的作用过大，可以服用中药来平肝补脾。也可根据五行学说选用穴位。例如，在"子"元素较弱的情况下，根据"补母"理论选择特定的穴位。在医学中，平衡的概念被广泛应用于生理学、病理学和治疗。

Ⅱ. Key Words 核心词语

1. Normal Activities of the Five Elements 五常

It refers to the relationship of the normal activities between promotion and inhibition of the matters as represented by the five elements.

指五行所代表的事物的正常生克制化关系。

2. Five Notes 五音

The note of a pentatonic scaled in ancient Chinese music，i. e. ，Gong，Shang，Jue，Zhi，and Yu.

中国古代音乐中的五个音阶——宫、商、角、徵、羽。

3. Five Voices 五声

It refers to the voices uttered by human weeping in different emotional states,i. e. ，shouting, laughing, singing, wailing and groaning.

指与人的精神活动有关而发出的呼、笑、歌、哭、呻五种声音。

4. Generation Among the Five Elements 五行相生

The term refers to the interrelationship of five elements in which each element engenders, strengthens, and promotes another in sequence. The order of generation is as follows：wood engenders fire, fire engenders earth, earth engenders metal, metal engenders water, and water engenders wood. In terms of generation relationship, each of the five elements contains both aspects of "generating" and "being generated". Traditionally, this kind of relationship is compared to the mother-child relationship. The element that generates is the mother, whereas the element that is generated is the child. Therefore, generation among the five elements means that one element engenders, strengthens, and promotes another element.

指的是五行之间相互滋生、助长和促进的关系。五行相生的次序是：木生火，火生土，土生金，金生水，水生木。在五行相生关系中，任何一行都有"生我"和"我生"这两方面的关系。传统上将五行相生的关系比喻为母子关系，即"生我"者为母，"我生"者为子。因此，五行相生，实际上通指五行中的某一行对另一行的滋生、助长和促进。

5. Restriction Among the Five Elements 五行相克

The term connotes the relationship of restraint and control among the five elements. Restriction among the five elements follows the sequence below: wood restricts earth, earth restricts water, water restricts fire, fire restricts metal, and metal restricts wood. In the restriction relationship, each of the five elements contains both aspects of "restricting" and "being restricted". According to the *Yellow Emperors Internal Canon of Medicine* (*Huangdi Nei Jing*), these two aspects are called "unconquered" and "not unconquered", i. e., "restricting" is equivalent to "unconquered" and "restricted" equals "not unconquered". Therefore, restriction among the five elements means one element restricts and brings another element under control.

指的是五行之间相互克制和相互制约的关系。五行相克的次序是木克土，土克水，水克火，火克金，金克木。在五行相克关系中，任何一行都具有"克我"和"我克"这两方面的关系。《黄帝内经》把相克关系称为"所胜"和"所不胜"的关系，即"克我"者为"所不胜"，"我克"者为"所胜"。因此，五行相克实际上指的是五行中的某一行对其所胜的某一行的克制和制约。

6. Inter-Invasion 相乘

It means that one excessively inhibits another beyond the normal extent, manifested as a disturbance of the normal harmony.

即五行相互克制太过，超过了正常的制约程度，是事物间的关系失却了正常协调的一种表现。

7. Inter-Insult 相侮

It refers to a reversal of inter-inhibition and is another manifestation of a disturbance of the normal harmony between matters. For example, metal normally inhibits wood. If, instead, wood inhibits metal, we would consider wood insulting metal. This abnormal phenomenon is "inter-insult".

即五行的反向克制，是事物间的关系失却了正常协调的另一种表现。如在正常情况下，是金克木；若木反过来克金，称侮金。这种反常情况便叫"相侮"。

8. Inhibition and Generation 制化

The five elements are not only mutually inhibiting but mutually generating. Inhibition exists in the process of generation and generation exists in the process of inhibition. These two processes regulate each other, thus maintaining a relative equilibrium.

说明五行之间不仅相互制约，而且相互化生。化生中有克制，克制中有化生，二者相辅相成，才能维持其相对平衡。

9. The Avoidance of Harm by Restraining Excesses 亢害承制

As considered by the theory of the five elements, there is not only generation on the one hand, but inhibition on the other hand. Generation without inhibition would lead to harmful extreme excesses, which must be restrained in order to maintain the normal relationship between matters.

五行学说认为,事物间既有化生的一面,又有克制的一面,若只有生而无克,势必亢盛至极而为害。因此必须抵御这种亢盛之气,令其节制,方能维持事物之间的正常关系。

10. To be Conquered 所胜

In the inter-inhibiting relationship of the five elements, conquering is synonymous with inhibiting. For example, in the expression "wood inhibits earth," earth is considered conquered by wood.

五行相克关系中,我克者为所胜。如木克土,又称土为木所胜。

11. Not to be Conquered 所不胜

In the inter-inhibiting relationship of the five elements, matters may not be conquered by inhibition. For example, in the expression "earth is inhibited by wood," it also means that wood can not be conquered by earth.

五行相克关系中,克我者为所不胜。如土被木克,又称木为土所不胜。

12. Conquering Activities of the Five Elements 五胜

In general it refers to the inter-inhibition of the five elements.

一般指五行相克。

13. The Offspring Principle 子气

In the inter-generating relationship of the five elements, the one which is generated by the other is called the offspring principle of the other. For example, "wood generates fire" means fire is the offspring principle.

在五行相生关系中,我生者,为子气。如木生火,火为子气。

14. The Maternal Principle 母气

In the inter-generating relationship of the five elements, the one which generates the other is called the maternal principle of the other. For example, "wood generates fire" means wood is the maternal principle.

在五行相生关系中,生我者,为母气。如木生火,木为母气。

15. A Maternal Disease Affecting Its Offspring 母病及子

The inter-generating relationship of the five elements is assigned to the five parenchymatous viscera. (The liver corresponds to wood, the heart to fire, the spleen to earth, the lung to metal, and the kidney to water.) When a maternal viscus is diseased and involves its offspring viscus, it is considered "a maternal disease affects its offspring." For example, when the liver is diseased and involves the heart, it is considered "a maternal disease affects its offspring."

用五行相生关系配属五脏。（肝属木、心属火、脾属土、肺属金、肾属水。）凡母脏有病累及子脏者,称之为"母病及子"。如肝有病累及心,就可称为"母病及子"。

16. An Offspring Stealing Its Maternal Principle 子盗母气

The inter-generating relationship of the five elements is assigned to the five parenchymatous viscera. (The liver corresponds to wood, the heart to fire, the spleen to earth, the lung to metal, and the kidney to water.) When an offspring viscus is diseased and involves its materal viscus, it is considered "an offsprs steals its materal principle." For example, when the lung is diseased and involves the spleen, it is consideread "an offspring steals its maternal principle."

用五行相生关系配属五脏。（肝属木、心属火、脾属土、肺属水。）凡子脏有病累及母脏者,称之为"子盗母气"。如肺有病影响到脾,就可称为"子盗母气"。

17. Wood Inclining to be Harmonious and Flourishing 木喜条达

Wood is used to represent the liver. The growth of a tree is employed to represent the physiologic tendency of the liver for harmony and flourishing rather than restraint.

木是肝的代名词。用树木生发的现象比喻肝喜调和畅达,不喜被压抑的生理特点。

18. Depression of Wood Generating Fire 木郁化火

Wood is used to represent the liver. When the liver is depressed, there would appear symptoms and signs of the liver fire, such as headache, dizziness, flushed face, redness of eyes, hemoptysis, hematemesis, anger, mania, etc.

木是肝的代名词。当肝气抑郁时,就会产生肝火症状,如头痛、眩晕、面红、目赤、呕血、咯血、发怒、发狂等。

19. Wood Fire Damaging Metal 木火荆金

Wood is used to represent the liver, and metal is used to represent the lungs. An excess of the liver fire may damage the lungs and would cause or aggravate the diseases of the lungs.

木是肝的代名词,金是肺的代名词。当肝火过旺时,可以损伤及肺,引起肺病或使肺病加重。

20. Depression of Wood Generating Wind 木郁化风

Wood is used to represent the liver, wind represents certain unsteadiness, abruptness, wandering, and other symptoms and signs. When the liver is depressed for a relatively long time, some wind symptoms, such as tremor, numbness of the extremities and of the tongue, dizziness or vertigo, and seizures may appear.

木是肝的代名词,风是某些摇摆、突然、游走不定等症状的代名词。当肝气抑郁较久时,就会产生一些风症,如震颤、肢体发麻、舌麻、眩晕、癫痫等。

21. The Flaring Nature of Fire 火性上炎

The burning nature of fire is used to exemplify the flaring characteristics of the pathogenic changes due to abnormal fire.

用火燃烧的象征,比喻火邪致病的病变表现也有向上的特点。

22. Blazing Fire Damaging Metal 火盛刑金

①When the liver fire becomes excessive, the lungs may be damaged. ② When the heart fire becomes excessive, the lung yin may be damaged, because metal represents the lungs.

①指肝火过旺时,损伤及肺;②指心火盛时,可耗伤肺阴,因金是肺的代名词。

23. Inability of Fire to Generate Earth 火不生土

Fire is used to represent the kidney yang (the vital fire). Earth represents the spleen. When the yang principle of the kidney is deficient and weak, and the vital fire is not vigorous, the spleen cannot receive the warmth of this yang principle. The processes of digestion, absorption, and transportation of nutriment and water will be impaired. The symptoms and signs due to weakness of the yang principle of the kidney and spleen will manifest as backache, chilliness of knees, intolerance to cold, anorexia, dyspepsia, dysuria, puffiness or edema, diarrhea before dawn, etc.

火是肾阳(命火)的代名词,土是脾的代名词。当肾阳虚弱,命火不足时,脾得不到阳气的温煦,消化、吸收、输布营养物质及水液的功能均会减退,因而可出现肾、脾阳气虚弱的症状,如腰酸、膝冷、畏寒、食欲不振、饮食不化、小便不利、浮肿、黎明前腹泻等。

24．Everything in Nature Grows out of the Earth 土生万物

Earth represents the spleen, which is the source of nutrition for building up the body, providing material basis for vital function, just as the earth is the source of everything in nature.

土是脾的代名词。用自然界万物滋生大地的现象,比喻脾为营养化生之源的生理特点。

25．Earth Liking Warmth and Dryness 土喜温燥

Earth represents the spleen, which is characterized by its inclination for warmth and dryness, and aversion to coldness and dampness. Warmth and dryness enhance the capability of transporting moisture by the spleen, while coldness and dampness impair the yang principle of the spleen, and, hence, reduce the capability of transporting moisture by the spleen.

土是脾的代名词。脾的生理特点是喜温喜燥,恶寒恶湿。因温和燥可使脾运化水湿的功能健旺,而寒和湿可以损伤脾阳,使脾运化水湿的功能减退。

26．Inhibition of Earth to Transport Water 土不制水

Earth represents the spleen. The spleen is too weak to transport water, so that moisture becomes stagnant and overflowing in the body. Symptoms like expectoration of whitish, frothy phlegm, obliguria, edema, and frequent loose stool will occur.

土是脾的代名词。即脾气虚不能运化水湿,而导致水湿在体内停滞或泛滥,出现吐稀白痰、小便不利、水肿、大便溏泄等。

27．The Metallic Pneuma Should be Clear and Descending 金气肃降

Metal represents the lungs. The pneuma(lung air) should be clear and descending rather than rising. If it rises abnormally, conditions like cough, shortness of breath or asthma, etc. will result.

金是肺的代名词。肺气以清肃下降为其生理特点,如肺气上逆,就会发生咳嗽、气喘等病症。

28．Chiliy Metal and Cold Water 金寒水冷

Metal represents the lungs, and water, kidney. It refers to weakness and coldness of the lungs and kidney.

金是肺的代名词,水是肾的代名词。"金寒水冷"即肺肾虚寒。

29．Water Flowing Downward 水性流下

The natural phenomenon that water always flows downwards is

employed to illustrate the downward characteristics of pathologic manifestation of illnesses due to an invasion of the body by excessive moisture.

用水往下流的自然现象,比喻水湿之邪侵犯人体致病的病理表现也有向下的特点。

30. Inadequate Water to Nourish Wood 水不涵木

Water represents the kidney yin, wood the liver. When the kidney yin is deficient, the liver cannot be nourished, and the liver yin will become deficient; thus, various disorders will result. This is similar to wilting and dryness of the tree when water does not nourish it.

水是肾的代名词,木是肝的代名词。当肾阴不足时,不能滋养肝,肝阴就亏乏,则会产生种种病症。如同水不能滋润树木,树木就要枯萎一样。

31. Lacking Water with Blazing Fire 水亏火旺

① Water refers to kidney water (the yin principle of the kidney), while fire, to the heart fire. An insufficiency of the kidney water will induce the heart fire to flare up, and symptoms such as anxiety and insomnia will occur. ②Water refers to the kidney water (the yin principle of the kidney), while fire, to the vital five (the yan principle of the kidney). An insufficiency of the kidney water will lead to an excess of the vital fire, and symptoms like exaggerated sexual desire and spermatorrhea will appear.

①水指肾水(肾阴),火指心火。当肾水亏乏时可导致心火偏盛,出现心烦、失眠等症。②水指肾水(肾阴),火指命火(肾阳)。当肾水亏乏时可导致命火偏亢,出现性机能亢进、遗精等病症。

32. Regulation Between Water and Fire 水火相济

Water refers to the kidney water, while fire, the heart fire. They regulate each other so as to keep physiologic dynamics in equilibrium.

水指肾水,火指心火。水火二者相互制约、相互作用以维持生理动态平衡。

33. Disturbance of the Regulation Between Water and Fire 水火不济

Water refers to the kidney water, while fire, to the heart fire. When the kidney water is deficient or the heart fire blazes, there is a loss of control by either of them. Disturbances of the equilibrium of the physiologic dynamics of both would result. And symptoms and signs like anxiety, insomnia, spermatorrhea, etc. will occur.

水指肾水,火指心火。肾水、心火二者只要一方失去制约,就会导致双方生理动态平衡失调,就会出现心烦、失眠、遗精等病症。

34. Seasonal Regulations 时令

① The usual climate in a season. ② The decree of the ancient government for agricultural and medical affairs, etc. set according to the seasons.

①每一季节的主要气候。②古代按季节制定的关于农事、医事等方面的政令。

35. Four Seasons 四时

Spring, summer, autumn, and winter.

春、夏、秋、冬四季。

36. Late Summer 长夏

The last month in summer.

夏季的最后一个月。

37. The Solar Terms 节气

A unit to predict the climate in four seasons in Chinese lunar calendar, with fifteen days in each solar term. There are twenty-four solar terms in a year, i. e., the Beginning of Spring, Rain Water, the Waking of Insects, the Spring Equinox, Pure Brightness, Grain Rain, the Beginning of Summer, Grain Full, Grain in Ear, the Summer Solstice, Slight Heat, Great Heat, the Beginning of Autumn, the Limit of Heat, Water Dew, the Autumnal Equinox, Cold Dew, Frost's Descent, the Beginning of Winter, Slight Snow, Great Snow, the Winter Solstice, Slight Cold and Great Cold.

中国农历推算四季气候的单位,每个节气有 15 天,一年共 24 个节气,即:立春,雨水,惊蛰,春分,清明,谷雨,立夏,小满,芒种,夏至,小暑,大暑,立秋,处暑,白露,秋分,寒露,霜降,立冬,小雪,大雪,冬至,小寒,大寒。

38. Triple Summer 三伏

The hottest time in a year.

指一年最炎热的时候。

39. Shichen (Time Interval) 时辰

A unit of time used in ancient times, equivalent to two hours.

中国古代的计时单位,一时辰相当于两小时。

40. Twelve Shichen 十二时

There are twelve shichen in a day, i. e., the first of the twelve Earthly

Branches, the second of the twelve Earthly Branches, the third of the twelve Earthly Branches, the fourth of the twelve Earthly Branches, the fifth of the twelve Earthly Branches, the sixth of the twelve Earthly Branches, the seventh of the twelve Earthly Branches, the eighth of the twelve Earthly Branches, the ninth of the twelve Earthly Branches, the tenth of the twelve Earthly Branches, the eleventh of the twelve Earthly Branches, and the last of the twelve Earthly Branches.

指昼夜有十二个时辰,即:子,丑,寅,卯,辰,巳,午,未,申,酉,戌,亥。

41. A Time Cycle 晬时

The time interval from a certain shichen of a day to the same time next day.

指一天的某一时辰到次日的同一时辰。

42. Five Movements and Six Climates 五运六气

The ancients combined the theory of the five elements with the changes of the six kinds of climate (wind, heat, warmth, dampness, dryness, and chills) to deduce the relationship between the changes of weather and the occurrence of disease in humans. This theory is somewhat similar to the modern climatological medicine and worthy of further investigation.

是古代运用五行学说,结合六种气候(风,火,热,湿,燥,寒)的转变,来推断每年气候变化与人体疾病发生的关系的理论。这一理论与现代气象医学有某些类似之处,值得进一步研究。

Ⅲ. Dialogues 情景对话

1. Dialogue 1 对话1

Student A: Hey, how you doing?
嗨,你好吗?

Student B: Not bad, just a little bit confused.
还不错,只是有点困惑。

Student A: What's the matter? You seem to have a big question mark on your face.
怎么了? 你的脸上似乎有一个很大的问号。

Student B：Oh, is it that obvious? If I turn out to be brain dead someday, tell the detectives that the five element theory is their guy.

哦,很明显吗? 如果有一天我脑死亡了,告诉侦探五元素理论就是罪魁祸首。

Student A：That's a serious accusation. I'm sure it won't come to that, 'cause I'm here to help.

这是严重的指控。我相信事情不会发展到那样的地步,因为我会帮你的。

Student B：Much obliged. You see, the correlations between the five elements and the zang-organs really give me a brain freeze. For starters, what does it mean by "wood tends to bend and straighten," and "liver likes orderly smoothness"? I just can't figure out the connections here.

非常感谢。你看,五行和五脏之间的相关性真的让我的大脑冻结了。对于初学者来说,"木头可以弯曲和拉直"和"肝脏喜欢有序的平稳"是什么意思? 我就是搞不清这里的联系。

Student A：Well, I think the former means wood has the characteristic to grow freely. It could bend or be straight, which also indicates the smoothness of the process. The latter refers to the free coursing function of the liver to ensure the free and smooth passage of qi. Can you make the connection now?

嗯,我认为前者是指木材具有自由生长的特性。它可以是弯曲的,也可以是直的,这也表明了这个过程的平稳性。后者指的是肝的自由流动,以确保气的自由顺畅流动。你现在能搞清这个联系吗?

Student B：Yes, a bit.

是的,有一点了。

Student A：How about earth and spleen?

土和脾是怎么回事?

Student B：From my point of view, these two are paired up because they both symbolize the source of transformation. To be more specific, it is the earth that turns seeds into crops, and the spleen is where food and water are transformed into qi and blood.

在我看来,这两个是成对的,因为它们都象征着转化的源泉。更具体地说,是土将种子转化为作物,而脾是食物和水转化为气血的地方。

Student A：That does explain a lot. What about metal then? It says that metal has the qualities of purification and elimination and it is associated with the lung.

这确实解释了很多。那么金属呢?据说金属具有净化和消除的特性,并且与肺有关。

Student B：You know the lung has the physiological function to ensure the purification and descending movement of lung-qi. To purify is to clean and eliminate impurities. In this sense, it is easy for us to make this assumption. Do you agree?

你知道肺具有保证肺气净化和下降的生理功能。净化就是清理和消除杂质。从这个意义上说,我们很容易做出这样的假设。你同意吗?

Student A：Yes, I do have a clearer picture in my mind now. Thanks a lot for the explanation.

是的,我现在脑子里确实有了更清晰的画面。非常感谢你的解释。

Student B：You're welcome. But this is only my personal interpretation. All the correlations are based on the observations of the wisdom through many generations. I think it is better to study their wisdom first. For this matter, sometimes comprehension can take a back seat.

不客气。但这只是我个人的解释。所有的相关性都建立在世代相传的智慧观察之上。我认为,首先研究他们的智慧更为重要。对于这个问题,有时候理解可以暂且搁置一旁。

2. Dialogue 2 对话 2

A：What's up?

怎么了?

B：I've been feeling under the weather lately.

我最近一直觉得不舒服。

A：Describe your symptoms to me please. Maybe I can help.

请把你的症状告诉我。也许我能帮上忙。

B：I feel pretty dizzy. My nose is very stuffy and my eyes are quite watery.

我觉得头很晕。我的鼻子堵得厉害，眼睛水汪汪的。

A：Do you feel cold?

你觉得冷吗？

B：Yes，a bit. I have been wearing short-sleeved T-shirts throughout the nice fall weather of Guangzhou. But today it just won't do. Oh, I cough from time to time too. And my throat feels kind of weird.

是的，有一点。我一直穿着短袖 T 恤衫度过广州宜人的秋季。但今天不行了。哦，我也时不时地咳嗽。我的喉咙感觉有点奇怪。

A：Do you bring up any phlegm when you cough?

你咳嗽时有痰吗？

B：Nope.

没有。

A：I see. I think you should take some cold cures and granules of SMC (xiasangju) for the liver cough.

我明白了。我认为你应该服用一些感冒药和夏桑菊颗粒治疗肝咳嗽。

B：Liver cough? But I'm thinking a lung problem. If I were seeing a western doctor right now, he'd probably have my lungs X-rayed.

肝咳嗽？但我在想是肺部的问题。如果我现在去看西方医生，他可能会给我做肺部 X 光检查。

A：The lung is just a small part of the bigger picture. The zang-organs are believed to be inter-related and are categorized analogically into five elements in traditional Chinese medicine. It is the harmonious relationship between them that contributes to balance or the healthy state of a person. Disharmony, on the other hand, generates imbalances from which diseases arise. In your case, even though the symptom manifests in the lungs, it doesn't mean the root cause lies only there.

肺只是大局的一小部分。中医认为，五脏是相互关联的，可以类比地分为五行。五脏之间的和谐关系维持一个人的平衡或健康状态。另一方面,不和谐会导致不平衡,从而引发疾病。按照你的情况,即使症状表现在肺部,也不意味着根本原因就在那里。

B: Then according to the theory, where else could it be?

那么根据这个理论,原因还能在哪里呢?

A: The lung is associated with metal, and the liver with wood, metal can overcome wood. So the purification and descending function of the lung inhibits the hyperactivity of liver-wood. However, depression or long-term frustration, for instance, can disturb the normal free coursing function of the liver and may eventually lead to liver-yang rising. In this scenario, wood becomes hyperactive and rebels against metal. When metal-qi is too weak to descend, it's forced to rise up leading to a cough, the clinical manifestation. That's why we need to have herbs like granules of SMC (xiasangju) to restore the balance.

肺属金,肝属木,金克木。因此,肺的净化和下降功能抑制了肝木的过度活跃。然而,例如,抑郁或长期沮丧会扰乱肝脏的正常自由流动功能,最终可能导致肝阳气上升。在这种情况下,木变得过度活跃,反抗金属。当金属气太弱而无法消退时,它会被迫上升,导致咳嗽,这是临床表现。这就是为什么我们需要像夏桑菊颗粒这样的草药来恢复平衡。

B: Thanks. Now I see the differences between the liver and the lung.

谢谢。现在我了解了肝和肺之间的区别。

Section 3　Key Concepts of Chinese Medicine: Zang-Fu Theory
第3节　中医文化关键概念:脏腑理论

I. Key Concepts 核心概念

Visceral manifestation is the outward revelation of internal organs through which physiological functions and pathological changes can be observed. It also refers to internal organs' corresponding things and phenomena in nature. Zang refers to the organs hidden inside human body while xiang refers to their external physiological and pathological signs as well as their anatomical images and their corresponding phenomena in nature. Visceral manifestation not only reveals the interconnections between internal organs and external phenomena, but also reflects a cognitive method of detecting the internal organs through their manifestations, which is an objective approach to assessing the changes of the internal organs by observing their external manifestations.

藏象是人体内脏及其表现于外的生理、病理征象,以及与自然界相通应的事物和现象。"藏"指隐藏于体内的脏器;"象"主要是指表现于外的生理病理现象,也涉及内在脏腑的解剖形象及其通应的自然界的物象。藏象既揭示了人体内在脏腑与外在现象之间的有机联系,又客观地反映了以象测脏的认识方法,即通过观察外在征象来研究内在脏腑的活动规律。

Zang-fu is a collective term of the five zang-organs, six fu-organs, and extraordinary fu-organs. The zang-fu theory evolved from ancient anatomy, through which the knowledge of shape, structure, and functions of zang-fu organs were obtained. It provided insights into the laws of functional activities of zang-fu organs and their relationships with such factors as meridians, physiques, orifices, and seasonal changes based on yin-yang and the five-element theory by means of observation, i. e., "detecting the internal organs through their manifestations". Therefore, the zang-fu theory features the holistic concept of traditional Chinese medicine. It constitutes an integrated system of functional activities with the focus on the five-zang organs, networked by meridians and collaterals, interconnected with the six fu-organs, the extraordinary fu-organs, tissues, and orifices, as well as corresponding to seasonal and climatic factors.

脏腑是人体内脏的总称,包括五脏、六腑和奇恒之腑。中医对于人体内在脏腑的认识,一方面借助于古代解剖学方法,以了解人体脏腑的结构及形态,推测其功能;另一方面,则是通过观察外在征象,借助于阴阳五行理论来研究内在脏腑的活动规律,以及脏腑与经脉、形体、官窍乃至自然界时令变化等的关系。由此建构了以五脏为中心,以经脉为联络通道,内系六腑、奇恒之腑以及各组织、官窍,外应四时的整体功能活动系统,形成了中医藏象理论有机整体观的特点。

Traditional Chinese medicine, shaped by Chinese philosophy and restricted by the historical conditions of the natural sciences, is quite different from modern western medicine in its conception of the structure of the human body. One of the most outstanding features of this conception is that of the human body as an integral whole. All component parts, including organs and tissues, are considered with respect to the whole body and to their close interrelationship. However, individual parts are ill-defined, especially from the modern anatomical point of view. This makes traditional Chinese medicine a unique system, one that at times seems fantastic and always resists easy comprehension. In fact, most of the traditional theories and principles are founded not upon anatomy but rather upon functional activities, either physiological or pathological, and rely particularly heavily on the notion of therapeutic effects. It should also be noted that all the traditional, physiological and pathological knowledge was not obtained by laboratory experimentation on isolated organs and systems but rather through the clinical observation of practitioners who viewed the human body as an organic whole.

中医受中国哲学的影响,受自然科学自身条件的制约,在人体结构的概念上与现代西方医学有很大的不同。这一概念最突出的特点之一是将人体视为一个整体。所有组成部分,包括器官和组织,都是从整个身体及其密切的相互关系来考虑的。然而,个别部位定义不清,尤其是从现代解剖学的角度来看。这使得传统中医成为一个独特的系统,有时看起来很神奇,总是难以理解。事实上,大多数传统理论和原理都不是建立在解剖学基础上的,而是建立在生理学或病理学的非生理活动基础上,并且在很大程度上依赖于治疗效果的概念。还应该注意的是,所有传统的生理学和病理学知识都不是通过对分离的器官和系统的实验室实验获得的,而是通过将人体视为有机整体的从业者的临床观察获得的。

In traditional Chinese medicine, internal organs are the core structure of the functions of the human body. The internal organs are divided into two categories, the zang and fu organs.

在中医学中,内脏是人体功能的核心部位。内脏分为两大类,脏和腑。

The heart is located in the chest, and is enclosed by the pericardium. The heart governs the circulation through the blood vessels, stores the spirit, and opens into the tongue. By means of its channel, it connects the small intestine with which it stands in interior-exterior relationship. Traditional Chinese medicine holds that the heart's principal functions are propelling the blood through the vessels and governing consciousness and mental activity. The importance of the heart is emphasized in *The Magic Pivot* (*Lingshu*), which states that the heart is the great governor of the five zang-organs and the six fu-organs and is the abode of the spirit. In clinical practice, cardiovascular diseases, many nervous and mental diseases, and conditions involving erosion of the tip of the tongue are all treated as heart diseases.

心脏位于胸部,由心包包裹。心脏主宰血脉,储存精神,并通向舌头。它通过其经络与小肠相连,两者构成了表里关系。中医认为,心脏的主要功能是通血管、调节意识和心理活动。《灵枢》强调了心脏的重要性:心大督五脏六腑,神居。临床上,心血管疾病、许多神经和精神疾病,以及涉及舌尖侵蚀的疾病都被视为心脏病。

II. Key Words 核心词语

1. Five Zang-Organs 五脏

It is a collective term of the heart, lung, liver, spleen, and kidney. The five zang-organs are also called five spiritual zang-organs due to their governing and participating roles in mental activities. The five zang-organs have the common physiological function of generating and storing essential qi. They are primarily involved in storing essential qi to nourish the whole body rather than transporting and eliminating food residues and wastes. Therefore, essential qi has to be abundant and move without blockage so that the nutrients can be distributed evenly. Otherwise, disorders may occur due to the stagnation. That's why the five zang-organs are characterized by storage without discharge and abundance without excess. Five zang-organs are not only closely related to each other, but also interconnected with their corresponding factors and phenomena in nature. They are the core of the theory of visceral manifestation.

是心、肺、肝、脾、肾的总称。由于五脏可主宰或参与人的精神活动,故又称为五神脏。五脏的共同生理功能是化生和贮藏精气。五脏主要贮藏精气,以营养全身组织器官,不参与水谷、糟粕的转输和排泄。因此,精气必须保持充满,运行流畅以不断地布散全身,才能发挥其营养作用,否则,壅实不通即为病态。故五脏的生理特点为藏精气而不泻,满而不能实。五脏之间不仅相互联系密切,而且与天地四时相通,从而形成了以五脏为中心的藏象学说。

2. Heart 心

As one of the five zang-organs, the heart is located in the thorax above the diaphragm and enveloped by the pericardium. It is primarily involved in governing the blood and vessels as well as housing the mind. Since its two physiological functions play significant roles in all activities of life, the heart is regarded as the "monarch of all the organs", "root of life", and "great governor of the five zang-organs and the six fu-organs". It pertains to fire in terms of five elements and relates to summer qi; therefore, it is yang within yang. It is related to the vessels, opens into the tongue, manifests its conditions in the luster of the face and associates with sweat in fluids and joy in emotions. It connects the heart meridian of hand-shaoyin which has an interior-exterior relationship with the small intestine meridian of hand-taiyang.

作为五脏之一,心居胸腔之内,膈膜之上,心包卫护其外。心的主要生理功能为主血脉与主神明。由于心的主血脉和主神明功能主宰着人体整个生命活动,故称心为"君主之官""生之本""五脏六腑之大主"。心在五行属火,为阳中之阳,通于夏气;在体合脉,开窍于舌,其华在面,在液为汗,在志为喜;其经脉为手少阴心经,与手太阳小肠经相互络属,互为表里。

3. Lung 肺

The lung, one of the five zang-organs, is located in the chest. There is one on the left side and one on the right. Since the lung is positioned higher than any other zang-fu organs in the body, it covers them all. The delicate lobe of the lung is vulnerable to the invasion of pathogenic factors such as cold, heat, dryness, and dampness. Associated with the nose, skin, and body hair, the lung is closely linked with the nature and susceptible to the invasion of pathogenic factors. Generally speaking, the lung governs dispersion, depuration, and descent. To be specific, it governs qi and respiration and regulates water passage; with all meridians and vessels converging in it, it assists the heart in promoting blood circulation. The lung pertains to metal in terms of the five elements. It is yin within yang and relates to autumn qi in nature. It is also related to the skin and nose, and manifests its conditions in the luster of the body hair. The lung is associated with nasal mucus in fluids and sorrow in emotions, and houses the corporeal soul. The lung meridian of hand-taiyin has an interior-exterior relationship with the large intestine meridian of hand-yangming.

肺为五脏之一,位于胸腔,左右各一。由于肺在脏腑中的位置最高,因此覆盖着五脏六腑。肺叶娇嫩,不耐寒、热、燥、湿诸邪之侵。肺上通鼻窍,外合皮毛,与自然界息息相通,易受外邪侵袭。肺的基本功能为主宣发肃降,由此派生出主气,司呼吸,通调水道,朝百脉,助心行血等功能。肺在五行属金,为阳中之阴,通于秋气;在体合皮肤,开窍于鼻,其华在毛,在液为涕,肺藏魄,在志为悲(忧)。其经脉为手太阴肺经,与手阳明大肠经相互络属,互为表里。

4. Spleen 脾

The spleen, located in the upper part of the abdomen, is one of the five zang-organs. Its basic functions include governing transportation and transformation, ascent, and blood, among which the transportation and transformation is the core. It is the function of transportation and transformation that helps provide essence for life activities. The spleen pertains to earth in five elements. It is extreme yin of yin and is related to late-summer qi in nature. The spleen is associated with muscles and limbs. It opens into the mouth, has its conditions manifested in the luster of lips, and houses consciousness. It is related to saliva in terms of fluids and thinking in terms of emotions. The spleen meridian of foot-taiyin has an interior-exterior relationship with the stomach meridian of foot-yangming.

脾为五脏之一,位于腹腔上部。脾的基本功能为主运化、主升举和主统血,其中以运化为核心,通过运化为机体生命活动提供精微物质。脾在五行属土,为阴中之至阴,通于长夏之气;在体合肌肉、主四肢,开窍于口,其华在唇,在液为涎,脾舍意,在志为思;其经脉为足太阴脾经,与足阳明胃经相互络属,互为表里。

5. Liver 肝

The liver, one of the five zang-organs, governs the coursing of qi and stores blood. Its physiology is characterized by ascent and movement. The liver prefers free activity and detests depression. It is yin in form but yang in function and is known as the unyielding zang-organ. The liver pertains to wood in five elements. It is yang within yin and is related to spring qi in nature. The liver is associated with sinews and eyes, and manifests its conditions in the luster of nails. It is related to tears in fluids, houses ethereal soul, and is linked with anger in emotions. The liver meridian of foot-jueyin has an interior-exterior relationship with the gall bladder meridian of foot-shaoyang.

肝为五脏之一,基本功能为主疏泄和主藏血。肝的生理特性为主升主动,喜条达而恶抑郁,体阴而用阳,被称为刚脏。肝在五行属木,为阴中之阳,通于春气;在体合筋,开窍于目,其华为爪,在液为泪,肝藏魂,在志为怒;其经脉为足厥阴肝经,与足少阳胆经相互络属,互为表里。

6. Kidney 肾

The kidney, located in the lumbar region on either side of the spine, is one of the five zang-organs. Its basic functions involve storing essence, dominating growth, development and reproduction, governing water, and receiving qi. The kidney stores the prenatal essence which could be transformed into kidney qi, i. e. , kidney yin and kidney yang. Kidney yin and kidney yang promote and coordinate the yin and yang of the whole body. They are the foundations of the yin and yang of zang-fu organs, and the source of life activities. Therefore, the kidney is the root of prenatal constitution. Pertaining to water in terms of the five-element theory, the kidney is yin within yin and corresponds to winter qi in nature. It is related to bones, opens into ears, anus, and genitals, associated with spittle in body fluids and fear in emotions, and stores will. Its conditions can be manifested in the luster of hair. The kidney meridian of foot-shaoyin has an interior-exterior relationship with the bladder meridian of foot-taiyang.

肾为五脏之一,位于腰部,脊柱两旁,左右各一。其基本功能为藏精,主生长、发育和生殖,主水,主纳气。由于肾藏先天之精,肾精化肾气,肾气分阴阳,肾阴与肾阳能促进、协调全身脏腑之阴阳,为脏腑阴阳之本,生命之源,故先天之本。肾在五行属水,为阴中之阴,通于冬气;在体合骨,开窍于耳与二阴,其华在发,在液为唾;肾舍志,在情志为恐。其经脉为足少阴肾经,与足太阳膀胱经相互络属,互为表里。

7. Six Fu-Organs 六腑

The six fu-organs is a collective term of the gall bladder, stomach, small intestine, large intestine, urinary bladder, and triple energizer (sanjiao). They are primarily involved in the digestion and transmission of food and water. They transport, discharge but do not store, characterized by the functions of unblocking and descending. These organs take in and digest food and water, absorb the essence, transmit the residues after decomposition, and finally remove wastes from the body. They cooperate and work in sequence to fulfill their respective functions. The six fu-organs are not supposed to be filled with food, water, and wastes. Otherwise, disorders will occur. The dysfunction of their transforming and transporting will make it difficult to digest food and water and further convert these substances into essence. Moreover, it will be difficult to remove waste substances and turbid qi from the body. All of the above may cause disorders of the five zang-organs.

六腑是胆、胃、小肠、大肠、膀胱、三焦的总称,具有出纳、转输、传化水谷的功能。六腑的生理功能是受盛和传化水谷。六腑的生理特点是传化物而不藏、以通为用、以降为顺。六腑受盛和传化水谷,排泄糟粕,必须及时把代谢后的糟粕排泄于体外,并不贮藏精气。六腑的传化,以一定的顺序先后,虚实更替,但六腑整体则不能被水谷糟粕充满,充塞滞满则为患。若六腑传化功能异常,水谷精微难以化生,体内废物及五脏浊气难以及时排出体外,则可导致五脏功能失常。

8. Gall Bladder 胆

The gall bladder, one of the six fu-organs and extraordinary organs, is located under the right side of the ribs and attached to the short lobe of the liver. It is a hollow muscular organ storing bile, the refined essence of human body. The stored bile should be excreted regularly; therefore, it is characterized with discharge without storage, which is why the gall bladder is one of the six fu-organs. The gall bladder also stores essence, but it is different from other fu-organs that transform food and water as well as discharge wastes. Therefore, it is also called the extraordinary organ. The physiological functions of the gall bladder involve storing and excreting bile and assisting the free flow of liver qi. The gall bladder meridian of foot-shaoyang has an interior-exterior relationship with the liver meridian of foot-jueyin.

胆为六腑之一,又属奇恒之腑,位于右肋下,附于肝之短叶间。胆为中空的囊性器官,内藏胆汁——人体的精气。胆所内藏的胆汁应适时排泄,具有泻而不藏的特性,故胆为六腑之一。又因其内藏精汁,与六腑传化水谷、排泄糟粕有别,故又属奇恒之腑。胆的生理功能是贮存、排泄胆汁,并助肝气之疏泄。胆的经脉为足少阳胆经,与足厥阴肝经相互络属,构成表里关系。

9. Stomach 胃

The stomach, one of the six fu-organs, is located in the middle energizer and can be divided into three parts, i. e. , the upper, the middle, and the lower part of gastric cavity. The upper part includes the cardia connecting to the esophagus and the lower part is the pylorus connecting to the small intestine, which provides the pathway for food and water into and out of the stomach. The stomach is indispensable to digesting and absorbing food and water. Its primary physiological functions involve receiving and decomposing the ingested food and drinks. The stomach and the spleen are both located in the middle energizer, pertaining to earth in the five elements. The stomach belongs to yang, namely yangming and dry earth, whereas the spleen pertains to yin, namely taiyin and damp earth. The stomach meridian of foot-yangming has an interior-exterior relationship with the spleen meridian of foot-taiyin.

胃为六腑之一,位于中焦,分上脘、中脘、下脘三部分。其上口为贲门,下口为幽门。贲门上连食道,幽门下通小肠,是饮食物出入胃腑的通道。胃是机体对饮食物进行消化吸收的重要脏器,主受纳、腐熟水谷。胃的生理功能是受纳与腐熟饮食物。胃与脾同居中焦,在五行中皆属土。胃为阳明燥土,属阳;脾为太阴湿土,属阴。经脉为足阳明胃经,与足太阴脾经为表里。

10. Small Intestine 小肠

The small intestine, located in the abdomen, is one of the six fu-organs. Its upper opening is connected with the stomach at the pylorus, and its lower one is connected with the large intestine at the ileocolic opening. The small intestine is a long, winding, and zigzagging tract organ divided into the duodenum, jejunum, and ileum. It plays an important role in digestion, absorption, and waste disposal, whose function is to receive the chyme and transform it, and to separate purified nutrients from turbid wastes. The small intestine meridian of hand-taiyang has an interior-exterior relationship with the heart meridian of hand-shaoyin.

小肠为六腑之一,位于腹中,上口在幽门处与胃相连,下口在阑门处与大肠相连。小肠是一个比较长的、呈迂曲回环叠积之状的管状器官,包括十二指肠、空肠和回肠,是机体消化饮食物,吸收其精微,下传其糟粕的重要脏器。小肠的生理功能是受盛、化物和泌别清浊。小肠的经脉为手太阳小肠经,与手少阴心经相互络属,构成表里关系。

11. Large Intestine 大肠

The large intestine, located in the abdomen, is one of the six fu-organs. It joins the small intestine at the ileocolic opening, and ends at the anus. The upper part of the large intestine is the hui (coiling) intestine, including the ileum and the upper colon in modern anatomy. The lower part is the guang (wide) intestine, including the sigmoid colon and the rectum. Like the small intestine, the large intestine is a hollow and zigzagging tract organ, primarily involved in water absorption of the remaining food residues, feces formation and defecation. The major function of the large intestine is to transmit the waste while absorbing water. The large intestine meridian of hand-yangming has an interior-exterior relationship with the lung meridian of hand-taiyin.

大肠为六腑之一,位于腹中。大肠上口通过阑门与小肠相接,下端出口为肛门。大肠的上段称为回肠,包括现代解剖学中的回肠和结肠上段;下段称为广肠,包括乙状结肠和直肠。与小肠一样,大肠也是一个管腔性器官,呈回环叠积之状,是对食物残渣中的水液进行吸收,形成粪便并有度排出的脏器。大肠的主要生理功能为传导糟粕和吸收水分。大肠的经脉为手阳明大肠经,与手太阴肺经相互络属,构成表里关系。

12. Urinary Bladder 膀胱

Urinary bladder, one of the six fu-organs, is a hollow muscular organ in the middle of the lower abdomen. It connects with the kidney in the upper through the ureters, and the urethra in the lower, and ends in an opening — the urinary meatus. Urinary bladder is responsible for temporarily storing and discharging urine. The urinary bladder meridian of foot-taiyang has an interior-exterior relationship with the kidney meridian of foot-shaoyin. The urine, temporarily stored in the urinary bladder after being processed by viscera, is separated into the refined material and the waste. The former is recycled in the human body, whereas the latter is discharged. Storage and discharge of urine depends on the qi transformation and securing function of the kidney. If the kidney fails to transform qi or secure urine, or the urinary bladder fails to control the urethral orifice, such symptoms will occur as dysuria, frequent urination, urinary urgency, enuresis, and urinary incontinence.

膀胱为六腑之一,位于小腹中央,是一个中空的囊状器官。其上有输尿管与肾相连,其下连尿道,开口于前阴。膀胱的生理功能是贮存津液和排泄尿液。膀胱的经脉为足太阳膀胱经,与足少阴肾经相互络属,构成表里关系。人体脏腑代谢后所形成的津液下达膀胱,在肾的气化作用下,升清降浊,清者被人体再吸收利用,浊者通过肾的气化作用,适时有度地排出体外。膀胱的存津液、排泄尿液功能,有赖于肾气的蒸化和固摄作用。若肾的气化和固摄作用失常,膀胱开阖失权,既可出现小便不利或癃闭,又可出现尿频、尿急、遗尿、小便失禁等。

13. Triple Energizer 三焦

Triple energizer, alternatively named the solitary fu-organ, is one of the six fu-organs. It is the largest in size among the zang-fu organs, including the upper energizer, the middle energizer, and the lower energizer. Triple energizer governs qi in the entire body and regulates water passage. The meridian of hand-shaoyang has an interior-exterior relationship with the pericardium meridian of hand-jueyin. Physicians of past generations held varied ideas about triple energizer in its form and substance. Some thought triple energizer pertained to six fu-organs and performed comprehensive functions. It was a large fu-organ located in the thoracic and abdominal cavity without an interior-exterior relationship with any of the five zang-organs. Others believed that triple energizer divided the internal organs into three parts. The upper energizer referred to the region above the diaphragm, the middle energizer in between the diaphragm and the navel, and the lower energizer below the navel.

三焦为六腑之一,是脏腑外围最大的腑,又称孤腑。三焦是上焦、中焦、下焦的合称。三焦的功能为主持诸气,通调水道。经脉为手少阳经,与手厥阴心包经为表里。历代医家对三焦的形态和实质有不同的认识。一种认为三焦为六腑之一,和其他脏腑一样是具有综合功能的器官,由于其与五脏无表里配合关系,是分布于胸腹腔的一个大腑。另一种认为三焦为划分内脏的区域部位,即膈以上为上焦,膈至脐之间为中焦,脐以下为下焦。

Ⅲ. Dialogues 情景对话

1. Dialogue 1 对话 1

Teacher: Good morning.
　　　　　早上好。

Student：Good morning.

　　　　早上好。

Teacher：Today, we are going to have a review of the zang-fu theory, mainly focusing on the knowledge of the heart. The class will be divided into two parts：firstly, the physiology and pathology of the heart; secondly, the relationship of the heart to the other organs. Now, let's begin.

　　　　今天我们来复习一下脏腑理论,主要讲心学。该课程将分为两个部分:首先,是心脏的生理学和病理学;其次,是心脏与其他器官的关系。现在,让我们开始吧。

Student：OK.

　　　　好的。

Teacher：To start with, do you still remember the function of the heart?

　　　　首先,你还记得心脏的功能吗?

Student：Yes. According to the *Plain Questions*（*Suwen*）, the heart governs the blood and vessels and the heart stores the spirit.

　　　　是的。《素问》说,心主血脉,心藏神。

Teacher：Great, the answer is correct. The first function emphasizes that all the blood and vessels of the body are subordinate to the heart. Although the blood is produced from the essence of grain and water assimilated by the stomach and spleen, it is the heart that ensures constant circulation of blood, maintaining the supply of nourishment to the whole body.

　　　　太好了,答案是正确的。第一个功能强调身体的所有血管都服从于心脏。虽然血液是由胃和脾吸收的谷和水的精华产生的,但是心脏确保血液的持续循环,维持对全身的营养供应。

Student：Yes, the first one is easy to understand. Can you give me more information about the second point? We know that in western medicine, the spirit or mental activity is related to the brain and has nothing to do with the heart, which is in contradiction with the Chinese concept.

　　　　是的,第一个很容易理解。关于第二点,你能给我更多的意见吗? 我们知道,在西方医学中,精神活动与大脑有关,与心脏无关,这与中医的观念不一致。

Teacher：I know what you mean. This is the difference between the two systems. Here, spirit refers to mental faculties. In western physiology, both consciousness and mental activity are considered functions of the brain, but in traditional Chinese medicine their different aspects are attributed to the heart. If the heart fulfills its functions normally and blood and qi are abundant, the spirit-mind is lucid, making the individual alert and responsive to the environment. If, however, the heart is diseased, the spirit may be disquieted and give rise to some signs, such as…?

我知道你的意思。这就是两种系统之间的区别。在这里,精神指的是心智能力。在西方生理学中,意识和精神活动都被认为是大脑的功能,但在中医中,它们的不同方面被归因于心脏。如果心功能正常,气血充足,精神就会清醒,使人对环境保持警觉和反应。然而,如果心脏有病,心灵可能会感到不安,并产生一些迹象,比如……?

Student：Such as vexation, susceptibility to fright and palpitation, restless sleep or profuse dreaming. Am I right?

比如烦恼、易受惊吓和心悸、睡眠不安或大量做梦。我说得对吗?

Teacher：Very good! Do you have any other questions?

很好! 你还有其他问题吗?

Student：How should I understand the statements "the heart opens into the tongue" and "the tongue is the sprout of the heart"? Are there any differences between these two concepts?

我应该如何理解"心向舌头开放"和"舌头是心的萌芽"这两个概念? 有什么区别吗?

Teacher：Actually, they are the same ones stated from different perspectives. These statements imply that disturbances of the heart are invariably reflected in the tongue. For example, in cases of pathological fire in the heart, the tip of the tongue becomes distinctly red and the tongue may become painful and ulcerated. We will discuss this during the class on four examination techniques in traditional Chinese medicine.

事实上,它们是从不同的角度说出来的相同概念。这些说法暗示着心灵的紊乱总是会在舌头上再次显现。例如,在心脏发生病理性有火的情况下,舌尖会明显变红,舌头可能会疼痛和溃疡。我们将在中医四大检查技术课上讨论这个问题。

Student：Oh, that's useful. Thank you very much for your help.

哦,那很有用。非常感谢你的帮助。

Teacher：You're welcome.

不客气。

2. Dialogue 2 对话 2

Teacher：Good morning everyone, welcome to my class.

大家早上好,欢迎大家来上课。

Students：Good morning.

早上好。

Teacher：Today, we are going to learn a new disorder and its treatment from the perspective of traditional Chinese medicine. I know most of you may have heard of this one, that is, gastritis. From the name we see that it means the inflammation of stomach mucous; pathologically, the disease may be diffuse, involving all parts of the stomach, or localized to a specific area. Clinically, we can classify gastritis into two types, who know the names?

今天,我们将从传统中医的角度来学习一种新的病症及其治疗方法。我知道你们大多数人可能都听说过这个,那就是胃炎。从名称上我们可以看出,它的意思是胃黏膜的炎症;在病理学上,这种疾病可能是弥漫性的,涉及胃的所有部位,或局限于特定区域。临床上,我们可以把胃炎分为两类,谁知道名字呢?

Student A：I know the answer. According to the cause of the disease, it can be divided into acute or chronic gastritis. The former is believed to be a self-limited disease, whereas the latter persists for a long period.

我知道答案。根据病因可分为急性或慢性。前者被认为是一种自我限制的疾病,而后者则持续很长一段时间。

Teacher：Very good! Does anyone know the symptoms of western-medicine-defined gastritis?

非常好！有人知道西医定义的胃炎的症状吗？

Student B：I'd like to answer this one. The western-medicine-defined gastritis is characterized by epigastric pain, nausea and vomiting, and in severe cases accompanied by hematemesis.

我想回答这个问题。西方医学定义的胃炎以上腹痛、恶心和呕吐为特征,严重时伴有吐血。

Teacher：Excellent!

太棒了！

Teacher：Now, from the perspective of traditional Chinese medicine, let's see how many causes can lead to gastritis. According to the book, we can find that there are five common causes. What are they? Any volunteers?

现在,从中医的角度来看,让我们看看有多少原因会导致胃炎。根据这本书,我们可以发现有五个常见的原因。它们是什么？有主动回答的吗？

Student C：The first is impairment of the spleen and stomach by improper diet; the second is attack of the stomach by hyperactive liver qi; the third is deficiency cold of the spleen and stomach; the fourth is blood stasis in the collateral; the fifth and final one is yin deficiency of the spleen and stomach.

一是饮食不当,脾胃受损;二是肝气上亢攻胃;三是脾胃虚寒;四是经方瘀血;五是脾胃阴虚。

Teacher：Good! So, from what we have learned you can easily conclude that the content is really different from the pathology based on the endoscopic and laboratory findings. In traditional Chinese medicine the diagnostic methods are all based on different clinical manifestations or as we call it, syndrome differentiation.

好！因此,根据我们所了解到的情况,我们很容易确定其内容与基于内窥镜和实验室结果的病理学确实不同。在传统中医中,诊断方法都是基于不同的临床表现,或者我们称之为辨证。

Student D：I think this diagnostic method is more scientific than the western one. It requires us to have more experience and the ability for comprehensive analysis.

我觉得这种诊断方法比西方的更科学。它要求我们有更多的经验和综合分析的能力。

Teacher：Yes, it really takes a long time to master.

是的,掌握它确实需要很长时间。

Section 4　Key Concepts of Chinese Medicine：Qi, Blood, Essence and Fluids
第4节　中医文化关键概念:气、血、精、液

I . Key Concepts 核心概念

Qi, blood, essence, and fluids are the basic elements of all human physiologic activities. Qi vitalizes the body, propels and warms, and is yang in nature. Blood and fluids are the sustenance of the body, nourishing and moistening the entire organism, and are yin in nature. Essence is the basis of physical development and reproduction. It is the stored surplus potential of the human body, and the basis of blood and fluid production. All changes that occur in the human body from birth to death result from the interaction of qi, blood, essence, and fluids.

气、血、精、液是人类一切生理活动的基本要素。气使身体充满活力,推动并温暖身体,本质上是阳。血和液是身体的营养,滋养和滋润整个机体,本质上是阴的。精本质是身体发育和生殖的基础。它是人体储存的剩余潜能,是血液和液体产生的基础。人从生到死的一切变化,都是气、血、精、液相互作用的结果。

Blood is the red fluid that nourishes the whole body. It is chiefly produced from nutrients absorbed from digested food. It provides nourishment to every part of the body and is propelled around the body by the action of qi. The main pathologies of blood are blood deficiency and blood stasis. When blood fails to perform its nourishing function, it is called the "insufficiency of the blood" or "blood deficiency". It is marked by a lusterless or withered-yellow complexion, a pale tongue, dizziness, heart palpitations, and a fine pulse. When the blood moves slowly or stops moving, this is called "blood stasis". Blood stasis accounts for bruises, varicose veins, abdominal masses, and many other conditions.

血液是滋养全身的红色液体。它主要是由消化后的食物的营养成分产生的。它为身体的每一个部位提供营养,并通过气的作用在身体周围推动。血液的主要病理是血虚血瘀。当血液不能起到滋养作用时,被称为"血不足"或"血亏"。其特点是面色无光泽或枯黄,舌头苍白,眩晕,心悸,脉搏细。当血液缓慢流动或停止流动时,被称为"血瘀"。血瘀是指瘀伤、静脉曲张、腹部肿块和许多其他情况。

Essence is a substance that is stored in the kidney. It is derived from two sources, from one's parents before birth, and from the nutrients ingested during the course of one's life. The concept of essence is used to explain reproduction, growth, development, and aging. Essence is susceptible to insufficiency. The manifestations differ according to the age at which the insufficiency appears. When essence is insufficient in young children, it causes problems of mental and physical development. When essence becomes insufficient in advancing years, it leads to signs of premature aging and early loss of mental faculties.

精是一种储存在肾脏中的物质。它有两个来源,一个是出生前的父母,另一个是一生中摄入的营养物质。精的概念主要用于解释生殖、生长、发育和衰老。精容易不足。出现功能不全的年龄不同,表现也不同。当幼儿的精不足时,会导致身心发展问题。当精在衰老时变得不足,就会导致过早衰老和早期丧失心智的迹象。

Fluids are a major element in the body. Fluids take specific forms such as saliva, gastric juice, tears, nasal mucus, sweat, and urine. Body fluids are formed from food and drink by the action of the stomach and spleen. They are distributed around the body principally by the action of the lung. By the action of the kidney, waste fluids are turned into urine, which is stored in the bladder for discharge. Fluid pathologies include various forms of insufficiency and accumulation. Insufficiency of the fluids can be the result of high fever or excessive vomiting and urination. Fluid accumulations take the form of edema, called "water swelling", or local accumulations in the chest, abdomen, and other parts of the body, generally called "phlegm".

液体是身体的主要成分。液体有特定的形式,如唾液、胃液、眼泪、鼻涕、汗液和尿液。体液是由食物和饮料在胃和脾的作用下形成的。它们主要通过肺的作用分布在全身。在肾脏的作用下,废液被转化为尿液,储存在膀胱中进行排泄。液体病理包括各种形式的功能不全和积聚。液体不足可能是由于高烧或过度呕吐和排尿造成的。液体积聚以水肿的形式出现,称为"水渍",或胸部、腹部和身体其他部位的局部积聚,统称为"痰液"。

II. Key Words 核心词语

1. Essence 精

Essence, a tangible and nutrient substance, is derived from the innate life substance from parents and nutrient substances that are acquired later from food and drinks. It is the origin of life and the most basic substance constituting human body and maintaining life activities. Essence could be understood in either a broad or a narrow sense. The former refers to all types of tangible and nutrient substances including blood, body fluids, marrow, and the nutrients from food and drinks, which are believed to constitute human body and maintain life activities. The latter refers to what is stored in the kidney, i. e. , kidney essence, including prenatal essence from conception and postnatal essence from food and drinks, which is believed to produce offspring and promote growth and development.

精是禀受于父母的生命物质与后天水谷精微融合而成的一种有形的精微物质,是生命的本原,构成人体和维持人体生命活动最基本的物质。精的含义有广义与狭义之分:广义之精,是指构成人体和维持人体生命活动的一切有形的精微物质,包括血、津液、髓以及水谷精微等;狭义之精,是指肾所藏之精,即肾精,包括禀受于父母的先天之精和后天水谷之精,具有繁衍后代、促进生长发育等作用。

2. Qi 气

The concept of qi includes three levels of meaning: ① An ancient philosophical concept, referring to the origin of everything in the universe and the substantial element that constitutes the soma and psyche. ② The substance, energy, and information that constitute the human body and maintain the life activities. Qi of human can be divided into yang qi and yin qi based on the nature; original qi, pectoral qi, nutrient qi, and defense qi based on the transformation; stomach qi, heart qi, liver qi, kidney qi, lung qi, spleen qi and visceral qi based on its function. ③Pathogenic qi, a type of qi that causes diseases.

气的含义可以概括为三个方面:一是中国古代哲学概念,指构成宇宙万物的实在本元,也是构成人类形体与化生精神的实在元素。二是构成人体、维持人体生命活动的物质、能量、信息的总称。人体生命之气随其性质有阳气、阴气之分,随其转化有元气、宗气、营气、卫气之别,随其功能活动有胃气、心气、肝气、肾气、肺气、脾气、脏腑之气等称谓。三是指导致人体发病的因素,即邪气。

3. Spirit 神

Spirit has three different meanings: ①the creator, master, and original source of everything in the universe; ②life activities including physiological functions and mental activities; and ③consciousness and mental activities such as cognition, emotion, and will. Governed by the heart, spirit in terms of life activities is primarily involved in human physiological functions and mental activities that pertain to five zang-organs respectively. Essence, qi, blood, and body fluids are the substantial foundations for spirit, which is the result of movements, changes, and interactions among the essential qi of zang-fu organs.

神有三种不同的含义:其一,指天地万物以及人体生命的创造者、主宰者和原动力。其二,指人体的生命活动,包括生理功能与心理活动。其三,指人的意识和心理活动,包括认知、情感与意志等活动。就人体生命活动而言,神主要指人的生理功能与心理活动,由心主管,而分属于五脏。神以精、气、血、津液作为物质基础,是脏腑精气运动变化和相互作用的结果。

4. Essential Qi 精气

Essential qi, a type of fine qi, is the material basis of human growth, development, and various functional activities. It includes reproductive essence, essence transformed from food and drinks, and the fresh air in nature.

精气是一种精灵细微之气,是人体生长、发育及各种功能活动的物质基础,包括生殖之精、饮食化生的精微物质和自然界的清气等。

5. Original Qi 元气

Original qi, also known as primordial qi, is the most essential and important qi of the human body and is the source qi that serves as the driving force for the activities of zang-fu organs. Transformed from the prenatal essence and nourished by the postnatal essence, it is distributed throughout the body via triple energizer (sanjiao). It internally permeates five zang-organs and six fu-organs and externally reaches the skin, striae, and interstices, promoting and stimulating the physiological functions of all organs and meridians. Original qi performs two physiological functions. First, it promotes and regulates growth, development, and reproduction. When the reproductive essence from parents combines and develops into an embryo, original qi comes into being. Second, original qi propels and regulates the physiological activities of zang-fu organs, meridians, as well as other organs and tissues when it flows to every part of the human body via triple energizer (sanjiao).

元气又称原气,是人体最基本、最重要的气,是人体生命活动的原动力,由先天之精所化,赖后天之精所滋养,通过三焦输布全身,内达五脏六腑,外至肌肤腠理,推动和激发人体各脏腑、经络等组织器官正常的生理活动。元气的生理功能主要有两个方面:其一,推动和调节人体的生长、发育和生殖。当父母的生殖之精结合形成胚胎时,即产生了胚胎个体内部的元气。其二,元气通过三焦,流布周身,推动并调节人体各脏腑、经络,以及其他器官和组织的生理活动。

6. Pectoral Qi 宗气

Pectoral qi refers to the qi in the chest transformed from the absorbed nutrients of food and drinks and the inhaled fresh air. It performs two functions：①facilitating breathing in the airway and promoting the breathing function of the lung; and ②permeating the heart and vessels to promote the flow of qi and blood and assist the blood circulation of the heart. Therefore, the exuberance or debilitation of pectoral qi is closely related to the circulation of qi and blood, the regulation of body temperature, the movement of limbs, and the strength of breath and voice.

宗气聚积于胸中,由水谷精微之气与肺吸入的大气汇聚而成。宗气的主要功能有二:一是走息道而行呼吸,推动肺的呼吸运动。二是贯心脉以行气血,促进心脏的血液循环。所以宗气之盛衰与人体的气血循环、寒温调节、肢体活动以及呼吸、声音的强弱均有密切关系。

7. Nutrient Qi 营气

Nutrient qi, also known as rong qi, flowing in the vessels with the function of nourishing, is extracted from the essence of food and drinks transformed and transported by the spleen and the stomach. It circulates in channels with blood and flows in the entire body via twelve regular meridians, conception vessel, and governor vessel. It is primarily involved in producing blood and nourishing human body. Nutrient qi, abundant in nutritive components, can produce blood when combined with body fluids; hence it is the primary substance for blood engenderment. It circulates in the body with blood and distributes nutrients to zang-fu organs and meridians, maintaining the normal physiological function.

营气又称荣气,指流动于脉中富有营养作用的气,由脾胃运化的水谷精微所化生。营气循行于经脉之中,与血液并行,通过十二经脉和任、督二脉运行于全身各个部分。其主要生理功能为化生血液及给全身提供营养。营气富含营养成分,与津液相结合而化生血液,是生成血液的主要物质基础。营气随血液运行于全身,输布于各脏腑、经络,发挥营养作用,维持正常的生理功能。

8. Defense Qi 卫气

Defense qi, intrepid and swift, is transformed from the nutrients of food and drinks, and originated from the spleen and the stomach. It reaches the upper energizer and flows swiftly outside the vessels. It is primarily involved in warming and nourishing the interior and the exterior of human body, protecting skin from exogenous pathogenic factors, nourishing interstices, and controlling the opening and closing of sweat pores. Being the primary source of heat, defense qi permeates the whole body, warms the muscles, skin, hair, and zang-fu organs to keep them lustrous and healthy, and maintains constant body temperature. It regulates sweat discharge by controlling the opening and closing of sweat pores.

卫气生于水谷,源于脾胃,出于上焦,行于脉外,其性刚悍,运行迅速流利,具有温养内外,护卫肌表,抗御外邪,滋养腠理,开合汗孔等功能。卫气是产生热量的主要来源,其流布于体表乃至周身,对肌肉、皮毛和脏腑发挥着温养作用,使肌肉充实,皮肤润泽,并维持人体体温的相对恒定。通过控制汗孔开合,可调节汗液的排泄。

9. Qi Transformation 气化

Qi transformation refers to various transforming changes caused by qi, i. e., metabolism and inter-transformation of essence, qi, blood, and body fluids, as well as the evolution of human life. Therefore, qi transformation is the metabolic process in human body whereby the substance and energy transformation takes place, and thus it is the root of life activities. Zang-fu organs play an indispensable role in activating and maintaining qi transformation, whose normal function depends on inter-regulation of physiological activities among zang-fu organs. Constant substance exchange between nature and human body is indispensable to maintaining life activities.

气化指产生各种变化的运动,具体表现为精、气、血、津液各自的新陈代谢及其相互转化,以及人体生命的演化等。所以气化实际上就是体内物质新陈代谢的过程,是物质转化和能量转化的过程,因而也是生命活动的本质所在。气化过程的激发和维系,离不开脏腑的功能;气化过程的有序进行,是脏腑生理活动相互协调的结果。人体生命活动的维持,需要不断地与自然界进行物质交换。

10. Qi Movement 气机

Qi movement refers to the movement of qi in all parts of the body including zang-fu organs and meridians. It motivates and propels the physiological functions of organs and tissues. Qi movement is manifested in such basic forms as ascending, descending, exiting, and entering (i. e., upward, downward, outward, and inward movement). There are many forms of qi movement, including the opposite forms of ascending and descending, exiting and entering, attracting and repulsing, diverging and converging. It is precisely because of the constant movement of qi that human body is able to exhale the stale and inhale the fresh, rasie lucidity and depress turbidity, be in an endless state of generating and transforming, and maintain normal metabolism and life activities. Balanced qi movement of ascending, descending, exiting, and entering is essential for maintaining life activities.

气机指气在全身各脏腑、经络等中的运动,激发和推动着人体各器官和组织的生理活动,其基本形式为升、降、出、入。气运动的形式多种多样,包括上升和下降、外出和内入、吸引和排斥、发散和凝聚等对立的形式。正是由于气的不断运动,人体才能吐故纳新、升清降浊、生化不息,并维持正常的新陈代谢及生命活动。气机升、降、出、入的协调平衡是保证生命活动正常进行的重要环节。

11. Acupoint 气穴

Acupoints, also called acupuncture point, are points on the surface of human body where meridian qi infuses, hence the Chinese name qixue (literally qi points). They are the points where qi of the zang-fu organs and meridians concentrates or passes, where needling can be applied, and where some diseases or pains are manifested or felt. The points, closely linked to zang-fu organs through meridians, can manifest the physiological and pathological changes in zang-fu organs. Various stimuli such as needling, moxibustion, and massage can be applied at acupoints to increase immunity against diseases, regulate deficiency and excess conditions, prevent and treat diseases, and in some cases aid diagnosis.

气穴，又称腧穴，为经脉之气输注的孔穴，因此中文名为气穴。气穴与脏腑、经络之气相通，是针刺治疗的刺激点，又是某些病痛的反应点。气穴通过经络与脏腑密切相关，它能反应各脏腑的生理或病理变化，通过针刺、艾灸、按摩等刺激，能够调动人体内在的抗病能力，调节机体的虚实状态，以达防治疾病的目的，有时还可以用作辅助诊断。

12. Set of Qi 气海

The sea of qi refers to danzhong where pectoral qi concentrates and originates. Danzhong refers to the central part of the chest where the lung is located, promoting breathing and governing the qi flow in the entire body. The lung, connecting all the vessels and meridians, can distribute the nutrients of food and drinks to replenish and nourish the entire body. Danzhong is the sea of qi where pectoral qi converges. It is alternatively named the upper sea of qi. The sea of qi is also the name of an acupoint located in the middle of the abdominal midline, i. e. , the upper sea of qi. It is indicated for collapse, syncope, abdominal pain, diarrhea, irregular menstruation, dysmenorrhea, uterine bleeding, leucorrhea, seminal emission, impotence, enuresis, and hernia.

气海指膻中，即宗气会聚、发源之处。膻中指胸中部位，肺居其中，行呼吸，主一身之气，肺朝百脉，能布散水谷精气，以充养全身，所以把膻中部位称为宗气汇聚之海，又称上气海。由于宗气积聚于胸中，故称胸中为气海。气海也指位于腹正中线的一个经穴名，即上气海。该穴主治虚脱、厥逆、腹痛、泄泻、月经不调、痛经、崩漏、带下、遗精、阳痿、遗尿、疝气等疾病。

13. Qi Deficiency 气虚

Qi deficiency refers to the weakness of healthy qi in human body. Two main reasons account for qi deficiency：①Insufficiency of qi transformation,

e. g. , the deficiency of prenatal essence may lead to the deficiency of original qi; spleen-stomach weakness may result in deficiency of essence from food and drinks; or the failure of lung in dispersing and descending may reduce the inhalation volume of fresh air. ② Excessive consumption of qi, e. g. , excessive lassitude, exogenously-contracted febrile diseases, or chronic consumptive diseases may lead to over-consumption of qi and consequently qi deficiency. Clinical manifestations of qi deficiency include listlessness, fatigue, disinclination to talk due to the lack of qi, dizziness, spontaneous sweating, pallor complexion, pale tongue, and feeble pulse.

气虚指人体的正气虚弱。造成气虚的原因主要有两方面：一是气的生化不足，如先天禀赋不足，元气衰少；或脾胃虚弱，水谷精气不足；或肺的宣降失常，清气吸入不足。二是气的消耗太多，如过于劳倦，或外感热病，或患慢性消耗性疾病，使气耗散过多而致虚亏。气虚的临床表现，以精神委顿、倦怠乏力、少气懒言、眩晕、自汗、面色苍白、舌淡、脉虚弱等症为特点。

Ⅲ. Dialogues 情景对话

1. Dialogue 1 对话 1

Teacher：Good morning everyone, welcome to my class.

　　　　大家早上好，欢迎大家来上课。

Students：Good morning.

　　　　早上好。

Teacher：Now, class begins. Firstly, I'd like to ask one student about the knowledge we studied last week. The question is what are fluids? Any volunteers?

　　　　现在开始上课。首先，我想问一个学生关于我们上周学习的知识。问题是什么是体液？有主动回答的吗？

Student A：I'd like to answer this question. The term "fluids" embraces all the normal fluid substances of the human body, such as sweat, saliva, stomach juices, urine, and other fluids secreted by or discharged from the body.

　　　　我想回答这个问题。"体液"一词包括人体所有正常的液体物质,如汗液、唾液、胃液、尿液和其他由身体分泌或排出的液体。

Teacher：Great! Can anyone summarize the physiological function of the fluids?

太好了! 有人能概括体液的生理功能吗?

Student B：The main functions of fluids are to keep the organs, muscles, skin, mucous membranes, and orifices adequately moistened, to lubricate the joints, and to nourish the brain, marrow, and bones.

体液的主要功能是保持器官、肌肉、皮肤、黏膜和孔口充分湿润,润滑关节,滋养大脑、骨髓和骨骼。

Teacher：The next question is, "where do the fluids come from?"

下一个问题是:"体液是从哪里来的?"

Student C：I know the answer. Body fluids are formed from food and drink by the action of the stomach and spleen.

我知道答案。体液是通过胃和脾脏的作用从食物和饮料中形成的。

Teacher：Good, do you know how the fluids are distributed throughout the human body?

很好,你知道体液是如何在人体内分布的吗?

Student C：I remember they are distributed around the body principally by the action of the lung.

我记得它们主要通过肺的作用分布在全身。

Teacher：So, how about the waste fluids?

那么,废液呢?

Student C：Eh? maybe by the action of the kidney?

嗯? 可能是肾的作用?

Teacher：Yes, by the action of the kidney, waste fluids are turned into urine, which is stored in the bladder for discharge. This is the same as western anatomy.

是的,通过肾脏的作用,废液会变成尿液,储存在膀胱中排出。这和西方解剖学是一样的。

2. Dialogue 2 对话 2

Teacher：The last one is，"who can tell me the difference between 'liquid'（jin）and 'humor'（ye）?"

最后一个问题是："谁能告诉我'津'和'液'的区别?"

Student D：I want to answer this question. Liquid refers to fluid that is relatively thin，mobile，and yang in quality，while humor denotes thicker and less mobile yin fluid. Am I right?

我想回答这个问题。津是指相对较薄、流动性强、具有阳气性质的液体，而液则是指较厚、流动性较差的阴液。我说得对吗?

Teacher：Marvelous! I think all of you really have reviewed well. Today we are going to talk about pathologies of the fluids. To start with，I will introduce two concepts to you，that is "damage to liquid" and "humor desertion". The former one refers to minor depletion of fluids，while the latter one means major depletion of fluids. Can you guess what causes can impair the fluids? Here I mean to reduce the amount of fluids in the human body.

太棒了! 我想你们都复习得很好。今天我们将讨论津液的病理特征。首先,我将介绍两个概念,即"津损"和"液脱"。前者是指液体的少量消耗,而后者则是指流体的大量消耗。你们能猜出是什么原因会损害体液吗? 这里我的意思是减少人体内的液体量。

Student E：Maybe great fever or long time of fever. Eh，a lot of sweating，a great amount of urination.

可能是高烧,也可能是长时间发烧。嗯,大量出汗,大量排尿。

Teacher：Anything else? How about the pathological conditions?

还有别的吗? 病理情况如何?

Student C：Such as vomiting and diarrhea which would cause great loss of fluids from our body.

比如呕吐和腹泻,这会导致我们身体的液体大量流失。

Teacher：Excellent! And we should also remember the most common causes are scorching of the fluids by heat evil or consumption of the fluids through lingering sickness.

太棒了！我们还应该记住，最常见的原因是热邪导致的液体灼热，或挥之不去的疾病导致的津液消耗。

Section 5　Four Examinations and Eight Principles
第5节　四诊八纲

Ⅰ. Key Concepts 核心概念

The neophyte Chinese physician encounters a patient in four stages. The four stages are called the four examinations, because each one focuses on a different way of recognizing signs in a patient. The physician completes each of the examinations, gathering signs to make the final "diagnosis".

初学中医的人遇到一个病人诊治一般有四个阶段。这四个阶段被称为四诊，因为每一次检查都侧重于识别患者体征的不同方式。中医师完成每一项检查，收集迹象，编织成最终的"诊断"。

Observing contains four aspects: spirit, complexion, physical conditions and actions. Traditional Chinese medicine believes that the five sense organs of the face are reflections of the five zang-organs. The eyes reflect the liver, the nose reflects the lungs, lips reflect the spleen, ears the kidneys and the tongue the heart. Thus, a doctor can tell just by looking at the face if there is any health problem internally.

望诊包括四个方面，分别为神、色、形、态。中医认为五官对应着五脏。眼对应肝，鼻对应肺，口对应脾，耳对应肾，舌对应心。因此，医生通过观看一个人的面部就能判断出人体内部是否有健康问题。

Wenzhen, or auscultation and olfaction in English, includes two aspects. First, TCM doctors will listen to the patient's voice to see if he has sufficient Qi. Second, TCM doctors will smell. If the patient has got poor digestion, or has been mentally ill, leading to bad breath, this is a manifestation of illness.

闻诊包括两个方面。第一个是听觉，通过听你说话的声音判断底气足不足。第二个是闻气味。如果患者消化或精神出现问题，导致口中产生异味，那么这就是一种疾病的表现。

Speaking of wenzhen, it's more likely to show the doctors' humanistic concerns. During the chat, you might feel relaxed as if you are not seeing a doctor.

问诊其实更能体现出中医的人文关怀。在问诊阶段的聊天过程中，医生会让你放松心情，从而感觉不到在看病。

At last, it's taking the pulse. Pulse-taking is the essence of TCM as well as a distinguishing feature of TCM. Cun, guan, and chi are placed on the left wrist from the outside to the inside. That is to say they represent different organs, namely heart, liver and kidney. Pulses on the right hand represent lung, spleen and vital gate.

最后是切脉。号脉是中医的精髓，也是中医的特色。左手从外往里数，对应着寸、关、尺，代表的脏器分别是心、肝、肾。而右手对应的则是肺、脾、命门。

The eight principal patterns are composed of four pairs of polar opposites：yin-yang, exterior-interior, deficiency-excess, and cold-hot. These eight principal patterns are actually a concrete subdivision of yin and yang into six subcategories. This division allows a clearer and more systematic approach to yin-yang theory and practice in traditional Chinese medicine. Yin and yang retain their primacy because of their broad and all-encompassing nature, while the other six patterns are finally subsumed in yin-yang patterns.

八种诊疗方式由阴阳、表里、虚实和寒热四对极性对立构成。这八种主要模式实际上是将阴阳具体细分为六个子类别。这一划分为中医阴阳理论和实践提供了一种更清晰、更系统的方法。阴阳因其广泛、包罗万象的性质而保持其首要地位，而其他六种模式最终被纳入阴阳模式。

Ⅱ. Key Words 核心词语

1. Four Examinations 四诊

望诊（wangzhen）：observation。

闻诊（wenzhen）：olfaction。

问诊（wenzhen）：inquiry。

切诊（qiezhen）：palpation。

2. Eight Principles 八纲

阴阳：ying-yang。

表里：exterior-interior。

虚实：deficiency-excess。

寒热：cold-hot。

Ⅲ. Dialogues 情景对话

1. Dialogue 1 对话1

Doctor：What brings you here today?

你哪里不舒服？

Patient：I feel terrible, doctor. I think I am running a fever and my neck and back are killing me.

我感觉很糟糕，医生。我想我发烧了，脖子和背部都快疼死了。

Doctor：Could you please place your palm facing up on this small pillow? I'd like to take a moment to feel your pulse.

你能把你的手掌朝上放在这个小垫子上吗？我想花点时间给你把脉。

(One minute later)

（一分钟后）

Doctor：Now please switch to the other palm.

现在请换到另一只手掌。

(Another minute passed)

（又过了一分钟）

Doctor：Your pulse feels as tight as a stretched cord and grows faint when pressed hard. We call this a floating pulse accompanied by a tight one. Do you dislike cold?

你的脉搏感觉像一根绷紧的绳子,用力按压会变得微弱。我们称之为浮动脉冲伴随着紧缩脉冲。你讨厌冷吗?

Patient：No complaints, from where I'm from, it is much colder than here in Guangzhou. So if you ask me, I'd say the winter here is very pleasant.

没有怨言,我的家乡比广州这里冷得多。如果你问我,我会说这里的冬天非常宜人。

Doctor：You know, cold is also an item that refers to a kind of physical discomfort rather than the weather. For example, if you feel chilled even in a hot summer and feel like adding thick clothes, it is a sign of illness.

你知道,冷也是一种身体不适,而不仅指天气。例如,即使在炎热的夏天,如果你也感到寒冷,想穿厚衣服,这就是生病的迹象。

Patient：Do you mean that I've caught a cold?

你是说我感冒了吗?

Doctor：Well, we want to be more specific. In traditional Chinese medicine, if the clothes keep the cold away we call that sensation no aversion to cold. If they fail, then it is called aversion to cold.

嗯,我们想说得更具体一些。在传统中医中,如果衣服御寒,我们称之为不畏寒。如果它们失败了,那就叫作恶寒。

Patient：Wow, I do shiver a lot as though I were not dressed. I thought that's just the typical reaction associated with a fever and didn't give it a second thought. Now that you mention it, I have a headache as well.

哇,我真的经常发抖,好像我没有穿衣服一样。我认为这只是发烧的典型反应,并没有多想。既然你提到了,我也头痛。

Doctor：Good, more of these details will definitely help me to assess your condition. Do you have a runny nose?

很好,更多的这些细节将极大地帮助我评估你的病情。你流鼻涕吗?

Patient：Sometimes, but more often my nose is stuffed and breathing is difficult.

有时候,但更多时候我的鼻子被堵住了,呼吸困难。

Doctor：OK，please stick out your tongue for a minute.

好的,请伸出舌头一分钟。

2. Dialogue 2 对话 2

Patient：I find this tongue diagnosis fascinating. What are you looking for in my tongue?

我觉得这个舌头诊断很有意思。你从我的舌头上能看出什么?

Doctor：Tongue diagnosis has a very long history in traditional Chinese medicine. By observing the tongue body, color and coating, for instance, we can acquire a lot of information on the patient's condition, especially in terms of the eight principles of patterns identification. In your case, for example, there's a thin, white tongue coating that displays exterior cold. It's quite reliable since these aspects of the tongue won't be affected by short-term activities like vigorous exercise or mood swings. Together with pulse diagnosis, another important area of the four examinations, the source of the illness could often be reflected.

中医舌诊有着悠久的历史。例如,通过观察舌体、颜色和舌苔,我们可以获得许多关于患者病情的信息,特别是在模式识别的八个原则方面。例如,在你的例子中,有一层薄薄的白色舌苔,显示出外寒。这是非常可靠的,因为舌头的这些方面不会受到短期活动的影响,比如剧烈运动或情绪波动。再加上四项检查中的另一个重要领域——脉搏诊断,通常可以反映疾病的来源。

Patient：Marvelous. So what are you going to do with my exterior cold?

太棒了。那么你打算怎么处理我的外寒?

Doctor：All of your symptoms suggest that cold as a pathogenic factor is fettering the exterior, so all I need to do is to dissipate external cold pathogen from the exterior portion of the body. Can you take herbs?

你所有的症状都表明,感冒作为一种致病因素正在束缚身体的外部,所以我所需要做的就是驱散体表的外寒邪气。你能吃草药吗?

Patient：I heard that herbs need to be cooked. But I have a pretty hectic schedule at work so that is out of the question.

我听说草药需要煮。但我的工作日程非常繁忙，所以这是不可能的。

Doctor：You won't need to. We now have these processed herbs that can be dissolved in boiling water for you to drink. But it certainly won't taste good.

不需要煮。我们现在有这些经过加工的草药，可以溶解在沸水中供你饮用。但是味道肯定不好。

Patient：That I won't mind. Thanks a lot, doctor.

我不会介意的。非常感谢，医生。

Doctor：You're welcome.

不客气。

Section 6　Abnormal Sweating
第6节　异常出汗

Ⅰ. Common Diseases 常见病症

1. Spontaneous Sweating 自发性出汗

Spontaneous sweating refers to excessive sweating during the daytime without such obvious factors as hot weather, too much clothing, emotional stimuli or physical exertion. It occurs in patients with either qi or yang deficiency. In patients with qi deficiency, sweating is aggravated by even minimal physical exertion, and is accompanied by other symptoms of qi deficiency, such as listlessness, shortness of breath and reluctance to speak. Spontaneous sweating due to yang deficiency is marked by intolerance to cold and cold limbs.

自发性出汗是指在没有天气炎热、衣服穿多、情绪刺激或体力消耗等明显因素的情况下，白天出汗过多。它发生在气虚或阳虚的患者身上。气虚患者即使体力消耗很小，出汗也会加重，并伴有其他气虚症状，如无精打采、气短和不愿说话。阳虚自汗的特点是不耐严寒，四肢冰冷。

2. Night Sweats 夜晚盗汗

The term night sweats denotes sweating that occurs during sleep and stops after awakening. This is usually caused by yin deficiency with exuberant fire, but may also be encountered when the heart blood is insufficient.

夜晚盗汗指的是在睡眠中出现并在醒来后停止出汗。这通常是由阴虚火旺引起的,但也可能在心血不足时遇到。

3. Local Sweating 局部出汗

Local sweating usually appears in the head, face, chest, hands, feet, armpits or genital area. Head and face sweating may occur in normal individuals under certain circumstances, for example, when they are eating dinner. Morbid sweating of the head and face is often encountered in those with yang deficiency. Local sweating in the thoracic region is due to either heart-spleen qi deficiency or heart-kidney yin deficiency. Sweaty hands and feet irrelevant to emotional stress may be a sign of dampness-heat in the spleen and stomach or deficiency of qi and yin. Morbid axillary and genital sweating are also most likely caused by yin deficiency or dampness-heat. Sweat due to yin deficiency is odorless, but not that due to dampness-heat.

局部出汗通常出现在头部、面部、胸部、手、脚、腋下或生殖器区域。在某些情况下,正常人可能会出现头部和面部出汗,例如在吃饭时。阳虚的人经常会出现头面大汗淋漓的症状。胸部局部出汗是心脾气虚或心肾阴虚所致。与情绪压力无关的手脚出汗可能是脾胃湿热或气阴两虚的迹象。病态的腋窝和生殖器出汗也很可能是由阴虚或湿热引起的。阴虚之汗无臭,湿热之汗则臭。

Ⅱ. Key Sentences 核心语句

(1) Does your sweating have anything to do with the environmental temperature? Do you sweat even when the weather is cold?
你出汗与周围的温度有关系吗? 天气冷时也容易出汗吗?

(2) When do you sweat? In the daytime or night-time?
一般是什么时间出汗? 白天还是夜间?

(3) Does your sweating have anything to do with wearing too much? Do you still sweat when you wear less?
你出汗与衣着过多有关系吗? 少穿些还照样出汗吗?

(4) Does your sweating have anything to do with physical activities? Do you sweat even without physical activities?

你出汗与体力活动有关系吗？不活动时也出汗吗？

(5) Are you particularly intolerant of wind while sweating?

出汗时特别怕风吗？

(6) Do you feel chills with cold extremities (hands and feet) while you are sweating?

你是否一面出汗，一面又感到寒冷、手脚发凉呢？

(7) Are you usually lethargic and tired, or even reluctant to speak?

你平时是否感到精神疲惫，连话都懒得说？

(8) You say that you sweat during sleep. Docs that happen every night?

你说你夜里睡觉时出汗，是每天夜里都这样吗？

(9) Do you sweat because you use too many blankets? Do you still sweat even with a lighter covering?

你出汗是不是因为被褥太厚了？少盖些也出汗吗？

(10) Does sweating continue after you wake up in the morning?

早上醒来还继续出汗吗？

(11) Do you take a nap during the daytime? Do you sweat during the nap?

白天睡午觉吗？睡午觉的时候出不出汗？

(12) Besides sweating during sleep, what other discomfort do you experience? Do you have palpitations and sleeping problems?

除了盗汗，还有没有别的不舒服的感觉？有没有心悸失眠等症状？

(13) Do you have a burning sensation in the palms of your hands and soles of your feet, or fever in the afternoon?

有没有手脚心发热或下午感到发热？

(14) (To male patients) Do you often have wet dreams?

（对男性病人）常有梦遗吗？

(15) You say that you often sweat from the head. Does it have anything to do with diet, such as hot and spicy food, hot beverages or alcohol?

你说你的头部特别容易出汗，和饮食有关系吗，比如吃辛辣的食物、喝热饮或饮酒？

(16) Besides head and face sweating, do you feel thirsty or emotionally

upset?

除了头面汗多,有没有心烦口渴等不适?

（17）Besides chest sweating, do you also experience palpitations, sleeping problems, soreness in the lower back and weakness in the knees?

除了前胸汗多,有没有心悸失眠、腰膝酸软之类的症状?

（18）Do you sweat a lot from the palms of your hands and soles of your feet? Does it happen whenever you are nervous? Do you still sweat after you calm yourself down?

你的手脚心汗多吗? 精神一紧张就出汗吗? 心情平静的时候也出汗吗?

（19）Besides sweating a lot from the palms of your hands and soles of your feet, do you have other symptoms, such as tiredness, lack of energy and decreased appetite?

你除了手脚心汗多,还有没有什么别的症状,比如疲倦乏力、食欲减退?

（20）You are aware of excessive sweating in the armpits. Are you also aware of a bad smell along with it?

你的腋下多汗,有没有不好闻的气味?

（21）Do you sleep soundly and have a normal appetite?

你的食欲和睡眠正常吗?

（22）You say that you sweat often from the genital area. Is it accompanied by urinary problems?

你说阴部多汗,是否伴有排尿的症状?

Ⅲ. Dialogues 情景对话

1. Dialogue 1 对话1

Doctor：Hello, how can I help you?

你好,有什么可以帮助你的?

Patient：I've been sweating a lot lately, especially when I'm sleeping at night, and I feel more than usual.

最近总是出汗,尤其是晚上睡觉的时候,而且感觉比平时多。

Doctor：I understand. When did your sweating start? Do you have any other discomfort symptoms?

明白了,你出汗的情况是什么时候开始的? 有没有其他不适的症状?

Patient：It started about a month ago and there was no other discomfort, but I felt like I was sweating too much.

大概一个月前开始的,没有其他不适,就是觉得出汗太多了。

Doctor：May I ask how your diet and daily routine are?

请问你平时的饮食和作息规律如何?

Patient：The diet is relatively normal, but I have been busy with work recently and may be staying up late.

饮食比较正常,但最近工作比较忙,可能有点熬夜。

Doctor：Do you feel dry mouth, thirst, or frequent urination?

有没有感觉口干、口渴,或者尿频的情况?

Patient：I'm a bit thirsty, but I don't have frequent urination.

口渴有点,但尿频倒没有。

Doctor：Do you have any abnormal sensations on your tongue? What color is the tongue coating?

你的舌头有没有异常的感觉? 舌苔是什么颜色?

Patient：I feel that the tongue coating is a bit yellow and the tongue is also a bit dry.

感觉舌苔有点黄,舌头也有点干。

Doctor：Based on your symptoms, you may have a condition of dampness and heat accumulation. I suggest you pay attention to adjusting your diet, avoid spicy and greasy foods as much as possible, drink more herbal tea, maintain a good daily routine, and avoid staying up late. I will prescribe a traditional Chinese medicine prescription for clearing heat and promoting dampness for you. You should take it on time and observe for a period of time. If the symptoms do not improve, please seek medical attention promptly.

根据你的症状,你可能患有湿热内蕴的病症。建议你注意调整饮食,尽量避免辛辣油腻的食物,多喝些凉茶,保持良好的作息规律,避免熬夜。我会给你开一服清热利湿的中药方子,你按时服用,同时观察一段时间,如果症状没有好转,请及时复诊。

2. Dialogue 2 对话 2

Doctor：Hello，may I ask if there is anything uncomfortable that needs to be seen?

你好,请问有什么不舒服的地方需要看诊吗?

Patient：Recently, I have been feeling sweaty and sometimes feel flustered.

最近老是觉得身体出汗,而且有时候感觉心慌。

Doctor：I understand. When is your sweating more pronounced? Are there any other accompanying symptoms?

了解,你这种出汗是在什么情况下比较明显?有没有伴随其他的症状?

Patient：It is more obvious when exercising or feeling nervous, and sometimes even feel dry mouth.

比较明显的是运动或者是紧张的时候,而且有时候还会觉得口干。

Doctor：Is there anything unusual with your tongue? What is the color of the tongue coating?

你的舌头有没有什么异样?舌苔颜色如何?

Patient：The tongue is a bit red with a thick layer of white coating.

舌头有点红,舌苔有厚厚的一层白色。

Doctor：Based on your symptoms, it may be caused by yang deficiency. I suggest you strengthen your exercise appropriately, maintain a good daily routine, and consume more mild yang tonifying foods, such as yam and goji berries. I will prescribe some traditional Chinese medicine to tonify yang for you. You should take it on time and pay attention to adjusting your diet and lifestyle. If the symptoms do not improve after being observed for a period of time, please return to the clinic in a timely manner.

根据你的症状,可能是阳虚引起的。建议你适当加强锻炼,保持良好的作息,多摄取一些温和的补阳食物,比如山药、枸杞等。我会给你开一些补阳的中药,你按时服用,同时注意调整饮食和生活习惯,观察一段时间后如果症状没有改善,请及时回诊。

Section 7　Cold and Flu
第 7 节　感冒和发烧

Ⅰ. Common Diseases 常见病症

1. High Fever 高热

High fever is often a reflection of the conflict between healthy qi and invading external pathogenic qi. Exuberance of yang constitutes the main mechanism. In clinical practice, fever resulting from external contraction is usually excess-heat in nature. Doctors need to identify whether the exterior or the interior portion of the body, as well as which viscus on bowel, is involved in these pathological changes. This is the key to finding out whether the patient suffers from chills in order to distinguish between exterior and interior syndrome patterns. A chilly sensation is bound to appear as long as an external pathogen invades the exterior part of the body. So, "if chills do not disappear, the exterior syndrome also remains."

高热往往反映了健康的气与入侵的外气之间的冲突。阳气过盛构成了主要机制。在临床实践中,由外部收缩引起的发烧通常是性质上的过热。医生需要确定身体的外部还是内部,以及肠道上的哪个内脏与这些病理变化有关。这是了解患者是否患有寒战的关键,以便区分外部和内部的综合征模式。只要外部病原体侵入身体就会有寒的感觉。因此,"如果寒战没有消失,外部综合征也会继续存在"。

High fever involving the interior is commonly encountered in the syndrome patterns of lung heat, stomach heat, bowel excess, gall bladder heat, dampness-heat of the spleen and stomach, dampness-heat of the large intestine, and dampness-heat of the bladder.

高热涉内,常见于肺热、胃热、肠盛、胆热、脾胃湿热、大肠湿热、膀胱湿热等证型。

2. Low Fever 低热

Low fever refers to a subjective feverish sensation with only mild elevation of body temperature, normally in the range of 37.5℃ to 38℃. Differentiation of syndrome patterns of low fever routinely starts from that between deficiency and excess. If a deficiency pattern is confirmed, the next step is to distinguish its subtypes, such as yin deficiency, yang deficiency and qi deficiency. Similarly, whether it is caused by qi stagnation, blood stasis or dampness-heat must be identified if pathogen excess is confirmed to be the basic character.

低热是指只有轻微体温升高的主观发烧感,通常在37.5℃至38℃之间。低热证型的辨证,通常从虚与实入手。如果确认了虚证,下一步则是区分其亚型,如阴虚、阳虚和气虚。同样,如果病原体过剩被证实是基本特征,则必须确定它是由气滞、血瘀还是湿热引起的。

3. Common Cold and Flu 普通感冒和流感

Among all the cases of external contraction, common cold and flu are the most frequently encountered. Apart from fever, patients who suffer from colds or flu may also experience other symptoms, such as stuffy or runny nose, sneezing, headache and aversion to cold. It is not difficult to identify the ailment, but syndrome differentiation is needed. The syndrome patterns of colds and flu include wind-cold, wind-heat, summer heat-dampness, and qi deficiency.

在所有的外部收缩病例中,普通感冒和流感是最常见的。除了发烧,感冒或流感患者还可能出现其他症状,如鼻塞或流鼻涕、打喷嚏、头痛和畏寒。鉴别病因并不困难,但需要辨证。感冒和流感的证型包括风寒、风热、暑湿和气虚。

Ⅱ. Key Sentences 核心语句

(1) Do you have a fever?
你发烧了吗?
(2) Have you taken your own temperature? Please let me take it again for you now.
自己量过体温吗? 现在再给你量一下体温吧。
(3) Do you feel chilly or hot?

你自己觉得身上发冷还是发热？

（4）Are you intolerant of wind?

怕风吗？

（5）Is your nasal discharge thin and clear or thick and sticky?

你流的鼻涕是清稀的还是黏稠的？

（6）Do you feel dryness in the mouth?

嘴里干吗？

（7）Do you have soreness in the throat?

喉咙疼吗？

（8）Have you sweated?

身上出过汗没有？

（9）Do you have a heavy cough?

咳嗽得厉害吗？

（10）Do you cough up sputum?

咳嗽有痰吗？

（11）Is the sputum white or yellow?

痰是白的还是黄的？

（12）Is the sputum thin or thick? Is it easy to expel?

痰是稀的还是稠的？容易咯出吗？

（13）Do you feel dizzy and groggy? Do you have tightness in the chest and nausea?

有没有感到头部昏昏沉沉,沉重发涨？是否感觉胸口烦闷,想要呕吐？

（14）How many days have you had this fever?

你发烧（发热）几天了？

（15）Did you feel chilly at the beginning?

开始时发冷（恶寒）吗？

（16）Are you still feeling chilly?

现在还发冷吗？

（17）Do fever and chills hit you alternately? Or do chills hit you first and then fever?

你的发烧和发冷是交替出现的还是从开始发冷之后就一直发烧？

（18）Do you have a stuffy or runny nose? Any soreness or pain in the throat?

有没有鼻塞流涕？咽喉疼不疼？

(19) Do you have dryness and a bitter taste in your mouth?

口干口苦吗？

(20) Do you feel continually thirsty during the fever?

发烧的时候一直都口渴吗？

(21) Do you have a desire for cold or hot drinks?

想喝冷水还是热水？

(22) Have you had any bowel movement since the fever started?

发烧以来排过大便吗？

(23) Did you sweat during the fever?

发烧时出过汗吗？

(24) Did the sweating bring down your body temperature?

出汗后体温下降了吗？

(25) (To patients with fever and jaundices) When did you realize that your eyes had turned yellow?

（对于出现黄疸的发热患者）你什么时候开始发现眼珠发黄了？

(26) Have you felt nauseous and vomited?

感到恶心吗？呕吐过吗？

(27) (To patients with fever and diarrhea) Have you noticed any blood and/or pus in your stools?

（对于发热兼有腹泻的患者）你有没有注意到大便中有脓血？

(28) Do you sill have the urge to empty your rectum right after a bowel movement?

有里急后重的症状吗？

(29) (To patients with fever and dysuria) Do you feel pain during urination?

（对于有发热兼有排尿症状者）你排尿时感到疼痛吗？

(30) What kind of pain is it?

是什么样的疼痛？

(31) How many times do you have to pass water (urine) each day?

你每天要排尿多少次？

(32) Have you noticed any change in your urine?

你注意到尿液有什么变化吗？

(33) Is your urine bloody?

尿里带血吗？

(34) Have you had any trouble with urination before?

你以前有过排尿异常吗？

(35) You say that recently you have developed a chronic low fever. Did you just feel that you had a fever or did you actually take your own temperature with a thermometer?

你说近来天天发低烧，是自己感觉发烧，还是用体温计量出来的？

(36) (If taken with a thermometer) Do you remember what the highest temperature was?

（如果是用体温计量的）你还记得最高是多少摄氏度吗？

(37) How many days have you had the fever?

你这样发烧多少天了？

(38) What triggered the fever originally? Has the fever been high? Or has it been low since the very beginning?

最初是什么原因引起的发烧？有没有发过高烧还是始终就是低烧？

(39) Does your fever come at a regular time every day?

你每天发烧的时间有规律吗？

(40) Does it come in the morning or in the afternoon?

是上午发烧还是下午发烧？

(41) Is your daily high temperature maintained at the same level?

每天的热度有大的变化吗？

(42) Do you feel really hot and want to wear less when your temperature goes up?

体温升高时，你是否的确感到发热而想减少衣着？

(43) Do you feel cold and want to wear more even when your temperature goes up?

有没有体温升高，你反而感到寒冷，想多穿点衣裳的情况？

(44) Where do you feel hot the most? All over your body, in the middle of the chest, or in the palms of your hands and soles of your feet?

你感觉发烧在身体什么部位最明显？全身、胸口还是手脚心？

(45) Do you sweat easily? Do you sweat even after very slight exertion?

容易出汗吗？有没有一动就出汗的现象？

(46) Does an emotional change affect your temperature? Do you get upset easily?

情绪对你的体温有影响吗？你容易生气着急吗？

(47) Does the fever affect your appetite?

发烧对你的食欲有影响吗？

(48) Does the fever affect your body weight?

发烧对你的体重有影响吗？

(49) Do you feel dry in the mouth when you have the fever? Do you want to drink much water?

你发烧时感到口渴吗？想不想喝水？

(50) Have you experienced a situation in which you only want to gargle with water but do not want to swallow it?

有没有只想含口水却不愿下咽的情况？

(51) Did you ever vomit water out right after drinking it?

有没有喝完水又立刻吐出来的情况？

(52) Besides low fever, do you have other symptoms, for example, any pain in the body?

除低烧之外同时还有其他的症状吗？比如身上有哪里疼痛。

(53) Does the illness affect your general heath a lot or not much? Do you feel tired all the time?

患病以来，是觉得对身体影响不大，还是影响很大？经常感觉疲倦乏力吗？

(54) Are you particularly susceptible to catching colds?

你比别人容易感冒吗？

(55) Each time you caught a cold, how many days did it last?

以前每次感冒，几天能好？

Ⅲ. Dialogues 情景对话

1. Dialogue 1 对话 1

Doctor：Hello, may I ask if there is anything uncomfortable that needs to be seen?

你好，请问有什么不舒服的地方需要看诊吗？

Patient：I have a fever, my body temperature has been above 38℃, and

I feel a headache and body soreness.

我发烧了,体温一直在38℃以上,而且感觉头痛、身体酸痛。

Doctor：I understand. How long do you think this fever has been going on?

明白了,你感觉这种发烧情况大概持续了多久?

Patient：It has been about two days now, and taking antipyretic medication will temporarily improve, but after a period of time, the fever will return.

大概两天了,吃了退烧药暂时会好一些,但过一段时间又会再次发烧。

Doctor：Please open your mouth and let me see your tongue.

请张嘴,让我看一下你的舌头。

(Patient extends tongue)

(患者伸出舌头)

Doctor：Your tongue looks a bit red. What about the tongue coating?

你的舌头看起来有点发红,舌苔呢?

Patient：A thin layer of white tongue coating.

舌苔有薄薄的一层白色。

Doctor：I need to feel your pulse, please extend your wrist.

我需要给你把脉,请伸出你的手腕。

(Doctor performs pulse diagnosis)

(医生进行脉诊)

Doctor：Your pulse is slightly floating, but also slightly weak. Based on your symptoms and pulse, you may have a cold caused by wind-heat. I suggest you drink more traditional Chinese medicine that can clear heat and detoxify, such as Forsythia suspensa and honeysuckle. At the same time, rest more, keep warm, and avoid eating spicy and stimulating foods. If symptoms persist or worsen, please seek medical attention promptly.

你的脉搏稍微有些浮,但也有些细弱。根据你的症状和脉象,你可能患有风热感冒。建议你多喝些清热解毒的中药,如连翘、金银花等,同时多休息,注意保暖,避免吃辛辣刺激性食物。如果症状持续或加重,请及时就诊。

2．Dialogue 2 对话 2

Doctor：Hello，may I ask if you have any discomfort or need medical attention?

你好，请问你有什么不适需要就诊吗?

Patient：I have been running a fever with a temperature of around 39℃. I feel weak all over and sometimes I have a dry cough.

我一直发烧，体温在 39℃左右，感觉全身无力，有时候会出现干咳。

Doctor：How long has this situation been going on?

这种情况持续多久了?

Patient：It has been about three days now. I have taken antipyretic medication，but the effect of reducing the fever is not very obvious.

大概有三天了，我吃了退烧药，但退烧效果不太明显。

Doctor：Please stick out your tongue and let me take a look.

请伸出舌头，让我看一下。

(Patient extends tongue)

(患者伸出舌头)

Doctor：Your tongue looks red. What about the tongue coating?

你的舌头看起来发红，舌苔呢?

Patient：The tongue coating is relatively thick with a yellow layer.

舌苔比较厚，有一层黄色。

Doctor：Now I need to feel your pulse，please extend your wrist.

现在我需要给你把脉，请伸出手腕。

(Doctor performs pulse diagnosis)

(医生进行脉诊)

Doctor：Your pulse is a bit smooth and slightly firm. Based on your symptoms and pulse，you may suffer from yin deficiency and excessive fire. I suggest you drink more water，rest more，and take some traditional Chinese medicine that nourishes yin and clears heat，such as zhimu and xuanshen. Try to avoid spicy and stimulating foods and maintain indoor air circulation. If the symptoms do not improve, please seek medical attention as soon as possible.

你的脉象有些滑数,稍微有点紧实。根据你的症状和脉象,你可能患有阴虚火旺的病症。建议你多喝水,多休息,同时可以服用一些滋阴清热的中药,如知母、玄参等。尽量避免辛辣刺激性食物,保持室内空气流通。如果症状无缓解,请尽快就诊。

Section 8   Changes in Appetite and Abnormal Taste in the Mouth

第8节 胃口改变及口气异常

Ⅰ. Common Diseases 常见病症

1. Anorexia (Loss of Appetite) 厌食症(食欲不振)

Anorexia or loss of appetite refers to lack of a desire to eat or subjective feeling of insipidity with reduced food intake. Anorexia occurs frequently along with spleen and stomach diseases. There are many factors that may induce anorexia, one of which is emotional disturbance, which may induce liver stagnation that invades the stomach, leading to anorexia. Overeating or intake of food that is hard to digest may also lead to anorexia via dyspepsia. Long-term over consumption of greasy and sweet food may injure the spleen and stomach via aggregation of dampness-heat, and result in anorexia. Anorexia may emerge as a sequel to other diseases.

厌食症或食欲不振是指食物摄入减少,缺乏进食欲望或主观感觉无味。厌食症常与脾胃疾病同时发生。可能诱发厌食症的因素有很多,其中之一是情绪障碍,情绪障碍可能诱发肝郁结侵犯胃部,导致厌食症。过量进食或摄入难以消化的食物也可能通过消化不良导致厌食症。长期过量食用油腻、甜食,可通过湿热聚集伤脾胃,导致食欲不振。厌食症可能是其他疾病的后遗症。

The syndrome patterns of anorexia commonly encountered clinically include liver-qi invasion of the stomach, dampness-heat accumulation in the spleen and stomach, yin deficiency of the stomach, qi deficiency of the spleen and stomach, deficiency-cold of the spleen and stomach, yang deficiency of the spleen and stomach, and dyspepsia.

临床上常见的食欲不振的证型有肝气犯胃、湿热积脾胃、胃阴虚、脾胃气虚、脾胃虚寒、脾胃阳虚、消化不良等。

2. Polyphagia (Excessive Appetite) 食欲过多

Polyphagia refers to increased appetite or excessive hunger. It describes a situation in which one feels hungry shortly after intake of food, regardless of the size and frequency of the intake. Diabetes is considered to be one of the main causes of polyphagia, and polyphagia is a major symptom of diabetics. That is why in traditional Chinese medicine diabetes is called consumption-thirst, in which consumption refers to polyphagia.

食欲过多是指食欲增加或过度饥饿。它描述了一种情况,即一个人在摄入食物后不久就感到饥饿,而不管摄入的量和频率如何。糖尿病被认为是多食症的主要原因之一,多食症是糖尿病患者的主要症状之一。这就是为什么在中医中糖尿病被称为消耗性口渴,其中消耗是指多食。

3. Abnormal Taste in the Mouth 口腔异味

Abnormal taste in the mouth always accompanies other symptoms, so it is usually ignored or complained of as a minor symptom. Nevertheless, quite a number of patients still come to clinics for it only. Abnormal taste in the mouth includes tastelessness, sticky or greasy taste in the mouth, as well as bitter, sweet, sour, salty, astringent, sticky and greasy coating in the mouth.

口腔异味总是伴随着其他症状,因此它通常被忽视或作为轻微症状来描述。尽管如此,仍有相当多的患者只是为此来诊所。口腔中的异常味道包括无味,口腔中的黏性或油腻味道,以及口腔中的苦、甜、酸、咸、涩、黏和油腻。

Ⅱ. Key Sentences 核心语句

(1) Besides a feeling of tastelessness, do you also feel a sticky and greasy coating in your mouth?

除了口淡,口中有没有发黏发腻的感觉?

(2) Has there been any change in your appetite?

你的食欲有没有受影响?

(3) How about your bowel movements? Are they normal? Have you experienced constipation or diarrhea?

你的大便情况如何？正常吗？是便秘，还是便溏？

（4） Are there any other digestive symptoms, such as abdominal distention (fullness) or nausea?

有没有其他消化道的症状，比如脘腹胀满或恶心欲吐等？

（5） Do you also feel tired, with a dry mouth and throat, and short of breath?

有没有咽干口燥、气短乏力之类的伴随症状？

（6） When did the anorexia start?

你的食欲从什么时候开始减退的？

（7） Do you have a dry mouth? If so, do you have a craving to drink water or other beverages?

你感到口干吗？想不想喝水或其他饮品？

（8） (To patients who complain of dryness of the mouth but do not have a craving for water or other beverages) Don't you want to drink water at all or do you feel uncomfortable after drinking?

（对于口干渴而不欲饮者）你是根本不想喝水还是喝了难受？

（9） Do you vomit what you drink right away?

喝了东西会不会立刻吐出？

（10） (To dry-mouth patients who have a craving for water) When do you feel thirsty the most during the day?

（对于口干渴而欲饮者）你在一天什么时候感到口渴最厉害？

（11） Do you feel dryness all over your body, for example, in the nose, lips and skin?

你有没有感到全身都干燥，比如鼻干、唇干、皮肤干燥等等？

（12） Do you cough? Do you have mucus in your throat?

你咳嗽吗？喉咙里有痰吗？

（13） Do you have a burning sensation in the palms of your hands and soles of your feet?

你有没有手脚心发热的感觉？

（14） Are your stools formed, soft, or loose?

大便是成形的，还是不成形甚至腹泻呢？

（15） Do you tend to put on weight because of eating a lot?

你会因为吃得太多而发胖吗？

（16） You do not look overweight at all. Have you lost some weight recently?

我看你并不胖,体重近来有没有减轻?

(17) If you keep losing weight despite an increased appetite, have you ever checked your blood glucose level?

如果食欲增强,体重反而在减轻,你有没有检查过血糖?

Ⅲ. Dialogues 情景对话

1. Dialogue 1 对话 1

Doctor：Hello，may I ask if you have any discomfort or need medical attention?

你好,请问你有什么不适需要就诊吗?

Patient：I have been losing my appetite lately, eating very little, and I also have no appetite when eating.

我最近总是没有胃口,吃东西特别少,而且吃饭时也没有食欲。

Doctor：How long has this situation been going on?

这种情况持续多久了?

Patient：It's been about a month now, and I've been trying to eat some food, but I always feel like I haven't had much sensation and my appetite is very poor.

大概有一个月了,我尝试吃一些食物,但总觉得吃了也没什么感觉,胃口很差。

Doctor：Please extend your tongue for me to take a look.

请伸出你的舌头,让我看一下。

(Patient extends tongue)

(患者伸出舌头)

Doctor：Your tongue has a thin coating with a hint of white. Now I need to feel your pulse, please extend your wrist.

你的舌苔薄薄的,有一点点白色。现在我需要给你把脉,请伸出手腕。

(Doctor performs pulse diagnosis)

(医生进行脉诊)

Doctor: Your pulse is a bit weak and slightly heavy. Based on your symptoms and pulse, you may suffer from spleen and stomach weakness, leading to loss of appetite. It is recommended that you adjust your diet and eat more digestible and mild foods, such as porridge, millet congee, and light vegetables. You can consider taking some traditional Chinese medicine that benefits qi and invigorates the spleen, such as Astragalus membranaceus and Codonopsis pilosula, to improve spleen and stomach function. Meanwhile, maintain a happy mood and avoid excessive fatigue.

你的脉搏有些细弱,稍微有点沉滑。根据你的症状和脉象,你可能患有脾胃虚弱,导致食欲不振。建议你调整饮食结构,多食用易消化、温和的食物,如稀粥、小米粥、清淡的蔬菜等。可以考虑服用一些益气健脾的中药,如黄芪、党参等,以改善脾胃功能。同时,保持心情愉快,避免过度疲劳。

2. Dialogue 2 对话2

Doctor: Hello, may I ask if there is any discomfort that requires medical attention?

你好,请问有什么不适需要就诊吗?

Patient: I haven't had much appetite lately. I feel full after eating a little, and I often have no appetite.

我最近吃东西没什么胃口,吃一点就觉得饱,而且经常没食欲。

Doctor: How long has this situation been happening?

这种情况出现多久了?

Patient: It has been about two months now. I have tried to eat some food, but I always feel that my appetite is not good and very poor.

大概有两个月了。我尝试吃一些食物,但总觉得胃口不好,食欲很差。

Doctor: Please let me take a look at your tongue.

请让我看一下你的舌头。

(Patient extends tongue)

（患者伸出舌头）

Doctor：Your tongue has a thick layer of white coating. Now I need to feel your pulse, please extend your wrist.

你的舌头有一层厚厚的白苔。现在我需要给你把脉,请伸出手腕。

(Doctor performs pulse diagnosis)

（医生进行脉诊）

Doctor：Your pulse is slightly dull and weak. Based on your symptoms and pulse, you may have dampness and turbidity accumulation, which affects the digestive function of the spleen and stomach, leading to anorexia. I suggest that you eat less raw, cold, and greasy foods, and more easily digestible and light foods, such as Job's tears, yam, etc. Consider taking some Chinese herbal medicines that can dispel dampness and invigorate the spleen, such as hawthorn and Poria cocos, to improve spleen and stomach function. At the same time, maintaining a regular lifestyle and avoiding excessive fatigue is also crucial for conditioning.

你的脉搏稍微有些沉滑,而且有点细弱。根据你的症状和脉象,你可能患有湿浊内蕴,影响了脾胃消化功能,导致厌食。建议你少吃生冷油腻的食物,多食用易消化、清淡的食物,如薏米、山药等。可以考虑服用一些化湿健脾的中药,如山楂、茯苓等,以改善脾胃功能。同时,保持规律的生活作息,避免过度疲劳,对调理也十分重要。

3. Dialogue 3 对话3

Doctor：Hello, may I ask if there is any discomfort that requires medical attention?

你好,请问有什么不适需要就诊吗?

Patient：Recently, I have been feeling very hungry and have a strong desire to eat. After finishing a meal, I quickly become hungry again.

最近我总是感觉非常饿,吃东西的欲望非常强烈,吃完一顿饭后很快就又饿了。

Doctor：How long has this situation been going on?

这种情况持续多久了？

Patient：It has been about a few weeks now, and I have been trying to control it, but I have always been unable to suppress my appetite.

大概有几个星期了，我尝试控制，但是总是无法抑制自己的食欲。

Doctor：Please extend your tongue for me to take a look.

请伸出你的舌头，让我看一下。

(Patient extends tongue)

（患者伸出舌头）

Doctor：Your tongue has a thick coating and some yellow. Now I need to feel your pulse, please extend your wrist.

你的舌苔厚厚的，有一些黄色。现在我需要给你把脉，请伸出手腕。

(Doctor performs pulse diagnosis)

（医生进行脉诊）

Doctor：Your pulse is slightly smooth and tight. Based on your symptoms and pulse, you may suffer from damp heat accumulation and spleen and stomach disorders, leading to overeating. I suggest you adjust your dietary structure, consume less greasy, spicy and stimulating foods, and consume more light and easily digestible foods, such as vegetables, fruits, whole grains, etc. You can consider taking some traditional Chinese medicine that clears heat and eliminates dampness, such as huanglian and zhizi, to promote digestion, clear heat and relieve summer heat. At the same time, maintaining a regular routine and moderate exercise can help balance yin and yang in the body, and also help control appetite.

你的脉搏稍微有些滑数，有点紧细。根据你的症状和脉象，你可能患有湿热内蕴、脾胃失调，导致食欲亢进。建议你调整饮食结构，少食用油腻、辛辣刺激的食物，多食用清淡易消化的食物，如蔬菜、水果、全谷类食物等。可以考虑服用一些清热利湿的中药,如黄连、栀子等,以促进消化、清热解暑。同时,保持规律的作息和适量的运动,有助于平衡体内的阴阳,对于控制食欲也有帮助。

4. Dialogue 4 对话 4

Doctor：Hello，may I ask if there is any discomfort that requires medical attention?

你好,请问有什么不适需要就诊吗?

Patient：Recently，I have noticed that the taste has become very strong，and I feel that everything I eat is not strong enough. I need to add a lot of seasoning to taste it.

最近我发现口味变得很重,吃什么东西都觉得淡,味不够,必须放很多调料才能尝到味道。

Doctor：How long did this situation last?

这种情况持续多久了?

Patient：It's been about a few months now，and I didn't pay much attention at first，but now I feel it's becoming more and more obvious.

大概有几个月了,一开始没太在意,但是现在感觉越来越明显了。

Doctor：Please extend your tongue for me to take a look.

请伸出你的舌头,让我看一下。

(Patient extends tongue)

(患者伸出舌头)

Doctor：There is a layer of white coating on your tongue，which may be a sign of heavy dampness in the body. Let me feel your pulse so that I can feel your physical condition.

你的舌头上有一层白苔,这可能是体内湿气较重的表现。再让我把一下脉,让我感受一下你的身体状况。

(Doctor performs pulse diagnosis)

(医生进行脉诊)

Doctor：Your pulse is slightly slippery，indicating heavy dampness.

Based on your symptoms and pulse, you may suffer from dampness, turbidity, and spleen stagnation. It is recommended that you eat less cold and greasy foods and more light foods that are easy to digest, such as congee, vegetables and fruits. You can consider some Chinese herbal medicines that can dispel dampness, such as Atractylodes, chenpi, etc., to promote spleen and stomach function and improve symptoms of heavy taste.

你的脉象稍滑,说明湿气较重。根据你的症状和脉象,你可能患有湿浊困脾的情况。建议你少食用生冷油腻的食物,多摄取一些易于消化的清淡食物,如粥、蔬菜、水果。可以考虑一些化湿的中药,如苍术、陈皮等,以促进脾胃功能,改善口味重的症状。

5. Dialogue 5 对话 5

Doctor：Hello, may I ask if there is any discomfort that requires medical attention?
你好,请问有什么不适需要就诊吗?

Patient：I have been feeling dry mouth lately and bad breath is very serious, and I haven't improved much by brushing my teeth and rinsing my mouth.
我最近总感觉口干,而且口臭得很厉害,我刷牙漱口都没太大改善。

Doctor：How long did this situation last?
这种情况持续多久了?

Patient：It's been about a few weeks now, and I thought it was a dental problem at one point, but I didn't find any obvious problem when I went to see the dentist.
大概有几个星期了,我一度以为是牙齿问题,但是去看牙医后也没发现明显的问题。

Doctor：Please extend your tongue for me to take a look.
请伸出你的舌头,让我看一下。

(Patient extends tongue)
(患者伸出舌头)

Doctor：Your tongue coating is a bit yellow, and the bad breath indicates that there may be some dampness and heat stagnation in your body. Let me feel your pulse so that I can feel your physical condition.

你的舌苔有些黄,而且口臭的情况说明体内可能有一些湿热郁结。再让我把一下脉,让我感受一下你的身体状况。

(Doctor performs pulse diagnosis)

（医生进行脉诊）

Doctor：Your pulse is slightly curved, which indicates that there may be some heat stagnation in the body. Based on your symptoms and pulse, you may have a condition of damp heat and bad breath. I suggest you drink plenty of water, maintain oral hygiene, and avoid spicy and stimulating foods. Consider some traditional Chinese medicines that can clear heat and detoxify, such as Coptis chinensis and Forsythia suspensa, to promote the elimination of dampness and heat, and improve symptoms of dry mouth and bad breath.

你的脉象稍弦,说明体内可能有一些郁热。根据你的症状和脉象,你可能有湿热口臭的情况。建议你多喝水,保持口腔卫生,避免辛辣刺激的食物。可以考虑一些清热解毒的中药,如黄连、连翘等,以促进湿热的排出,改善口干口臭的症状。

Section 9　Pain
第 9 节　疼痛

I. Common Diseases 常见病症

1. Headache 头痛

As one of the commonest symptoms, headache occurs in many diseases, both acute and chronic. Here, however, headache is discussed only when it is taken as a patient's chief complaint.

头痛是最常见的症状之一，发生在许多疾病中，包括急性和慢性疾病。然而，这里只讨论被视为患者主诉的头痛。

The locations of headaches may include the forehead, as well as the temporal, parietal and occipital regions. Headache caused by external contraction is characterized by a sudden onset with a sensation of pulling, throbbing, burning, distending or heaviness. On the other hand, headache caused by an internal injury often makes a patient suffer from a sustained intermittent pain with a slow onset. The sensation of the pain may be hollow, dull or muddy, and the headache may be induced or aggravated by mental and physical stress.

头痛的部位可能包括前额、颞叶、顶叶和枕叶区域。外部收缩引起的头痛的特点是突然发作，有拉、悸动、灼热、膨胀或沉重的感觉。另一方面，内伤引起的头痛通常会使患者遭受持续的间歇性疼痛，但发作缓慢。疼痛感可能是空洞的、沉闷的或浑浊的，精神和身体压力可能会引起或加重头痛。

Headaches due to external contraction can be further classified into wind-cold headache, wind-heat headache and wind-dampness headache; and those due to internal injury into liver-yang headache, qi-deficiency headache, blood-deficiency headache, blood-static headache, and phlegm-turbidity headache.

外缩头痛又可分为风寒头痛、风热头痛和风湿头痛，内伤者分为肝阳头痛、气虚头痛、血虚头痛、血瘀头痛、痰浊头痛。

2. Shoulder Pain 肩痛

Shoulder pain refers to the pain that comes from a shoulder joint and its surrounding tissues. Shoulder pain usually impedes the activity of the arm, and any forced action of the arm is bound to aggravate the pain. Its common causes include wind-cold infection and phlegm-dampness invasion. It can also be caused by a sprain that leads to blood stasis.

肩痛是指来自肩关节及其周围组织的疼痛。肩部疼痛通常会阻碍手臂的活动，手臂的任何强迫动作都势必会加剧疼痛。其常见病因有风寒感染和痰湿侵袭。它也可能是由扭伤导致的瘀血。

3. Epigastric Pain (Stomachache) 上腹痛 (胃痛)

Stomachache, or epigastric pain, refers to the pain occurring in the upper abdomen adjacent to the precordial region. The main mechanism involves invasion of the stomach by pathogenic cold, injury of the stomach by improper food intake, dysfunction of the stomach due to emotional disorder, and weakness of the spleen and stomach. Invasion of the stomach by cold may induce congealment, and hence pain. Dietary irregularity and improper food intake, including excessive consumption of greasy and sweet food, may lead to stagnation of undigested food in the stomach, hindering the function of qi and resulting in stomachache. Anger or depression may hurt the liver, giving rise to qi stagnation. Disordered liver qi may affect the stomach, leading to stomachache. Internal injury due to overstrain or weakness of the spleen and stomach due to a prolonged disease may lessen the yang qi of the middle energizer (the spleen and stomach), leading to undernourishment of the stomach. As a result, pathogenic cold is generated internally in the middle energizer, and hence the pain of deficiency cold. Furthermore, long-term stagnation of qi usually results in blood stasis. Both qi stagnation and blood stasis may impede the function of the middle energizer, leading to stomachache.

胃痛,或称上腹痛,是指发生在上腹部靠近心前区的疼痛。其主要机制涉及邪寒侵胃、食入不当伤胃、情志紊乱致胃功能障碍、脾胃虚弱等。感冒侵袭胃部可能引起充血,从而引起疼痛。饮食不规律,食物摄入不当,包括过多食用油腻和甜食,可能导致未消化的食物在胃里停滞,阻碍气的功能,导致胃痛。愤怒或抑郁可能会伤害肝脏,导致气滞。肝气紊乱可能会影响胃,导致胃痛。积劳成疾致内伤,或久病脾胃虚弱,可使中焦(脾胃)阳气减弱,导致胃营养不良。结果,致病性感冒在中焦内部产生,从而产生虚寒之痛。此外,长期气滞通常会导致瘀血。气滞血瘀都可能阻碍中焦的功能,导致胃疼。

In summary, stomachache can be generally classified into deficiency and excess patterns according to the pathomechanisms. Obstruction or stagnation of the qi function belongs to the excess pattern, and the resulting pain appears by the rule of thumb: "Wherever there is obstruction, there is pain. " Deficiency of the spleen and stomach indicates lack of nourishment. Deficiency-pattern pain occurs because "wherever there is undernourishment, there is pain. "

总之,根据发病机制,胃痛通常可分为虚证和实证。气功能的阻塞或停滞属于实证,由此产生的疼痛根据经验法则出现:"哪里有阻塞,哪里就有疼痛。"脾胃虚说明缺乏营养。虚证疼痛的发生是因为"哪里有营养不良,哪里就有疼痛"。

4．Abdominal Pain 腹痛

Abdominal pain refers to pain that occurs in the region below the epigastrium and above the pubis. Doctors need to rule out abdominal pain from surgical conditions first. Abdominal pain from non-surgical conditions is usually comparatively mild with mild tenderness and a soft abdomen, and occurs without fixed location. Abdominal pain, however, is severe, and occurs at fixed location with obvious tenderness, muscular tension and rebound tenderness. In the case of female patients, doctors also need to look into the possibility of gynecological pain, which is associated with menstruation, vaginal discharge, pregnancy and childbirth. Only abdominal pain stemming from internal medical conditions will be discussed here. Improper food intake, emotional disorder and cold-catching are the common factors inducing abdominal pain. Clinically, it may be classified into the following syndrome patterns: cold obstruction, dampness-heat, deficiency cold, food stagnation and qi depression.

腹痛是指发生在上腹部以下和耻骨上方的疼痛。医生首先需要排除手术条件引起的腹痛。非手术条件下的腹痛通常是轻微的,伴有轻微压痛和腹部绵软,发生在没有固定位置的情况下。然而,手术条件引起的腹痛是严重的,发生在固定位置,有明显的压痛、肌肉张力和反跳压痛。对于女性患者,医生还需要研究妇科疼痛的可能性,妇科疼痛与月经、阴道分泌物、怀孕和分娩有关。这里只讨论由内科疾病引起的腹痛。饮食摄入不当、情绪障碍和感冒是引起腹痛的常见因素。临床上可分为以下几种证型:寒阻、湿热、虚寒、食滞、气郁。

5．Hypochondriac Pain 胁痛

Hypochondrium refers to either of the superolateral regions of the abdomen, lateral to the epigastric region, and overlying the costal cartilages. Pain occurring in one or both hypochondriac regions is called hypochondriac pain, and is different from chest pain and epigastric pain. Since both the liver and gall bladder meridians pass through the hypochondriac regions, hypochondriac pain is closely associated with liver and gall bladder disorders. Clinically, hypochondriac pain is often caused by emotional stress that leads to liver-qi stagnation and even blood stasis, or by either exogenous or endogenous dampness undergoing heat transformation. In all those cases, the pain is due to obstruction of qi-blood flow, and hence is excessive in nature. Hypochondriac pain can also take place when liver yin is deficient due to chronic disease or overexertion and fatigue. In those cases, the pain is due to undernourishment, and hence is deficient in nature. Generally, qi stagnation produces distending or scurrying pain, while blood stasis often leads to severe or stabbing pain. As for patients with the deficiency pattern, the pain is mostly chronic and dull.

季肋区是指腹部的上外侧区域,位于上腹部区域的外侧,并覆盖在肋软骨上。发生在一个或两个季肋区的疼痛称为胁痛,与胸痛和上腹痛不同。由于肝胆经都经过季肋区,胁痛与肝胆疾病密切相关。临床上,胁痛往往是由情绪应激导致肝气郁结甚至瘀血引起的,或者是由外感或内生湿化热引起的。在所有这些情况下,疼痛是由于气血流动受阻,因此本质上是实。慢性病肝阴虚或用力过猛、乏力时也可发生胁痛。在这些情况下,疼痛是由营养不良造成的,因此本质上是虚。一般来说,气滞会引起腹胀或急骤疼痛,而血瘀往往会导致剧烈或刺痛。对于虚证患者来说,疼痛大多是慢性和无症状的。

6. Lumbago (Lower Back Pain, Low Back Pain) 腰痛

Lumbago refers to pain in the lumbar region. The causal factors of lumbago are either exogenous or endogenous. The exogenous factors include pathogens like wind, cold, dampness and heat, as well as trauma. The subsequent lumbago is excessive in nature. The endogenous factors include aging and chronic illness, both of which may lead to consumption of kidney qi. Lumbago thus caused is deficient in nature. Lumbar pain due to bony lesions of the lumbar vertebrae is outside the category of lumbago, and hence it is often necessary to take an X-ray film of the lumbar vertebrae for diagnosis.

腰痛指的是腰部的疼痛。腰痛的病因既有外源性因素,也有内源性因素。外源性因素包括风、寒、湿、热等病原体以及创伤。如此产生的腰痛本质上是实。内源性因素包括衰老和慢性病,两者都可能导致肾气消耗。这样造成的腰痛本质上是虚。由腰椎骨病变引起的腰椎疼痛不属于腰痛,因此通常需要拍摄腰椎的 X 光片进行诊断。

7. Arthralgia (Joint Pain) 关节痛

Arthralgia refers to pain in one or more joints, the latter of which may occur simultaneously. A variety of causes may lead to arthralgia. Wind, cold or dampness may invade the body when healthy qi is insufficient. Those pathogenic factors may stay in the body for a long period of time to generate heat. When wind, cold, dampness or heat blocks the meridians that control the joint(s), the flow of qi and blood to the relevant joint(s) is blocked, and arthralgia occurs. Clinically, doctors need to distinguish among those pathogenic factors and the degree of insufficiency of healthy gi (liver-kidney deficiency or qi-blood deficiency).

关节痛是指一个或多个关节的疼痛,后者可能同时发生。多种原因可能导致关节痛。当正气不足时,风、寒或湿可能侵入身体。这些致病因素可能会在体内停留很长一段时间以产生热量。当风、冷、湿或热阻断了控制关节的经络时,流向相关关节的气和血液就会受阻,从而出现关节痛。临床上,医生需要区分这些致病因素和正气不足的程度(肝肾亏虚或气血亏虚)。

Ⅱ. Key Sentences 核心语句

(1) How long have you been suffering from abdominal pain?
你的腹痛有多长时间了?

(2) Have you ever suffered from the same pain before?
以前发作过吗?

(3) Did it happen suddenly or gradually?
是慢慢发生的还是急剧发生的?

(4) Is the pain alleviated when you press the abdomen with your hands?
用手按压腹部能不能使腹痛减轻?

(5) Is the pain alleviated when you warm the abdomen with a hot pad?
用热的东西焐焐腹部能不能使腹痛减轻?

(6) Do you feel dryness in the mouth? Do you have an urge to drink water?
你感觉口干吗? 想不想喝水?

(7) Have you had the experience of having a dry and bitter mouth but not wanting to drink water?
有没有口干口苦,却不愿意喝水这种情况?

(8) Are you intolerant of a cold environment? Are your hands and feet always cold?
你怕冷吗? 手脚是不是经常冰凉?

(9) Do you want to relieve the bowels when you have abdominal pain?
腹痛起来想不想大便?

(10) Do you feel relaxed in the abdomen after a bowel movement, or do you still feel the urge to evacuate?

大便后觉得腹部轻松了,还是仍然感到里急后重?

(11) Is there a strong stool odor?

大便有没有特别酸臭的气味?

(12) Can you find undigested food in the stools?

大便里有没有许多未消化的食物?

(13) Is your abdominal pain alleviated or aggravated after taking food?

吃点东西能使腹痛减轻还是加重?

(14) Does your abdominal pain have anything to do with emotional changes? Is it aggravated when something or someone bothers you?

腹痛与精神情绪有什么关系吗? 有没有一生气着急腹痛就加剧的情况?

(15) Besides pain, do you also have abdominal fullness?

除了腹痛,腹胀吗?

(16) Do you belch or break wind very often?

有没有嗳气、矢气(放屁)之类的症状?

(17) Is your pain alleviated after you belch or break wind?

嗳气、矢气(放屁)之后,腹痛能减轻吗?

(18) How long have you been suffering from joint pain?

你的关节疼痛已经多久了?

(19) Did it start suddenly or gradually?

起病急不急?

(20) What triggered the pain? Did you catch a cold or become exposed to a windy environment? Or did you ever get drenched by rain? Or was there any other reason?

关节疼痛是怎么引起的? 受风受寒了? 被雨淋着了? 还是有什么其他的原因?

(21) In which joint or joints do you feel the pain?

都有哪个或哪些关节作痛?

(22) (If there is pain in multiple joints) Is the pain fixed at one location or does it move?

(如有多处关节疼痛)疼痛是固定的还是到处移动的?

(23) Do you feel better with a hot compress? How about a cold compress?

患病的关节是敷热毛巾舒服些还是敷冷毛巾舒服些？

(24) How long have you been suffering from headaches?

你患头痛多久了？

(25) Does it take place suddenly or gradually?

是突然发生的还是慢慢发生的？

(26) Which part of the head does the pain come from? Can you point it out to me?

你的头部都有哪里疼痛？指给我看看可以吗？

(27) Can you describe your headache? For example, do you feel as if your head were pin-pricked, or as if tightly wrapped with a piece of cloth? Is the pain sharp or dull?

能够形容一下头痛的感觉吗？比如说，像锥刺那样，或像用布紧裹那样？是剧烈疼痛还是隐隐作痛？

(28) Do weather changes affect your headache? Does your headache get more serious on windy or rainy days?

你的头痛与天气有关系吗？刮风下雨会不会使头痛加重？

(29) Is there any correlation between your emotions and headache?

情绪对你的头痛有影响吗？

(30) Does your headache affect your emotions or your emotions affect your headaches?

是头痛影响你的情绪，还是情绪影响你的头痛？

(31) Besides headache, do you have pain elsewhere, such as a sore throat or joint pain?

除了头痛，身体还有其他部位的疼痛吗？比如咽痛、关节疼痛。

(32) Besides headache, do you feel dizzy with blurred vision?

除了头痛还有头晕眼花的症状吗？

(33) Have you ever suffered from a head injury?

头部受过外伤吗？

(34) Please describe the injury in detail.

请具体描述一下外伤的经过。

(35) Do you sleep well at night? Does your headache affect your sleep?

你夜间睡眠好吗？头痛有没有影响睡眠？

(36) Have you noticed any change in your physical condition? Do you suffer from fatigue or unwillingness to participate in physical activity?

近来你的体力有没有变化？有没有感到疲倦乏力，不愿意活动？

(37) Does physical exercise alleviate or aggravate your headache?

活动活动身体对你的头痛有影响吗？是使头痛减轻还是加重？

(38) Do you feel nauseous during an attack of headache?

头痛发作时有没有恶心、想要呕吐的感觉？

(39) How long have you had this shoulder pain?

你的肩痛有多久了？

(40) Does it hurt badly? What kind of pain is it? Slight，dull, pricking (or stinging) or sharp?

疼得厉害吗？怎么个疼法？微痛，隐痛，刺痛，还是剧痛？

(41) What caused your shoulder pain? Was it coldness or an injury?

最初是怎么疼起来的？是因为受凉还是由受伤引起的？

(42) (If caused by cold) How and when was the shoulder exposed to coldness?

(如与受凉有关)是怎样受凉的？什么时候？

(43) (If caused by an injury) How did you injure the shoulder?

(如与受伤有关)是怎样伤着肩膀的？

(44) When did it happen?

这是什么时候的事情？

(45) Does the shoulder pain have any impact on the movement of your arm? Try to raise your arm.

肩痛对手臂的活动有影响吗？你把手臂向上抬一下试试。

(46) Do you feel cold in that shoulder?

患侧的肩部有寒冷的感觉吗？

(47) Have you ever applied a hot compress to that shoulder?

有没有试过热敷？

(48) Did the hot compress relieve the pain?

热敷有用吗？

(49) What other treatments have you had? Did they help?

有没有用其他方法治疗过？有效吗？

(50) (To patients with recent onset of acute stomachache) When did the

stomachache start?

（对近期急性发作者）你的胃痛是从什么时候开始的？

(51) Was there any obvious cause for your stomachache? For example, catching a cold, taking a large amount of cold drinks, overeating, or getting into an argument with someone?

你的胃痛有明显诱因吗？比如受寒了，或喝了大量冷饮，或暴饮暴食，或和人吵架了？

(52) Can the stomachache be alleviated by drinking hot water?

喝点热水能使胃痛减轻吗？

(53) Does it help to alleviate the pain to warm your stomach area with a hot-water bag?

胃脘部热敷（例如用热水袋）能使胃痛减轻吗？

(54) Is the pain alleviated or aggravated when you press the stomach area with your hands?

用手按压胃脘部能使胃痛减轻还是加重？

(55) Do you feel nauseous? Have you vomited?

想吐吗？吐过吗？

(56) What did you vomit, undigested food or acid fluid? Did you feel better after you vomited?

都吐了些什么？是未消化的食物还是酸水？吐后胃痛有没有减轻？

(57) Do you belch often?

经常打嗝吗？

(58) Is there any foul breath along with the belches?

打嗝时有酸臭的气味冒上来吗？

(59) (To patients with chronic stomachache) Do you have a lot of pressure at work? Do you take meals at regular times?

（对慢性胃痛患者）你的工作紧张吗？有固定的时间进餐吗？

(60) Do you drink alcohol often?

你经常饮酒吗？

(61) What kind of alcohol do you drink? And how much do you drink each time?

你都喝什么酒？每次喝多少？

(62) Do you eat hot and spicy food on a regular basis?

你经常吃辛辣的食物吗？

(63) Does your daily diet include a lot of food that is difficult to digest?

平日的膳食中不好消化的食物多吗？

(64) Can you describe your stomach pain? Is it a dull pain that lasts off and on, a burning pain that runs like a fire, or a distending pain that gives you both pain and a stuffiness or fullness sensation?

你能形容一下胃痛的感觉吗？是丝丝拉拉地隐隐作痛，火烧火燎地烧灼疼痛，还是满闷痞塞地胀痛？

(65) Does heartburn or acid reflux come along with your stomachache?

胃痛是否伴有烧心泛酸等症状？

(66) Do you have a dry mouth and throat with a burning sensation in the chest, palms of your hands and soles of your feet? Do you also have constipation?

有口燥咽干、手脚心烦热的情况吗？大便干燥吗？

(67) Does your stomachache have anything to do with emotional changes? Is it aggravated whenever you are upset?

胃痛与心情变化有关系吗？每次烦心的时候是不是加重了？

(68) Have you ever vomited blood or have you had tarry stools?

有没有吐过血或排出过黑色发亮的大便？

(69) Please point out the painful area.

请你指出疼痛的部位。

(70) It is hypochondriac pain (pain in the ribs). Is the pain on both sides or only on one side?

你这个是胁痛。你是一侧疼还是两侧都疼？

(71) How long have you had this pain?

疼痛的时间有多久了？

(72) Is it getting worse, better, or staying the same?

是越来越重，还是逐渐减轻，还是没有变化？

(73) Can you figure out how the pain started? For example, did it start after a fit of temper?

你能回忆起开始疼痛有什么明显的诱因吗？比如说是不是与人争吵生气后开始疼的？

(74) Can you tell me what the pain feels like? Is it stabbing, distending or scurrying pain? Or just a mild dull pain? Is it fixed in location or does it often move?

你能描述一下疼痛的感觉吗？是刺痛，胀痛，窜痛，还是隐隐作痛？是固定在一点上还是常有移动？

(75) Is the painful area tender when you press it?

痛处有明显的按压痛吗？

(76) Do you feel better when pressing the painful area?

用手按压能使疼痛减轻吗？

(77) Is the pain persistent or on and off?

是持续疼痛，还是时轻时重？

(78) Is it worse during the day or during the night?

一天之中，是白天疼痛较重，还是夜间疼痛较重？

(79) Besides the hypochondriac pain (pain in the ribs), do you have any digestive problems, such as nausea and vomiting?

除胁痛之外，有没有消化方面的障碍，例如恶心呕吐？

(80) Does your mouth feel dry and bitter?

感到口干口苦吗？

(81) Is there any change in your general condition? Are you feeling weaker? Have you had dizzy spells?

全身状况有什么变化吗？是不是愈来愈虚弱？感到过头晕吗？

(82) How long have you had this lumbar pain?

你患腰痛多久了？

(83) Can you remember how the pain started, for example, after catching a cold, following an injury, due to excessive fatigue, and so on?

还记得初起的原因吗？比如说受凉、受伤、过劳等等？

(84) Have you had an X-ray taken of your lumbar vertebrae (lower back bones)?

你照过腰部的 X 光片吗？

(85) Can you describe the pain? Is it a stabbing pain or dull pain or just soreness?

能描述一下是怎么个疼法吗？刺痛，隐痛，还是酸痛？

(86) Do you feel cold or hot in the painful area?

腰痛的地方是发凉还是发热？

(87) Is the pain limited to the lower back? Any involvement of other joints?

是单纯的腰痛吗？其他关节也疼吗？

(88) Is the pain related to weather changes? Is it worse in cold or hot weather? How about on rainy days?

你的腰痛与天气变化有关系吗？天冷时加重还是天热时加重？阴雨天会不会加重？

(89) Are you able to move your lower back? Can you try to move it now?

能活动活动腰吗？请你活动一下看看。

(90) Does the pain get worse when you move your back，or the other way around?

活动之后腰痛是减轻还是加重？

(91) What happens when you press the lower back with your hands? Is the pain alleviated or aggravated?

用手按按能有效吗？是能使腰痛减轻还是越按越痛？

(92) Does the lower back pain affect your walking?

腰痛影响你走路吗？

(93) Do you feel your legs are as strong as before while walking?

走路时两条腿和以前一样强劲吗？

(94) Is the lumbar pain still there when you lie down?

躺着休息的时候还腰痛吗？

(95) Is massage of the painful joint helpful? Do you feel better when pressing or rubbing it? Or does the pain get worse if you do so?

痛处能用手按揉吗？揉揉按按能减轻疼痛，还是越按揉疼痛越重？

(96) There is no redness or swelling of the joint now. Was it reddened and swollen at the outset?

你现在的患病关节不红不肿，开始时红肿过吗？

(97) Do you feel feverish?

身上有发热的感觉吗？

(98) Are you intolerant of a windy or cold environment?

怕风吹吗？怕冷吗？

(99) Can you move the painful joint? Please try to move.

疼痛的关节能活动吗？请你动动看。

(100) Is the pain alleviated or aggravated after the movement?

活动后疼痛是加重还是减轻？

Ⅲ. Dialogues 情景对话

1. Dialogue 1 对话 1

Doctor：Hello，may I ask what is the condition of your headache?
你好,请问你头痛的情况是怎样的?

Patient：Headache mainly occurs on the forehead and both sides，feeling a bit heavy.
头痛主要在额头和两侧,感觉有点沉重。

Doctor：Do you have any other symptoms when you have a headache，such as dizziness，nausea，or blurred vision?
头痛的时候有没有其他症状,比如头晕、恶心,或者视物模糊?

Patient：Sometimes I feel a bit dizzy，but there is no particularly noticeable nausea.
有时候会觉得有点头晕,但没有特别明显的恶心感。

Doctor：Okay, I will check your tongue coating and pulse to see if it is caused by an imbalance of qi and blood. Please stick out your tongue and let me take a look.
好的,我会检查一下你的舌苔和脉搏,看看是不是气血不调引起的。请伸出舌头,让我看一下。

2. Dialogue 2 对话 2

Doctor：Hello, how did the shoulder pain start?
你好,请问肩膀疼痛是怎么开始的?

Patient：Perhaps due to long working hours in the office，the shoulders are often in a fixed position.
可能是办公室工作时间长,肩膀经常处于一个固定的姿势。

Doctor：Is the nature of pain dull or piercing?
疼痛的性质是钝痛还是刺痛?

Patient：It feels like a sense of soreness and swelling，especially at night.

像是一种酸胀的感觉,尤其是在晚上比较明显。

Doctor：Okay, I will check your shoulders and neck to see if the pain is caused by muscle tension.

好的,我会检查一下你的肩部和颈部,看看是不是肌肉紧张导致的疼痛。

3. Dialogue 3 对话 3

Doctor：Hello, please tell me about your abdominal pain.

你好,请告诉我你的腹痛情况。

Patient：Abdominal pain mainly occurs in the lower abdomen, sometimes feeling like throbbing pain.

腹痛主要在下腹部,有时候感觉像是一阵一阵的抽痛。

Doctor：Is there any accompanying symptom of abdominal pain, such as nausea, vomiting, and decreased appetite?

腹痛有没有伴随其他症状,比如恶心、呕吐、食欲减退?

Patient：Occasionally feeling nauseous, but not vomiting, and appetite is also okay.

偶尔会感觉恶心,但没有呕吐,食欲也还好。

Doctor：Okay, I will examine your abdomen and also observe your tongue coating to see if it is caused by organ dysfunction.

好的,我会检查一下你的腹部,同时观察一下你的舌苔,看看是不是脏腑功能失调引起的。

4. Dialogue 4 对话 4

Doctor：Hello, please describe your condition of flank pain.

你好,请描述一下你的胁痛情况。

Patient：The feeling of flank pain is under the ribs, sometimes even more pronounced after eating.

胁痛感觉在肋骨下面,有时候在进食后会感觉更明显。

Doctor：Does flank pain come with digestive problems, such as hiccups and acid reflux?

胁痛有没有伴随着消化问题,比如打嗝、反酸?

Patient：Sometimes burping occurs, but acid reflux is not common.
有时候会打嗝,但反酸的情况不常见。

Doctor：Okay, I will examine your flank and also observe your tongue coating to see if it is caused by abnormal gastrointestinal function.
好的,我会检查一下你的胁部,同时观察一下你的舌苔,看看是不是胃肠功能异常引起的。

5. Dialogue 5 对话5

Doctor：Hello, please tell me about your lower back pain.
你好,请告诉我你的腰痛情况。

Patient：Lower back pain mainly occurs in the lumbar spine and sometimes feels stiff.
腰痛主要在腰椎部位,感觉有时候僵硬。

Doctor：Did the lower back pain radiate to other areas, such as the lower limbs?
腰痛有没有扩散到其他部位,比如下肢?

Patient：Occasionally, pain radiates towards the thighs.
偶尔会感觉痛向大腿方向扩散。

Doctor：Okay, I will check your waist and also observe your tongue coating to see if it is caused by insufficient qi and blood.
好的,我会检查一下你的腰部,同时观察一下你的舌苔,看看是不是气血不足引起的。

6. Dialogue 6 对话6

Doctor：Hello, please describe your joint pain.
你好,请描述一下你的关节痛情况。

Patient：Joint pain mainly occurs in the wrist and knee, sometimes feeling particularly stiff.
关节痛主要出现在手腕和膝盖,有时候觉得特别僵硬。

Doctor：Has there been any cold or sports injury to joint pain?
有没有受凉或者运动受伤导致关节痛的情况?

Patient：No obvious cold or injury, just sudden joint pain.

没有明显的受凉或者受伤，就是突然间感觉关节疼。

Doctor：Okay, I will check your joints and also observe your tongue coating and pulse to see if it is caused by rheumatism or insufficient qi and blood.

好的，我会检查一下你的关节，同时观察一下你的舌苔和脉搏，看看是不是风湿或气血不足引起的。

Section 10　Head, Body, Chest and Abdomen Complaints

第 10 节　头部、身体、胸部和腹部不适

Ⅰ. Common Diseases 常见病症

1. Dizziness 头晕

Dizziness refers to either a vexing sensation of unsteadiness accompanied by blurred vision and a feeling of movement within the head, or an illusion that the environment on one's own body is revolving. Dizziness may be caused by a variety of factors, such as emotional disturbance, improper diet, hemorhage, trauma or overstrain. It takes place in the brain. The mechanisms involve insufficient nourishment of the brain, which is caused by deficiency of qi and blood or deficiency of liver-kidney yin, and upward invasion of the head by liver yang, phlegm fire, or static blood.

头晕是指一种令人烦恼的不稳定感，伴随着视力模糊和头部运动的感觉，或者是一种感觉自己身体上的环境在旋转的错觉。头晕可能由多种因素引起，如情绪障碍、饮食不当、出血、创伤或过度训练。它发生在大脑中。其机制包括气血不足或肝肾阴不足引起的脑营养不足，以及肝阳、痰火或静血向上对头部的侵犯。

2. Deafness and Tinnitus 耳聋和耳鸣

Deafness refers to partial or total loss of hearing. Tinnitus refers to the perception of a sound where there is no sound in the environment. It may sound like a cicada chirping, a bell ringing, water running, or wind blowing. Of course those are the traditional Chinese descriptions for the quality of tinnitus, which may simply be replaced by hissing, ringing, roaring, or buzzing, respectively.

耳聋是指部分或全部听力丧失。耳鸣是指在环境中没有声音的情况下对声音的感知。它可能听起来像蝉鸣、铃声、水流或刮风。当然,这些都是中国对耳鸣性质的传统描述,可以简单地分别用嘶嘶声、铃声、咆哮声或嗡嗡声代替。

A variety of factors may lead to deafness or tinnitus, via different mechanisms. Pathogenic wind-heat caught during external contraction may invade the auricular orifice, leading to deafness or tinnitus. Anger damages the liver, and so does depression, as they induce liver fire. Liver fire due to either anger or depression may move upward to invade the ears, resulting in tinnitus and deafness. Excessive consumption of alcohol and intake of greasy food may induce aggregation of dampness to form phlegm. Stagnant phlegm may turn into fire, and the resulting phlegm fire may move up and obstruct the ears, leading to impaired hearing and tinnitus. Constitutional weakness, malnutrition due to a prolonged disease, or excessive sexual activity may exhaust the kidney essence, leading to deficient vitality in the sea of marrow (the brain), and consequently tinnitus and deafness. Fatigue and improper food intake, including excessive intake of cold food, may damage the spleen and stomach. Consequently, impaired transformation and transportation ability of the spleen or spleen yang deficiency may occur. The former may lead to insufficient supply of qi and blood to the auricular orifice, while the latter may lead to insufficient power to transport clear qi up to the ears.

多种因素可能通过不同的机制导致耳聋或耳鸣。在外收缩过程中,邪风热可能侵入耳廓,导致耳聋或耳鸣。愤怒会损害肝脏,抑郁也会损害肝脏,因为它们会诱发肝火。愤怒或抑郁引起的肝火可能向上移动侵犯耳朵,导致耳鸣和耳聋。饮酒过量,饮食油腻,可引起湿气聚集,形成痰。痰郁结可化为火,由此产生的痰火可能向上移动,阻塞耳朵,导致听力受损和耳鸣。体质虚弱、长期疾病导致的营养不良或过度性活动可能会耗尽肾精,导致骨髓(大脑)缺乏活力,从而导致耳鸣和耳聋。疲劳和不适当的食物摄入,包括过量摄入冷的食物,都可能损害脾胃。因此,可能出现脾的转化和运输能力受损或脾阳虚。前者可能导致耳孔气血供应不足,而后者可能导致将清气输送到耳朵的力量不足。

3. Aphthae (Oral Ulcers) 口疮

Aphthae are small ulcers in the mouth. There are two types of aphthae, excess and deficient pattens，caused by excess fire and deficiency fire，respectively. As a rule of thumb，excess fire is commonly found in acute cases，and deficiency fire in chronic ones. Excess fire is transformed from the overwhelming heat accumulated in the spleen and stomach，which results from the habitual intake of hot and spicy food，and alcoholic beverages，as well as barbecued and fried food with strong flavors. Yin-deficiency fire normally results from obsessive worrying，and can also be found in the late stage of febrile diseases. In addition，aphthae may also be attributed to spleen-stomach qi deficiency，which occurs in those suffering from overfatigue or long-standing maladies.

口疮是口腔中的小溃疡。口疮有两种类型——实证和虚证，分别由实火和虚火引起。根据经验，实火多见于急性病例，虚火多见于慢性病例。实火是由脾胃中积聚的过多热量转化而来的，这是由于习惯性摄入辛辣食物、酒精饮料以及味道浓烈的烧烤和油炸食物造成的。阴虚火通常是由强迫症引起的，在温病晚期也可发现。此外，口疮也可归因于脾胃气虚，脾胃气虚发生在那些过劳或患有长期疾病的人身上。

4. Gingival Swelling and Pain (Painful Swollen Gums) 牙龈肿胀疼痛

Gingival swelling and pain or painful swollen gums refers to redness, swelling and pain of the tissiue surrounding the bases of the teeth but without ulceration. Gingival swelling and pain results from fire（heat），which can be divided into two categories：fire of excess type and fire of deficiency type. The first may be derived from the pathogenic heat in an external contraction of wind-heat，or from stomach heat due to excessive consumption of hot and spicy food. The second originates in the kidney when there is a deficiency of kidney yin.

牙龈肿胀疼痛是指牙齿基部周围组织的红肿和疼痛，但没有溃疡。牙龈肿痛由火（热）引起，可分为两类：上火型和虚火型。第一种可能来源于风热外缩时的邪热，也可能来源于过量食用辛辣食物引起的胃热。第二种来源于肾阴不足时的肾脏。

5. Oppression in the Chest (Chest Tightness) 胸部压迫（胸闷）

Oppression in the chest or chest tightness refers to a feeling of obstruction, stuffiness or fullness in the chest. It is usually encountered in excess syndromes and induced by wind-cold or pathogenic heat externally，or by stagnant qi and static blood retained in the chest internally.

胸部压迫或胸闷是指胸闷、闷胀的感觉,多见于证候过盛,外感风寒或邪热,内蕴气滞、血滞所致。

6. Angina Pectoris（Chest Impediment with Heart Pain）心绞痛（胸痹心痛）

Angina pectoris is called chest impediment with heart pain in Chinese medicine. It refers to a condition marked by brief paroxysmal attacks of smothering discomfort or pain in the middle of the sternum or left submammary area. In mild cases, patients occasionally feel short and mild discomfort in the chest, described as heaviness, smothering, choking, or dull aches. In severe cases, sharp, fleeting pain or intense, suffocative pain is complained of.

心绞痛在中医上被称为胸痹心痛。它是指胸骨中部或左胸骨下区短暂发作的窒息性不适或疼痛。在轻度病例中,患者偶尔会感到胸部短暂而轻微的不适,表现为沉重、窒息、呼吸困难或隐隐作痛。在严重的病例中,会出现强烈的、稍纵即逝的疼痛或剧烈的、令人窒息的疼痛。

The main mechanism involves the impediment of the heart vessel by turbid phlegm, static blood, stagnant qi or congealing cold, when healthy qi is insufficient. In clinical practice, doctors need to rule out epigastric pain, chest pain and hypochondriac pain. Epigastric pain usually occurs in the upper abdomen, and is characterized by a sensation of distension, prolonged duration and local tenderness. Chest pain is often exacerbated by deep breathing, exercising, or turning the body, and is accompanied by respiratory symptoms such as coughing and panting. Hypochondriac pain occurs mostly on the right side and is characterized by tenderness beneath the ribs.

其主要作用机制是当正气不足时,痰浊、血滞、气滞、寒凝而阻心。在临床实践中,医生需要排除上腹痛、胸痛和胁痛。胃痛通常发生在上腹部,其特征是腹胀、持续时间延长和局部压痛。深呼吸、锻炼或转动身体通常会加剧胸痛,并伴有咳嗽和喘息等呼吸道症状。胁痛主要发生在右侧,其特征是肋骨下方有压痛。

7. Palpitations 心悸

The term palpitations denotes the awareness of abnormally rapid and strong beating of the heart which leads to uneasiness. Palpitations can be subdivided into fright palpitation and fearful throbbing. Fright palpitation is ascribed to fright or anger, and is characterized by paroxysmal attacks. Fright palpitation is a mild symptom, with the sufferer normally in good health. Fearful throbbing is not caused by fear, but the awareness of severe heart palpitations usually alarms the sufferer. Persisting throughout the day, fearful throbbing can be brought on by fatigue, and even a little overstress may lead to a strong reaction. Fearful throbbing is a severe symptom, and the sufferer is usually in poor health.

心悸一词表示意识到异常快速和强烈的心跳并导致不安。心悸可分为惊恐心悸和恐惧悸动。惊恐心悸可归因于恐惧或愤怒,并以阵发性发作为特征。惊恐心悸是一种轻微的症状,患者健康状况良好。恐惧悸动不是由恐惧引起的,但严重心悸的意识通常会让患者恐慌。恐惧悸动持续一整天,可能由疲劳引起,甚至一点点过度的紧张也可能导致强烈的反应。恐惧悸动是一种严重的症状,患者通常身体状况不佳。

Palpitations are either excess or deficient. Deficiency-pattern palpitations are caused by impaired nourishment of the heart due to deficiency of yin and yang including qi and blood. Excess-pattern palpitations may be attributed to disturbance of the heart by sluggish flow of qi and blood due to phlegm-heat, retained fluid or static blood.

心悸要么实证,要么虚证。虚证心悸是由于气血等阴阳两虚,使心的营养受到损害而引起的。实证心悸可归因于痰热、滞液或瘀血引起的气血不畅,扰乱了心脏。

8. Cough 咳嗽

Cough is the most commonly encountered symptom in lung diseases. It is due to failure of qi to descend and be diffused in the lung and the consequent reverse upward movement of qi. Dysfunction of the lung may also be induced by disorders of other viscera.

咳嗽是肺部疾病中最常见的症状。这是由于气不能下降并在肺中扩散,从而导致气逆上运动。肺功能紊乱也可能是由其他脏器的紊乱引起的。

In clinical practice, doctors need to know the details, about the coughing that a patient complains about, such as its onset, duration, time, rhythm, quality of sound, and other accompanying symptoms as well as exacerbation factors. Except for the quality of its sound, which may be distinguished by listening, other information needs to be acquired via inquiries. Of the accompanying symptoms, expectoration of sputum is the most relevant.

在临床实践中,医生需要了解患者主诉的咳嗽的细节,如发作、持续时间、时间、节奏、声音特质、其他伴随症状以及加重因素。除声音的特质可以通过聆听来区分外,其他信息都需要通过询问来获取。在伴随症状中,咳痰是最相关的。

There are two main categories of cough — cough caused by external contraction and that due to internal injury. The former is acute with short duration of illness, and may be accompanied by chills, fever, and runny nose. The latter is chronic and recurrent, and may be accompanied by shortness of breath. Clinically, externally contracted cough can be classified into wind-cold cough, wind-heat cough, wind-dryness cough and lung-heat cough. Accordingly, cough due to internal injury can stem from lung qi deficiency, lung yin deficiency, accumulation of phlegm-dampness in the lung, and liver fire invasion of the lung.

咳嗽主要有两类,一类是由外部收缩引起的,另一类是由内部损伤引起的。前者是急性的,病程短,可能伴有发冷、发烧和流鼻涕。后者是慢性的,反复发作,并可能伴有呼吸急促。外感咳嗽临床上可分为风寒咳嗽、风热咳嗽、风燥咳嗽和肺热咳嗽。相应地,内伤咳嗽可源于肺气虚、肺阴虚、痰湿积肺和肝火侵肺。

9. Dyspnea (Panting) 呼吸困难(气喘)

Dyspnea or panting refers to difficult or labored respiration. In severe cases, the patient has to breathe through the mouth, with the shoulders lifted and the nostrils flaring, and is unable to lie flat. In clinical practice, doctors need, first of all, to distinguish between deficiency and excess patterns of dyspnea. The excess pattern is characterized by acute onset, coarse, deep and prolonged respiration with particular difficulty in exhalation. The deficiency pattern shows the common features of gradual onset, shortness of breath relief with deep inspiration and worsening with physical activity, and weak voice. Dyspnea of the excess pattern normally takes place in the lung, where accumulated pathogenic qi impairs the ventilating function. Obstruction of the lung by wind, cold, phlegm-heat, or phlegm turbidity is commonly encountered. Dyspnea of the deficiency pattern occurs in the lung and/or the kidney. In other words, deficiency of either the lung qi or the kidney gi may lead to dyspnea. Dyspnea may also be induced by retained fluid that attacks the heart and the lung. In this case, both palpitations and dyspnea are the chief complaints of the patient.

呼吸困难或气喘是指呼吸困难或费力。在严重的情况下,患者必须通过嘴呼吸,肩膀抬起,鼻孔张开,无法平躺。在临床实践中,医生首先需要区分呼吸困难的虚证和实证。实证的特点是急性发作,呼吸粗糙、深长,呼气特别困难。虚证表现为逐渐发作、深吸气时呼吸急促缓解、体力活动时加重和声音微弱的共同特征。实证型呼吸困难多发于肺,邪气郁积,影响通气功能。风、寒、痰热或痰浊常阻肺。虚证型呼吸困难发生在肺和/或肾。换句话说,肺气不足或肾气不足都可能导致呼吸困难。呼吸困难也可能是由攻击心脏和肺部的滞留液体引起的。在这种情况下,心悸和呼吸困难都是患者的主诉。

10. Wheezing (Asthma) 喘息(哮喘)

Wheezing, also called asthma, refers to a condition marked by paroxysmal episodes of labored breathing accompanied by a whistling sound. The main reason is the presence of retained phlegm in the lung. The onset is usually precipitated by a change in weather, improper food intake, emotional disorder or overfatigue. When the retained phlegm is agitated, blockage of the air passage with spasm occurs, and hence the wheezing (asthma). To identify its syndrome patterns, doctors need to distinguish between cold phlegm and heat phlegm in acute cases, and determine whether there is deficiency of the lung, the spleen or the kidney when dealing with patients at the stage of remission.

喘息,也称为哮喘,是指一种以阵发性呼吸困难并伴有口哨声为特征的疾病。主要原因是肺部有滞留的痰。发病通常是由天气变化、食物摄入不当、情绪障碍或过度疲劳引起的。当滞留的痰被搅动时,就会出现气道堵塞和痉挛,从而出现喘息(哮喘)。为了确定其证型,医生需要在急性病例中区分冷痰和热痰,并在治疗病情缓解期的患者时确定是否存在肺、脾或肾虚。

11. Acid Reflux (Acid Regurgitation) 胃酸反流(反酸)

Acid reflux or acid regurgitation refers to a condition in which the acid content of the stomach flows backward up the esophagus and the pharynx, followed by re-swallowing of the gastric contents, leading to a sour taste in the mouth along with heartburn, a burning feeling in the lower part of the sternum. Acid reflux may be induced by emotional changes as well as improper food intake. Clinically, patients with liver qi invasion of the stomach, food stagnation, or cold-dampness obstruction often have such a complaint.

胃酸反流或反酸是指胃中的酸含量向后流到食道和咽部,然后重新吞咽胃中的内容物,导致口腔中有酸味和胃灼热,胸骨下部有灼烧感。胃酸反流可能是由情绪变化以及食物摄入不当引起的。临床上,肝气侵胃、食滞、寒湿壅塞的患者常有这样的主诉。

12. Eructation (Belching) 嗳气(打嗝)

Eructation refers to the act of expelling gas noisily from the stomach out through the mouth. Occasional belching especially after meals is not a pathological symptom. However, frequent belching may result from liver qi invasion of the stomach or deficiency of spleen-stomach qi. Belching with the release of an unpleasant odor is often due to food accumulation in the stomach. Belching is different from hiccupping. The former originates in the stomach, producing a sound that lasts longer; while the latter comes from the pharynx and larynx, producing a sound that is sharp and short.

嗳气(打嗝)是指通过口腔将气体从胃里大声排出的行为。偶尔打嗝,尤其是饭后,不是一种病理症状。然而,经常打嗝可能是由于肝气侵胃或脾胃气虚所致。打嗝并释放出难闻的气味通常是由于食物在胃里堆积造成的。打嗝和呃逆不同。前者起源于胃,产生的声音持续时间更长;而后者来自咽部和喉部,产生的声音尖锐而短暂。

13. Epigastric Upset (Gastric Discomfort) 胃不适

Epigastric upset or gastric discomfort refers to an unpleasant feeling somewhat between hunger and fullness or between pain and comfort in the epigastric region. It often occurs with other symptoms such as belching, acid reflux, nausea, retching, and epigastric pain. Improper food intake, stomach heat, stomach cold, as well as disharmony of the liver and stomach may all induce epigastric upset or gastric discomfort.

胃不适是指上腹部饥饿和饱腹之间或疼痛和舒适之间的不适感。它常伴有其他症状,如打嗝、反酸、恶心、干呕和上腹痛。食物摄入不当,胃热,胃寒,以及肝胃不和,都可能引起上腹部不适或胃不适。

14. Nausea 恶心

Nausea refers to the unpleasant feeling of an imminent desire to vomit. Both stomach cold and stomach heat may induce nausea. Nausea induced by the former usually lasts for a long time, during which deficiency manifestations appear. Nausea induced by the latter demonstrates the opposite characteristics: short course with no deficiency manifestations.

Nausea in the case of stomach yin deficiency is often followed by violent vomiting, which usually occurs in patients at the late stage of a febrile disease or after a major surgery. Any food or drink may be immediately vomited up upon intake.

恶心是指即将呕吐的不适感。胃寒和胃热都可能引起恶心。前者引起的恶心通常持续很长时间,在此期间会出现虚的表现。后者引起的恶心表现出相反的特征:病程短,没有虚的表现。胃阴虚患者恶心后常伴有剧烈呕吐,通常发生在温病晚期或大手术后。任何食物或饮料一经摄入可立即呕吐。

Nausea in the case of disharmony of the liver and stomach results from invasion of the stomach by stagnant liver qi. It may be accompanied by the symptoms that manifest liver qi stagnation, such as a sensation of oppression in the chest, hypochondriac pain, bitterness in the mouth, and dryness in the throat.

肝胃不和时的恶心是由肝气郁结侵犯胃引起的。可能伴有肝气郁结的症状,如胸闷、胁痛、口苦、咽干等。

Nausea in the case of dyspepsia is usually attributed to gluttony. Patients who suffer from dyspeptic nausea usually have a history of overeating and overdrinking. Besides nausea, other dyspeptic symptoms may appear, such as belching, foul breath and acid reflux.

消化不良患者的恶心通常归因于贪食。患有消化不良恶心的患者通常有过量饮食和过量饮酒的病史。除了恶心,还可能出现其他消化不良的症状,如打嗝、口臭和反酸。

15. Retching 干呕

Retching is vomiting without vomitus or only with a little amount of mucus. Retching is different from both nausea and vomiting. Nausea is merely the feeling of being about to vomit, producing neither sound nor vomitus, while vomiting produces both. Retching, however, only produces a sound.

干呕是指没有呕吐物或只有少量黏液的呕吐。干呕不同于恶心和呕吐。恶心只是一种即将呕吐的感觉,既不会发出声音也不会呕吐,而呕吐会同时发出声音和呕吐。然而,干呕只会发出声音。

Retching results from a failure of stomach qi to descend, occurring in patients with stomach heat, stomach cold, liver depression, or food stagnation.

胃热、胃寒、肝郁或食滞的患者，胃气不降，引起干呕。

16．Vomiting 呕吐

Vomiting refers to involuntary oral expulsion of gastric contents, which is induced by reversed upward movement of stomach qi. Very often, nausea precedes or accompanies vomiting.

呕吐是指胃气逆上运动引起的胃内容物不自主地经口排出。通常情况下，恶心先于呕吐或伴随呕吐。

A variety of factors may induce vomiting, such as contraction of the six external pathogenic factors, internal injury, improper diet, disharmony of emotions, and weakened functions of viscera and bowels. Vomiting occurs in both excess and deficiency syndrome patterns. In the excess patterns vomiting is induced via the invasion of the stomach by external pathogenic factors, improper diet, retained phlegm-fluid, stagnant qi, etc. In the deficiency patterns, the stomach loses proper nourishment due to deficiency of qi, yang, or yin. In any case, vomiting is caused by disharmony of the stomach functions that makes the stomach qi move upward in a reverse manner.

诱发呕吐的因素多种多样，如外六邪收缩、内伤、饮食不当、情绪不和、内脏功能减弱等。呕吐既有实证型，也有虚证型。在实证型中，呕吐是由外邪犯胃、饮食不当、痰液滞留、气滞等引起的。在虚证型中，胃因气虚、阳虚或阴虚而失去适当的营养。无论如何，呕吐是由于胃功能不协调，使胃气逆上运动引起的。

Ⅱ．Key Sentences 核心语句

(1) How long have you been suffering from dizziness?

你患头晕的毛病多久了？

(2) Is this the first time, or has it happened before?

是第一次发作还是过去也发作过？

(3) How would you describe your dizziness? Do you have a sensation of fainting, blurred vision or spinning (vertigo)?

你能具体描述一下头晕的症状吗？是仅仅感到头部昏沉，看东西昏花，还是觉得天旋地转？

(4) Besides dizziness, do you have any other discomfort, for example,

headache or ringing in the ears?

除了头晕还同时感到有什么其他不舒服吗,例如头痛、耳鸣?

（5）Do you also feel any tightness in the chest or nausea?

有没有同时感到胸闷恶心?

（6）Is your sense of taste normal? Have you ever felt your mouth dry and had a bitter taste?

嘴里的感觉和往常一样吗? 有没有觉得口干口苦?

（7）Do you have any idea of the cause(s) of your dizziness? Is it because of anger, fatigue or any other reason?

你认为你的头晕是什么原因引起的? 因为着急生气,工作过于劳累,还是什么其他的原因?

（8）Have you ever had a blow to the head?

头部过去受过外伤吗?

（9）Do you drink alcohol regularly? Do you think that the dizziness has something to do with that?

你平时饮酒吗? 这次头晕和饮酒有没有关系?

（10）Does dizziness affect your sleep?

头晕发作后对睡眠有影响吗?

（11）How is your sleep affected by dizziness? Do you feel lethargic or sleepy during an attack of dizziness? Do you sleep peacefully or is your sleep disturbed by stressful dreams?

头晕是怎样影响睡眠的? 头晕发作期间是昏昏沉沉想睡觉吗? 睡得踏实,还是常做噩梦?

（12）Do you have a mild temper, or are you easily upset?

你平时的脾气好吗? 容易生气着急吗?

（13）How long have you been suffering from chest tightness?

你感到胸闷有多久了?

（14）Did it start suddenly or gradually?

是突然发生的,还是逐渐发生的?

（15）Is your chest tightness serious? Does it bother your breathing just a little bit, or do you have a serious discomfort as if your chest were heavily compressed?

你的胸闷严重吗? 只是感到呼吸有些费力,还是很难受,胸膛好像被重物压住了那样?

(16) Was there any cause for the tightness，such as a bout of anger?

发生胸闷有什么诱因吗，比如发生了让你愤怒的事情？

(17) Do you cough up sputum（mucus）?

有痰吗？

(18) Besides tightness，do you have any pain in the chest?

除了胸闷，胸部疼痛吗？

(19) Do you feel the pain in front of the heart or in the lateral side(s) of the chest?

是心口部位疼痛还是侧胸部疼痛？

(20) Do you also have dizziness and blurred vision along with chest tightness?

胸闷的时候感到头晕眼花吗？

(21) Has there been any change in your temperament since you started to suffer from dizziness?

患病以来脾气有什么变化吗？

(22) Do you have such symptoms as night sweats and a burning sensation in the palms of your hands and soles of your feet?

有没有夜间盗汗和手脚心发热的症状？

(23) Do you have such symptoms as memory loss，soreness in the lower back and weakness in the legs?

有没有感到记忆力减退和腰膝酸软的症状？

(24) How long have you been suffering from tinnitus（hearing noises in your ears）? Did it happen suddenly or gradually?

你感到耳鸣多久了？ 是突然出现的还是渐渐发生的？

(25) Has your hearing ability been affected?

听力有影响吗？

(26) Is your hearing ability seriously affected?

对听力的影响很明显吗？

(27) What is the noise like? Is it a hissing sound, or a roaring one like waves breaking on a shore?

耳鸣的声音像什么？ 像夏天的蝉鸣还是像潮水那样的轰鸣？

(28) Do you hear the noise all the time? Or is it intermittent?

耳鸣的声音是始终如一的，还是有时轻有时重？

(29) Is there any difference in the noise between daytime and nighttime?

Is it worse at night?

耳鸣的声音白天和晚上一样吗？晚上是不是会加重？

(30) Did you also have flu symptoms when you first experienced tinnitus?

耳鸣刚开始时有没有感冒的症状？

(31) Does tinnitus or deafness have anything to do with your emotions? Does the attack become more intense when you get upset?

耳鸣耳聋与心情有关系吗？有没有恼怒生气之后加重的情况？

(32) Does tinnitus or loss of hearing have anything to do with your body positioning? Do you suddenly feel hollow when you stand up from a crouching position，while the ringing in the ears and deafness become worse?

耳鸣耳聋与体位有关系吗？有没有发生过蹲下站起来的时候耳朵里会突然感到空虚、耳鸣耳聋加重的情况？

(33) Do you have a blocked sensation in your ear(s)，with dizziness, oppression in the chest and coughing with mucus?

耳朵里有没有堵闷的感觉,伴随头昏沉重、胸闷、咳嗽多痰的症状？

(34) Do you have a sensation of fullness or pain in your ear(s)?

耳朵里发胀或者耳朵里疼痛吗？

(35) Does tinnitus or loss of hearing have anything to do with tiredness? Do you feel chronically tired?

耳鸣耳聋和劳累有关系吗？身体经常感到倦怠吗？

(36) Do you have dizziness with blurred vision or a sore lower back and limp knees?

有没有头晕眼花、腰膝酸软的症状？

(37) Did you suffer from any oral ulcer before? Is this the first time or does it happen frequently?

你以前患过口疮吗？这是第一次,还是以前也常常发生？

(38) Does it hurt badly? Does it affect your chewing and swallowing food?

疼得厉害吗？影响不影响你吃饭？

(39) Have you noticed any particular cause for the ulcer, for example, any unpleasant experience or stress at work that disturbs your rest?

这次长口疮有什么明显的诱因吗，比如，生活上有不如意的事情或工作特别紧张，影响休息？

（40）Can you describe your diet? Do you like hot and spicy food? Do you drink alcohol regularly? Do you eat barbecued food often?

能否说一下你的饮食习惯？喜欢吃辛辣食品吗？经常饮酒吗？常吃烧烤吗？

（41）Does the ulcer affect your sleep?

口疮影响你的睡眠吗？

（42）Besides pain，do you have any other abnormal feelings，such as thirst and a craving for cold beverages?

嘴里除疼痛外还有没有其他的感觉，比如口渴、想喝冷饮？

（43）Do you have a burning sensation，especially in the palms of your hands and soles of your feet?

有没有发热，特别是手脚心发热的感觉？

（44）How about your bowel movements? Do you experience constipation or diarrhea?

大便的情况如何？稀软还是干硬秘结？

（45）How is your urination? Is it normal? Is the amount reduced，or has the color turned dark?

小便呢？正常吗？尿量减少，或者颜色加深了吗？

（46）How long have the gums been swollen and painful?

你的牙龈肿痛几天了？

（47）Was the onset acute or gradual?

是逐渐发生的还是突然发生的？

（48）How is the pain? Is it just some endurable mild pain，or an intense pain that you cannot stand?

你的牙龈疼到什么程度？是只有一点轻微疼，可以忍受，还是剧烈疼痛，难以忍受？

（49）Do you have any symptoms of infection（external contraction），such as fever and chills?

你有没有发热恶寒之类的感染症状？

（50）Do you like hot and spicy food?

你平时喜欢吃辛辣的食物吗？

（51）Did you eat hot and spicy food just before your gingival pain started?

发病前有没有吃辛辣的食物？

(52) Do you feel thirsty and have a craving for cold water or other cold beverages? Are you constipated? Is your breath foul?

你有没有口渴想喝冷饮,大便秘结,口气臭秽等情况？

(53) Do you have dizziness, tinnitus, a sore lower back and limp legs, or heat sensation in the chest, palms of your hands and soles of your feet?

你平时有没有头晕耳鸣、腰酸腿软、五心烦热？

(54) How about night sweating?

有没有夜间盗汗的症状？

(55) How long have you been suffering from chest tightness?

你感到胸闷有多久了？

(56) Did it start suddenly or gradually?

是突然发生的,还是逐渐发生的？

(57) Have you caught a cold recently? Did you get a fever with chills? Did you cough and have difficulty in breathing?

最近感冒了没有？ 有没有发热恶寒的症状？ 有没有咳嗽气喘的症状？

(58) I have noticed that you often let out a long deep breath. Do you feel relieved afterwards?

你不时地叹气,是不是长出一口气,胸闷就能减轻？

(59) Can you point out the location of the pain?

请你用手指点一下疼痛的部位。

(60) Does your pain have anything to do with breathing or turning of the body?

疼痛与呼吸或转动身体有关系吗？

(61) Is it connected with coughing?

与咳嗽有关系吗？

(62) Is the pain fixed at one location, or does it move?

疼痛的部位是固定不变的还是变来变去不固定的？

(63) Is the pain localized at the precordial area and behind the sternum, or does it radiate to other areas?

疼痛只限于胸骨后和心前区,还是向他处放散？

(64) Which part of the body does the pain radiate to?

疼痛都往哪里放散?

(65) Is the pain intense? Can you describe the pain? Is it dull, smothering, bloating, burning, stinging, squeezing, or stabbing?

疼痛发作时疼得厉害吗? 你能形容一下疼痛的感觉吗? 是隐隐作痛,闷痛,胀痛,灼痛,刺痛,绞痛,还是痛如刀割?

(66) Do you know the cause of each heart pain, for example, fatigue, emotional agitation, weather changes, or windy or cold environment?

每次心痛发作有什么诱因吗,比如身体劳累,情绪激动,天气骤变,遇到风寒?

(67) Does the pain often attack you on rainy days?

遇到阴雨天会不会容易发病?

(68) Do you sweat during the heart pain?

心痛发作时出汗吗?

(69) Are you prone to sweating? Do you sweat even when the weather is not hot at all, when you do not wear enough, or when you are not doing any physical exercise?

平时容易出汗吗? 天气不热,衣着不多,不运动时也会出汗吗?

(70) Do you have palpitations or shortness of breath?

有心悸气短之类的症状吗?

(71) Do you have a burning sensation in the palms of your hands and soles of your feet? Do you sweat at night?

平时有没有手脚心发热和夜间盗汗的情况?

(72) Are you especially intolerant of coldness? Are your hands and feet usually cold or warm?

平时比别人怕冷吗? 手脚经常是热的还是凉的?

(73) Do you normally cough up mucus?

平时咳嗽吐痰吗?

(74) How long have you been suffering from palpitations?

你感到心悸多久了?

(75) Did your first attack of palpitations come suddenly or gradually?

第一次心悸是突然发生的还是渐渐显现的?

(76) Have you noticed any cause for your palpitations, for example,

have you ever been extremely frightened or extremely tired, or up all night for many days?

发生心悸有什么诱因吗,比如说受了惊吓,过于劳累,或者接连熬夜,没有睡好觉?

(77) Is there any change in your physical condition? Are you as energetic as before? Or do you feel tired?

体力有什么变化没有? 和以前一样精力旺盛吗? 有没有感到疲倦?

(78) Is there any change in your mental condition? Are the palpitations making you listless?

精神状态有什么变化没有? 心悸让你无精打采吗?

(79) Have you had anything wrong with your chest, for example, have you had a choking sensation in the chest or a chest pain?

胸口有什么异常的感觉吗,比如说胸口发闷或者有时候感到疼痛?

(80) Do you sleep normally at night? Do the palpitations make you sleepless or awaken you with nightmares?

夜间睡眠好吗? 有没有因为心悸而失眠,或者做噩梦?

(81) Normally, do you always have cold extremities (hands and feet) or have a feverish feeling in the palms of your hands and soles of your feet? In comparison with the past or with others, are you particularly averse to cold or heat?

平常你的手脚是凉的还是手脚心发热? 与病前比较或者与其他人比较,你是怕冷还是怕热?

(82) Do you have any change in sweating? Are you more liable to sweating than before?

出汗有什么变化吗? 有没有比以前容易出汗?

(83) Do you sweat in the daytime or at night?

是白天活动时容易出汗,还是夜间睡觉时出汗?

(84) (If sweating during sleep at night) Does the sweating stop as soon as you wake up?

(如果夜间睡觉时出汗)醒来是不是就不出汗了?

(85) Is there any change in the volume of your urine? Has your daily volume of urine increased or decreased?

小便有变化吗? 比以前多了还是少了?

(86) Besides palpitations, do you have any other problems, for

example, dizziness or constipation?

除心悸之外，还有什么其他不适吗，比如说头晕目眩或者大便秘结？

(87) How long have you been suffering from coughing? Did it happen before?

你咳嗽多久了？以前有咳嗽的老毛病吗？

(88) (In an acute case with no history of recurrent cough) Is your coughing caused by a flu? Did you have a stuffed-up or running nose before the coughing started?

（对于新近发病，过去无反复咳嗽的患者）你的咳嗽是不是感冒引起的？咳嗽之前有没有鼻塞流涕的症状？

(89) (In a case of flu) Do you have a fever? How about chills and sweating?

（如有感冒）发烧了吗？全身发冷吗？有没有出汗？

(90) Do you have a dry, itchy or sore throat? To what extent is your throat sore? Does it hurt when you swallow?

喉咙发干、发痒，还是感到疼痛？疼到什么程度？咽东西疼吗？

(91) Do you cough to expel mucus (sputum)? Does the mucus (sputum) come out easily?

有痰咯出吗？容易咯出吗？

(92) Do you cough up a lot of sputum?

痰多吗？

(93) Is your sputum thin or sticky (viscous)? Is it white or yellow in color?

痰是稀薄的还是黏稠的？是白色的还是黄色的？

(94) Have you coughed up blood or bloody sputum?

有没有痰中带血的情况？

(95) Have you experienced dryness in the mouth, nose, lips and throat? So dry that drinking water is not helpful at all?

有没有感到口、鼻、唇、咽全都十分干燥，连饮水也无济于事？

(96) Does your chest hurt when you cough?

咳嗽时胸痛吗？

(97) (In a chronic recurrent case) Is your cough persistently recurring? (Does your cough come and go repeatedly?) Does it seem to be

getting worse?

（对于长期反复发病的患者）你的咳嗽是反复发作的吗？是不是越来越重？

(98) (In the case of repeated aggravation) Was there any reason for the aggravation each time, for example, do you easily catch a cold even when there is only a mild change of weather?

（如果是反复加重）每次加重有什么诱因吗，比如说，天气稍有变化，你就会特别容易感冒？

(99) Does the coughing fit come back when you are tired, angry or worried?

身体劳累了或者生气着急了会不会使咳嗽再犯？

(100) When do you cough the most heavily during the day?

一天之中什么时候咳嗽最重？

(101) Have you had a weight loss accompanied with your coughing?

除了咳嗽，体重有没有减轻？

(102) Does your cough change with your emotions?

咳嗽与情绪有关吗？

(103) How long have you been suffering from dyspnea (difficult or labored breathing)? Did it start recently, or a long time ago?

你患气喘病多久了？是最近几天才有的，还是已经很久了？

(104) (In acute cases) Did you catch a cold right before you found trouble breathing?

（对于新病气喘者）发生气喘之前有没有受凉感冒？

(105) (If the patient caught a cold) Did you have a fever with chills?

（如曾感冒）当时有没有恶寒发热？

(106) Do you sill have a fever? Are you sweating?

现在还有没有发热？身上出汗吗？

(107) Do you cough to bring up mucus (sputum)?

你咯痰吗？

(108) Is the amount of sputum large? Is it easy to cough up the sputum?

痰量多还是少？容易咯出来吗？

(109) Do you feel relieved right after you cough up sputum? Or do you still have a blocked feeling in the chest afterwards?

痰咯出来是不是立刻就痛快了，还是仍然觉得胸中不爽快？

(110) (In chronic cases) Are you apt to sweat with no obvious cause? Do you find that you cannot tolerate a windy environment? Do you easily catch colds?

（对于久病气喘者)你平时常出虚汗吗？是不是害怕吹风？容易感冒吗？

(111) Do you have a sore lower back and limp legs? Are your hands and feet always cold?

你平时感到腰酸腿软,手脚发凉吗？

(112) Do you often have palpitations?

你经常感到心慌心跳吗？

(113) (In cases of edema of the lower limbs) How long have you been suffering from edema of the lower limbs? Did edema come along with difficult breath?

（对于下肢浮肿者)你的腿肿多久了？与气喘同时发生的吗？

(114) Did you notice any change in your urine volume after the onset of edema?

腿肿的同时,小便量有变化吗？

(115) Is this the first time you have suffered from such an asthmatic symptom? Or has it happened before?

你是第一次发生哮喘,还是以前就曾经发作过？

(116) Is there an obvious cause that you know of for the wheezing, for example, catching a cold in cold weather or eating something unusual? Or have you ever suffered a mental trauma or became overtired?

你发生哮喘有什么明显的诱因吗,比如天气凉,受寒了？吃了什么特殊的食物？精神受了什么刺激？身体过于疲劳？

(117) Are you allergic to anything?

你对什么东西过敏吗？

(118) (To patients suffering an attack) Do you feel cold or hot now?

（对于发作期的患者)你现在觉得身上发冷还是发热？

(119) Do you have mucus in your throat? Can you cough it up easily?

喉咙里有痰吗？容易咯出来吗？

(120) Is it because there is not much mucus or because it is too sticky to bring up?

是因为痰少还是因为痰稠不容易咯出?

(121) Are you thirsty? Do you have a desire to drink cold or hot water?

口渴吗? 想喝凉的还是热的?

(122) (To patients in remission) Are you often short of breath? (Do you often experience shortness of breath?)

(对于缓解期患者)你平时感到气短吗?

(123) Do you have a sputum problem all the time? Is it a lot?

你平时有痰吗? 痰多吗?

(124) Do you catch cold easily?

你容易感冒吗?

(125) Is your wheezing connected with colds?

每次哮喘发作与感冒有关吗?

(126) How is your appetite in general?

你平时的食量如何?

(127) Are you prone to diarrhea?

容易腹泻吗?

(128) How is your physical condition when you are not wheezing?

你不犯病时体力如何?

(129) Do you have a sore lower back and limp legs, dizziness, or tinnitus?

你有腰酸腿软、头晕耳鸣的症状吗?

(130) How long have you been suffering from acid reflux? Does it happen frequently?

你犯反酸的毛病有多久了? 常犯吗?

(131) Do you know what caused the acid reflux that you are now suffering from? For example, was there anything unpleasant at work or in your everyday life, that upset you? Did you eat or drink too much?

这次犯病有什么诱因吗,比如说工作和生活上发生了什么令你生气的事情,或是饮食上有过暴饮暴食等?

(132) Besides acid reflux, do you have any other digestive problems? For example, have you had an impaired appetite sometimes, or even total loss of appetite? Have you suffered from belching, sometimes with foul breath?

你除了反酸,还有其他消化方面的症状吗,比如不想进食甚至厌食,嗳气甚至嗳气酸腐?

(133) How is your appetite? Does acid reflux affect it?

你的食欲如何? 反酸影响你的食欲吗?

(134) Do you have any unusual feeling in your stomach? For example, a replete or burning sensation?

胃里有什么异常的感觉没有,比如闷胀或烧灼的感觉?

(135) Do you have a dry mouth or throat? Do you have a bitter taste in your mouth?

有没有感觉到口干咽干,甚至口中发苦?

(136) Do you feel any discomfort in your rib areas (hypochondriac regions)?

胸胁部有什么不适没有?

(137) How long have you been suffering from frequent belching (burping)? Did it start recently, or has it been like that for a long time?

你频繁嗳气(打嗝)多久了? 是新得的病还是长期就有?

(138) Normally, do you belch (burp) only after meals, or regularly without any reason?

一般是吃完饭后嗳气(打嗝),还是平时就时常嗳气(打嗝)?

(139) Is your belching accompanied by an odor, such as sour and fetid?

打嗝有没有气味,比如酸味、臭味?

(140) How do you rate your appetite from "very good" to "poor"?

饮食情况怎么样? 是食欲很好,还是不想吃饭?

(141) Do you have any discomfort in the epigastric or hypochondriac regions (in the stomach or rib areas)?

胃脘胁肋这些部位有什么不舒服吗?

(142) Is your discomfort alleviated after belching (burping)?

嗳气(打嗝)之后不舒服的感觉能减轻吗?

(143) Do you have normal bowel movements? Do you have constipation or expel stools that are abnormally smelly?

大便正常吗? 有没有便秘或者大便的气味异常酸臭?

(144) Is there any change in your general health condition? For example, do you feel tired easily?

身体情况有变化吗，比如感到疲倦乏力吗？

(145) How long have you had discomfort in your stomach?

你感到胃里不舒服，嘈杂不安有多久了？

(146) Do you know what triggered off the discomfort? Overeating or eating spoiled food? Or did it start as a result of an emotional disturbance?

有什么诱因吗？暴饮暴食，吃多了？吃变质的食物了？还是因为什么事情生气了？

(147) Does your stomach discomfort have anything to do with food temperature? Does it get worse after eating cold food and better after eating warm food? Or just the opposite?

你胃里嘈杂不舒服的感觉和饮食温度有关系吗？是吃冷的东西加重，吃热的减轻，还是相反，吃冷的感觉好些？

(148) Besides discomfort in your stomach, do you have acid reflux?

除胃里嘈杂不舒服之外，向上反酸吗？

(149) Do you feel nauseous? Have you ever vomited?

感到恶心吗？有没有吐过？

(150) Did your stomach feel better after vomiting?

呕吐过后胃里有没有舒服些？

(151) Do you often belch? Is there unpleasant breath when you belch?

打嗝吗？打上来的嗝有没有不好闻的气味？

(152) Has anyone complained that you have foul breath? Or have you found that you have foul breath by yourself?

自己或者别人闻到你口中有臭味吗？

(153) Besides stomach discomfort, do you feel oppression or fullness in the chest? Or do you have a pain in your rib areas?

除胃部不舒服外，胸中有没有感到胀闷，两胁有没有疼痛？

(154) How long have you been suffering from nausea?

你感到恶心有多久了？

(155) Did it happen suddenly or gradually?

是突然发生的，还是逐渐发生的？

(156) Is there any obvious reason for your nausea? For example, did you get into an argument or a fight and get upset or even furious? Or did you eat improper food or overeat?

出现恶心的症状有什么明显的原因吗,比如说病前曾与人生气争吵,或暴饮暴食吃坏了?

(157) Did you vomit? Was your vomiting violent?

呕吐过吗? 吐得厉害吗?

(158) Besides nausea, do you also have a stomachache? Do you have other symptoms such as acid reflux and stomach discomfort?

除了恶心,还有胃痛吗? 还有反酸、嘈杂这类的不适吗?

(159) Has your nausea anything to do with the warmth or coldness of food and drinks? For example, do you feel better after taking warm soup or a cold drink?

恶心与饮食温度有关系吗,比如说喝点热汤舒服些呢,还是喝点冷饮好些呢?

(160) Has there been any change in your appetite? How do you describe the change? Is it a mild reduction or a total loss of appetite?

对食欲有影响吗? 怎么样的影响? 是稍有影响还是影响严重,根本不愿进食?

(161) Do you have any abnormal sensation in the mouth, such as a bitter or sour taste?

嘴里感觉到有什么异常的味道吗,比如苦味、酸味?

(162) Are your stools loose or hard and dry?

大便是稀溏的还是干结的?

(163) When did you start to feel nauseous? Did you vomit? Did anything come out?

你是什么时候开始想吐的? 吐了没有? 有东西吐出来吗?

(164) What do you think is the cause? Is it because you ate some contaminated food or because something unpleasant made you upset?

你认为是什么原因引起的? 是因为吃了不干净的食物,还是因为有什么事情影响了你的情绪?

(165) Do you feel dryness in your mouth while retching? Do you have an urge to drink water?

干呕的时候感到口渴吗? 想不想喝水?

(166) Do you have any discomfort in the pit of your stomach? Do you have any discomfort in your stomach? Do you have any abdominal

pain?

心窝处有什么不舒服吗？肚子难受吗？疼吗？

(167) Is there any special odor accompanying retching? For example, any unpleasant sour odor?

有没有特殊的气味干呕上来,例如酸臭的气味？

(168) Do you know the cause of the most recent vomiting? Was it that you were upset? Did anything unpleasant happen before the vomiting?

你知道这次呕吐是什么原因引起的吗？是不是因为生气着急引起的？呕吐前有什么不愉快的事情发生吗？

(169) (To women of child-bearing age) When was your last period?

(对于育龄女性)你上次来例假是什么时候？

Ⅲ. Dialogues 情景对话

1. Dialogue 1 对话 1

Doctor：Hello, may I ask if there is any discomfort?

你好,请问有什么不适？

Patient：I have been feeling dizzy lately, and sometimes when I stand up, I feel dizzy.

最近总是感到头晕,有时候站起来就觉得晕乎乎的。

Doctor：Understood. There may be multiple reasons for dizziness, and I need to know your specific situation. Have you had any special life or work pressure recently?

了解。头晕可能有多种原因,我需要了解一下你的具体情况。最近有没有特别的生活或工作压力？

Patient：Recently, I have been busy with work and sometimes I do feel a bit tired.

最近工作比较繁忙,有时候确实感觉有些累。

Doctor：Okay, let me check your pulse and tongue coating first to gain a more comprehensive understanding of your physical condition.

好的,我先检查一下你的脉象和舌苔,以便更全面地了解你的体质状况。

(Doctor's examination completed)

（医生检查完毕）

Doctor：Your pulse is slightly weak, and the tongue coating is a bit thin
　　　　and white. This may be related to the poor circulation of qi and
　　　　blood in your body. Additionally, your work pressure may also
　　　　be a factor leading to dizziness.

　　　　你的脉象略弱，舌苔有些薄白，这可能与你的体内气血运行不畅
　　　　有关。另外，你的工作压力可能也是导致头晕的一个因素。

Patient：So how should we treat it?

　　　　那该怎么治疗呢？

Doctor：I will prescribe a Chinese medicine for you to help adjust your qi
　　　　and blood, and enhance your physique. At the same time, you
　　　　should pay attention to rest and maintain a regular schedule. To
　　　　avoid prolonged continuous work, it is advisable to engage in
　　　　stress relieving activities such as walking or deep breathing.

　　　　我会给你开一服中药方，帮助你调整气血，增强体质。同时，你要
　　　　注意休息，保持规律的作息时间。避免长时间连续工作，可以适
　　　　当进行一些舒缓压力的活动，比如散步或深呼吸。

Patient：How do I take traditional Chinese medicine?

　　　　中药需要怎么服用？

Doctor：I will prescribe a prescription for you. Please boil it according to
　　　　the instructions, and take it in batches. Meanwhile, if dizziness
　　　　does not improve or other symptoms appear, please let me
　　　　know promptly.

　　　　我会开给你药方，请按照说明煎煮后分次服用。同时，如果头晕
　　　　的情况没有改善，或者出现其他症状，及时告诉我。

Patient：Okay, I will follow the doctor's advice. Thank you, doctor.

　　　　好的，我会按照医生的建议去做的。谢谢医生。

Doctor：You're welcome. I hope you recover soon. If you have any
　　　　other questions, feel free to contact me.

　　　　不客气，希望你早日康复。如果有其他问题，随时联系我。

2．Dialogue 2 对话 2

Doctor：Hello，may I ask if there is any discomfort?

你好,请问有什么不适?

Patient：Recently，my ears have been buzzing and sometimes I feel very harsh. I don't know what's going on.

最近耳朵老是嗡嗡响,有时候感觉很刺耳,不知道是怎么回事。

Doctor：Understood. Tinnitus may be a symptom caused by various reasons. Have you had any colds or other physical discomfort during this period?

了解。耳鸣可能是多种原因引起的症状。在这段时间内,你有没有感冒或其他身体不适的情况?

Patient：No cold，no other discomfort in the body.

没有感冒,身体其他地方也没什么不适。

Doctor：Okay，let me first check your pulse and tongue coating to understand your overall physical condition.

好的,我先检查一下你的脉象和舌苔,了解一下你的整体体质。

(Doctor's examination completed)

(医生检查完毕)

Doctor：Your pulse is relatively normal，and there is no abnormality in your tongue coating. But tinnitus may be related to poor circulation of qi and blood in the body. Are you under a lot of work and life pressure?

你的脉象较正常,舌苔也没有异常。但耳鸣可能与体内的气血运行不畅有关。你的工作和生活压力大吗?

Patient：Recently，I have been quite busy with work and may be under some pressure.

最近工作确实比较忙碌,可能有一些压力。

Doctor：I understand. I suggest you adjust your schedule and maintain a regular lifestyle. In addition, I will prescribe a Chinese medicine prescription for you to regulate your qi and blood, and enhance your body's resistance.

明白了。我建议你调整作息,保持规律的生活习惯。此外,我会

　　　　　给你开一服中药方,以调理你的气血,并增强身体的抵抗力。

Patient：How do I take traditional Chinese medicine?

　　　　　中药需要怎么服用?

Doctor：I will provide you with detailed medication instructions. Please take it according to dosage and time. In addition，avoiding excessive fatigue and maintaining a comfortable mood can also help alleviate the symptoms of tinnitus.

　　　　　我会开给你详细的用药说明,请按照剂量和时间进行服用。另外,避免过度疲劳,保持心情舒畅,对于缓解耳鸣的症状也有帮助。

Patient：Okay, I will follow the doctor's advice. Thank you, doctor.

　　　　　好的,我会按照医生的建议去做的。谢谢医生。

Doctor：You're welcome. I hope your tinnitus improves soon. If you have any other questions，feel free to contact me.

　　　　　不客气,希望你的耳鸣早日好转。如果有其他问题,随时联系我。

3．Dialogue 3 对话 3

Doctor：Hello，may I ask if there is any discomfort?

　　　　　你好,请问有什么不适吗?

Patient：Recently, there have been some sores in the mouth that I feel very uncomfortable.

　　　　　最近口腔里老是有一些疮,感觉很不舒服。

Doctor：Understood. Oral ulcers may be caused by dampness and heat, poor qi and blood flow, or unstable emotions in the body. Do you have any special dietary or lifestyle habits recently?

　　　　　了解。口腔溃疡可能是由体内湿热、气血不畅或情绪不稳引起的。你最近有什么特别的饮食或生活习惯吗?

Patient：Recently, I have been under a lot of work pressure and my diet may be slightly irregular.

　　　　　最近工作压力大,饮食可能稍微不规律。

Doctor：I understand. I will check your pulse and tongue coating to understand your physical condition.

明白了。我会检查一下你的脉象和舌苔，了解一下你的身体状况。

(Doctor's examination completed)

(医生检查完毕)

Doctor：Your pulse is slightly slender and the tongue coating is yellow, which may indicate an accumulation of dampness and heat. I will prescribe a Chinese medicine prescription for you to help clear heat and detoxify, and I suggest that you adjust your diet to avoid spicy and stimulating foods.

你的脉象偏弦细，舌苔偏黄，看起来可能是湿热内蕴。我会给你开一服中药方，帮助清热解毒，建议你调整饮食，避免辛辣刺激的食物。

Patient：How do I take traditional Chinese medicine?

中药需要怎么服用？

Doctor：I will provide you with a detailed explanation of the medication method. Please take it on time and in the appropriate amount. In addition, trying to maintain a happy mood and avoid emotional fluctuations can also help alleviate oral ulcers.

我会详细给你说明用药方法，请按时按量服用。此外，尽量保持心情愉快，避免情绪波动，对于口腔溃疡的缓解也有帮助。

Patient：Okay, I will follow the doctor's advice. Thank you, doctor.

好的，我会按医生的建议去做。谢谢医生。

Doctor：You're welcome. I hope you recover soon. If you have any other questions, feel free to contact me.

不客气，希望你早日康复。如果有其他问题，随时联系我。

4. Dialogue 4 对话 4

Doctor：Hello, may I ask if there is any discomfort?

你好，请问有什么不适吗？

Patient：Gingival swelling and pain, feeling very uncomfortable while eating.

牙龈肿痛，吃东西时感觉很不舒服。

Doctor：I understand. Gum swelling and pain may be caused by

dampness, heat, qi stagnation, and blood stasis in the body. Do you have any oral hygiene habits in your daily life?

了解。牙龈肿痛可能是由体内湿热、气滞血瘀等引起的。你平时有没有口腔卫生方面的习惯?

Patient：Maybe I haven't paid much attention to brushing my teeth and rinsing my mouth recently.

可能最近没怎么注意刷牙漱口。

Doctor：Okay. I will check your pulse and tongue coating to understand your physical condition.

好的。我会检查一下你的脉象和舌苔,了解一下你的身体状况。

(Doctor's examination completed)

(医生检查完毕)

Doctor：Your pulse is relatively smooth, and the tongue coating is a bit yellow and greasy, which may be due to the accumulation of dampness and heat. I will prescribe a Chinese medicine prescription for you to help clear heat and detoxify, and I also suggest that you strengthen oral hygiene.

你的脉象较滑,舌苔有些黄腻,可能是湿热内蕴。我会给你开一服中药方,帮助清热解毒,同时建议你加强口腔卫生。

Patient：How do I take traditional Chinese medicine?

中药需要怎么服用?

Doctor：I will provide a detailed explanation of the medication method. Please take it on time and in the appropriate amount. In addition, maintaining oral hygiene, rinsing your mouth frequently, and avoiding spicy and irritating foods can help alleviate symptoms.

我会详细说明用药方法,按时按量服用。此外,保持口腔清洁,多漱口,避免辛辣刺激的食物,有助于症状缓解。

Patient：Okay, I will pay attention to that. Thank you, doctor.

好的,我会注意的。谢谢医生。

Doctor：You're welcome. I hope you recover soon. If you have any other questions, feel free to contact me.

不客气,希望你早日康复。如果有其他问题,随时联系我。

5．Dialogue 5 对话 5

Doctor：Hello，may I ask if there is any discomfort?

你好，请问有什么不适吗?

Patient：Recently，I have been experiencing chest pain and feel a bit like colic．

最近心口疼痛，感觉有点像是绞痛。

Doctor：Understood．Angina may involve issues such as insufficient qi and blood，qi stagnation and blood stasis．Have you had any recent emotional fluctuations or high work pressure?

了解。心绞痛可能涉及气血不足、气滞血瘀等问题。你最近有没有情绪波动或工作压力大的情况?

Patient：I have been under some work pressure recently and may be feeling a bit down．

最近确实有一些工作上的压力，可能有点情绪低落。

Doctor：I understand．I will check your pulse and tongue coating to understand your overall condition．

明白了。我会检查一下你的脉象和舌苔，了解一下你的整体状况。

(Doctor's examination completed)

(医生检查完毕)

Doctor：Your pulse is relatively slender，the tongue is slightly red，and the tongue coating is thin and white，which may be caused by insufficient qi and blood．I will prescribe a traditional Chinese medicine prescription for tonifying qi and nourishing blood for you，and I suggest that you adjust your mood and maintain a good daily routine．

你的脉象较弦细，舌质稍红，舌苔薄白，可能是气血不足引起的。我会给你开一服补气养血的中药方，并建议你调整情绪，保持良好的作息。

Patient：How do I take traditional Chinese medicine?

中药需要怎么服用?

Doctor：I will provide a detailed explanation of the medication method．

Please take it according to the dosage and time. Meanwhile, avoiding strenuous exercise and maintaining a stable mood are also important for relieving angina.

我会详细说明用药方法,请按照剂量和时间进行服用。同时,避免剧烈运动,保持心情平稳,对于心绞痛的缓解也很重要。

Patient：Okay, I will follow the doctor's advice. Thank you, doctor.

好的,我会按医生的建议去做。谢谢医生。

Doctor：You're welcome. I hope you recover soon. If you have any other questions, feel free to contact me.

不客气,希望你早日康复。如果有其他问题,随时联系我。

6. Dialogue 6 对话 6

Doctor：Hello, may I ask if there is any discomfort?

你好,请问有什么不适?

Patient：I have been feeling palpitations lately, sometimes very noticeable.

最近总是感觉心悸,有时候特别明显。

Doctor：I understand. Palpitations may be related to the imbalance of qi and blood in the body. Have there been any changes in your recent lifestyle habits?

了解。心悸可能与体内的气血不调和有关。你最近的生活习惯有什么变化吗?

Patient：Recently, I have been busy with work and may not sleep well at night.

最近工作比较忙,可能晚上睡眠不太好。

Doctor：Okay, I will check your pulse and tongue coating to gain a more comprehensive understanding of your physical condition.

好的,我会检查一下你的脉象和舌苔,以便更全面地了解你的身体状况。

(Doctor's examination completed)

(医生检查完毕)

Doctor：Your pulse is slightly weak and the tongue coating is slightly thin, which may be due to insufficient qi and blood. I will prescribe a Chinese medicine prescription for you to regulate qi and blood, and I suggest that you pay attention to rest and maintain a regular schedule.

你的脉象稍弱,舌苔稍薄,可能是气血不足。我会给你开一服中药方,调理气血,同时建议你注意休息,保持规律的作息时间。

Patient: How do I take traditional Chinese medicine?

中药需要怎么服用?

Doctor: I will provide you with a detailed explanation of the medication method. Please take it on time and in the appropriate amount. In addition, adjusting lifestyle habits and avoiding excessive fatigue can also help alleviate palpitations.

我会详细给你说明用药方法,请按时按量服用。另外,调整生活习惯,避免过度劳累,对于心悸的缓解也有帮助。

Patient: Okay, I will follow the doctor's advice. Thank you, doctor.

好的,我会按医生的建议去做。谢谢医生。

Doctor: You're welcome. I hope you recover soon. If you have any other questions, feel free to contact me.

不客气,希望你早日康复。如果有其他问题,随时联系我。

7. Dialogue 7 对话 7

Doctor: Hello, may I ask if there is any discomfort?

你好,请问有什么不适?

Patient: Recently, I have difficulty breathing, especially at night, and feel chest tightness.

最近呼吸困难,尤其是晚上,感觉胸闷。

Doctor: Understood. This may be related to spasms in the airways. Do you have any obvious triggering factors, such as allergens or climate change?

了解。这可能与气道的痉挛有关。你有没有明显的诱发因素,比如过敏原或气候变化?

Patient: I have found that I am allergic to some pollen, and it becomes more severe when the weather changes greatly.

我发现自己对一些花粉过敏,而且天气变化大的时候会更严重。

Doctor：Okay, I will check your pulse and tongue coating to gain a more comprehensive understanding of your symptoms.

好的,我会检查一下你的脉象和舌苔,以更全面地了解你的症状。

(Doctor's examination completed)

(医生检查完毕)

Doctor：Your pulse is tight and your tongue coating is a bit thin and white, which may be caused by airway spasms. I will prescribe a Chinese medicine prescription for you to help relieve spasms and I suggest that you avoid contact with allergens.

你的脉象较紧,舌苔有些薄白,可能是气道痉挛引起的。我会给你开一服中药方,帮助缓解痉挛,并建议你避免接触过敏原。

Patient：How do I take traditional Chinese medicine?

中药需要怎么服用?

Doctor：I will provide a detailed explanation of the medication method. Please take it on time and in the appropriate amount. In addition, try to avoid contact with allergens and keep indoor air fresh, which can help alleviate asthma.

我会详细说明用药方法,请按时按量服用。另外,尽量避免接触过敏原,保持室内空气清新,有助于哮喘的缓解。

Patient：Okay, I will follow the doctor's advice. Thank you, doctor.

好的,我会按医生的建议去做。谢谢医生。

Doctor：You're welcome. I hope you recover soon. If you have any other questions, feel free to contact me.

不客气,希望你早日康复。如果有其他问题,随时联系我。

8. Dialogue 8 对话 8

Doctor：Hello, may I ask if there is any discomfort?

你好,请问有什么不适?

Patient：Recently, I have been feeling acid water surging up in my stomach and sometimes even vomiting.

最近总是感觉胃里有酸水往上涌,有时候还会呕吐。

Doctor：Understood. This may be related to gastric acid reflux. Are there any irregularities in your diet and lifestyle habits?

了解。这可能与胃酸反流有关。你的饮食和生活习惯有没有什
么不规律的地方？

Patient：Maybe I have been eating spicy food frequently lately and I also like to have late night snacks.

可能最近经常吃辣的,也喜欢晚上吃夜宵。

Doctor：Okay, I will check your pulse and tongue coating to understand your physical condition.

好的,我会检查一下你的脉象和舌苔,以了解你的身体状况。

(Doctor's examination completed)

(医生检查完毕)

Doctor：Your pulse is slightly curved and the tongue coating is slightly yellow, which may be caused by an increase in stomach heat. I will prescribe a traditional Chinese medicine formula for clearing heat and reducing fire for you, and I suggest that you adjust your diet to avoid spicy food.

你的脉象稍弦,舌苔稍黄,可能是胃火上升引起的。我会给你开一服清热降火的中药方,建议你调整饮食,避免辛辣的食物。

Patient：How do I take traditional Chinese medicine?

中药需要怎么服用?

Doctor：I will provide a detailed explanation of the medication method. Please take it on time and in the appropriate amount. In addition, adjusting dietary structure and avoiding late night snacks are also important for relieving acid reflux and vomiting.

我会详细说明用药方法,请按时按量服用。另外,调整饮食结构,避免夜宵,对于胃酸反流和呕吐的缓解也很重要。

Patient：Okay, I will follow the doctor's advice. Thank you, doctor.

好的,我会按医生的建议去做。谢谢医生。

Doctor：You're welcome. I hope you recover soon. If you have any other questions, feel free to contact me.

不客气,希望你早日康复。如果有其他问题,随时联系我。

Section 11   Sleep Disorders and Mental Impairments
第 11 节   睡眠障碍和精神障碍

I . Common Diseases 常见病症

1. Insomnia (Sleeplessness) 失眠

Insomnia or sleeplessness refers to inability to obtain adequate sleep. It may be manifested in different forms: difficulty in getting to sleep, tendency to wake during the night and difficulty in getting back to sleep, or tendency to sleep on and off throughout the night. In severe cases, patients may stay awake all night. A variety of factors contribute to insomnia, and the pathogenesis may involve imbalance between the kidneys. Of all those imbalances, such as the liver, the gall bladder, the spleen, the stomach, and either yin and yang or qi and blood in some visceral organs, uneasiness of the mind (the heart) is considered to be the "ultimate" factor in insomnia. Anxiety, worry, fear and fright may all lead to insomnia when a certain level of uneasiness is reached. Clinically, inquiry may help discriminate the conditions of the viscera in terms of insufficiency or excess. In excess conditions, the common patterns include mental agitation by heart fire, liver fire, or phlegm heat, while in deficiency conditions mental uneasiness may be due to yin deficiency with exuberant fire, deficiency of both the heart and the spleen, and qi deficiency of the heart and the gall bladder.

失眠是指无法获得充足的睡眠。它可能表现为不同的形式:难以入睡,夜间易醒,难以再度入睡,或整夜睡得断断续续。在严重的情况下,患者可能彻夜难眠。多种因素导致失眠,其发病机制可能涉及肾脏失衡。在所有这些失衡中,如肝、胆、脾、胃,以及某些内脏器官的阴阳或气血失衡,内心的不安(心脏)被认为是导致失眠的"最终"因素。当达到一定程度的不安时,焦虑、担忧、害怕和恐惧都可能导致失眠。在临床上,探究可能有助于区分内脏的不足或过剩情况。过剩的情况常见心火、肝火、痰热激神,虚者则可能是阴虚火旺、心脾两虚、心胆气虚所致。

2. Somnolence (Sleepiness or Drowsiness) 嗜睡

Somnolence refers to a state of being ready to fall asleep regardless of daytime or night-time. In many cases, somnolent patients may be able to go back to sleep shortly after waking. Somnolence is different from clouding of consciousness. Unlike those who suffer from clouded consciousness and experience a chronic sensation of mental clouding, somnolent patients are mentally clear when awake.

嗜睡是指无论白天还是晚上都准备入睡的状态。在许多情况下,嗜睡的患者可能在醒来后不久就能重新入睡。嗜睡与意识模糊是不同的。与那些意识模糊并经历慢性精神模糊感的患者不同,嗜睡患者在清醒时精神清晰。

Somnolence may be due to encumbrance of the spleen yang by dampness or deficiency of both the heart and the spleen. It may also be due to decline of kidney yang or insufficiency of kidney essence. In the case of head trauma, blood stasis in the brain may also give rise to somnolence.

嗜睡可能是湿阻脾阳或心脾两虚所致。也可能是肾阳气下降或肾精不足所致。在头部有创伤的情况下,大脑中的瘀血也可能导致嗜睡。

3. Amnesia (Forgetfulness) 遗忘症

Amnesia refers to loss of memory, which leads to forgetfulness in daily life. To be discussed here is the type of amnesia induced by the decline of the brain function, during which the memory is gradually lost. Congenital amnesia is excluded.

遗忘症是指在日常生活中失去记忆,从而导致健忘。这里要讨论的是由大脑功能下降引起的遗忘症,在这期间记忆逐渐丧失。先天性遗忘症除外。

The heart stores the spirit and governs all the mental activities, while the kidney stores essence and communicates with the brain. The spleen governs thought and ideation. So amnesia is closely associated with conditions of the hearing, the spleen and the kidney. Qi-blood deficiency of the heart and spleen, essence deficiency of the kidney, and disturbance of the heart by phlegm-turbidity may all lead to amnesia.

心藏神,统辖一切心性活动;肾藏精,通脑;脾主思。所以遗忘症和听觉、脾脏和肾脏的状况密切相关。心脾气血不足、肾精亏虚、痰浊扰心等都可能诱发遗忘症。

Ⅱ. Key Sentences 核心语句

（1）When did you discover that your memory was not as acute as before?

从什么时候开始你感到记忆力不如以前了？

（2）Are you losing memory very fast?

你的记忆力减退发展得快不快？

（3）Do you have a hard time recalling events in the remote past, or those of the recent past, or even things you just did?

是想不起来远期发生的事情了，还是容易忘记近期的事情甚至刚刚做过的事情？

（4）Do you sleep well at night?

你夜里睡眠好吗？

（5）Do you feel energetic during the daytime?

白天精神好吗？

（6）Have you felt any bout of dizziness or tinnitus recently?

近来有没有头晕耳鸣之类的症状？

（7）Have you experienced other symptoms such as oppression in the chest and nausea?

近来有没有胸闷恶心之类的症状？

（8）How long have you been suffering from insomnia?

你患失眠多久了？

（9）Please describe how your insomnia occurs and how serious it is. Do you find it hard to fall asleep or easy to wake up during the night and hard to return to sleep? Have you ever been "up all night"? And how often is that?

请你具体描述一下失眠的情况和程度。是入睡困难还是睡而易醒不能再睡？有没有彻夜未眠过？这样的情况常发生吗？

（10）Do you often have dreamful sleep? Are you often woken early by nightmares?

睡眠中做梦多吗？常被噩梦惊醒吗？

（11）Do you know the cause(s) of your insomnia? For example, are you disturbed by something unpleasant, problematic, or alarming during work or life?

你自己知道失眠的原因吗？比如说,你会因为工作上或生活上一些令人不快的事情、难以解决的事情或担心害怕的事情而烦心吗?

(12) Have you noticed any changes in your emotions since you began to have problems sleeping? For example, are you getting more and more easily agitated? Or do you get angry more often? Or are you increasingly worried about anything?

失眠以来,你的心情有什么变化吗？比如说,你是不是越来越容易感到烦躁？是不是遇事容易生气？或者感到恐惧,总怕有祸事降临?

(13) Have you noticed any changes in your memory because of insomnia? Do you forget things more easily?

失眠对你的记忆力有明显的影响吗？是不是容易忘事了?

(14) Are you aware of any dryness or a bitter taste in your mouth?

你感到口干口苦吗?

(15) If you do not sleep well at night, do you feel tired the next day?

你夜里睡不好觉的话,白天感到困倦吗?

(16) Do you suffer from dizziness or a headache when you wake up?

睡醒后感到头晕或头痛吗?

(17) How about your appetite? Do you experience chest congestion, stomach distension (bloating or fullness sensation), acid reflux (regurgitation), or belching?

你的食欲怎么样？有没有胸闷、胃胀、反酸、嗳气之类的不适?

(18) How about your bowel movements recently? Do you suffer from constipation or diarrhea?

你的大便情况近来怎么样？有没有便秘,或者大便溏薄?

(19) Any changes in urination? For example, do you have to get up frequently at night for urination, and have you observed that your urine has become darker?

小便有变化吗？比如夜间尿多了或者尿色变深了吗?

(20) Do you have a heat sensation in the palms of your hands and soles of your feet?

你感到手脚心发热吗?

(21) Do you have any other discomfort or symptom(s)?

你还有什么其他不适吗？

(22) Do you often take sleeping pills?

你常服用安眠药吗？

(23) Are the sleeping pills effective?

安眠药有效吗？

(24) How many hours do you sleep every day?

你一天能睡几个小时？

(25) When you get up, do you feel high-spirited or drowsy?

起床后感到精神焕发还是仍然昏昏欲睡？

(26) Can you fall asleep in the daytime? And under what circumstances? For example, can you fall asleep during a meeting or a conference, or while you are watching TV?

白天犯困吗？你在什么情况下就能睡着？比如在开会、研讨、看电视时会睡着吗？

(27) Do you experience dizziness or headache while you are awake?

你在清醒时有没有头晕头痛之类的症状？

(28) Have you noticed any change in your memory?

记忆力有什么变化吗？

(29) Are you as energetic as before at work?

工作的精力和以前一样吗？

(30) Is there any change in your power of reasoning and analysis?

思考和分析问题的能力有变化吗？

(31) Do you think that you have less tolerance of coldness than others?

你认为你比其他人怕冷吗？

(32) Are your hands and feet always cold or warm?

平时手脚是凉的还是热的？

(33) How are your lower back and legs? Have you experienced conditions such as soreness in the lower back and edema of the legs?

你的腰腿怎么样？有没有腰痛或者小腿浮肿等情况？

(34) Do you have a good appetite? Has there been any change in it?

胃口好吗？饭量与病前比较有什么变化吗？

(35) Has there been any change in your sense of taste? For example, have you been aware of any lack of taste or stickiness and

greasiness in your mouth?

嘴里的感觉有什么变化吗？比如说有没有感觉口中无味或口中黏腻？

（36）（To young and middle-aged women）Have you experienced anything abnormal in your periods?

（针对中青年女性）你的月经有什么异常的情况吗？

（37）Did you experience any head trauma before the onset of drowsiness （before you first suffered from drowsiness）?

嗜睡发病前头部受过外伤吗？

（38）Do you have any other abnormal sensations?

你自己感觉还有什么其他异常？

Ⅲ. Dialogues 情景对话

1. Dialogue 1 对话 1

Doctor：Hello，may I ask if there is any discomfort that requires medical attention?

你好，请问有什么不适需要就诊吗？

Patient：It has been difficult to fall asleep recently，and lying in bed at night can actually make me more alert，affecting my daily life.

最近总是很难入睡，晚上躺在床上反而会变得更加清醒，影响了我的日常生活。

Doctor：How long did this situation last?

这种情况持续多久了？

Patient：It has been about a month now. I have tried drinking some sleeping pills，but the effect is not very good.

大概有一个月了。我试着吃过一些安眠药，但效果不太好。

Doctor：Please extend your tongue for me to take a look.

请伸出你的舌头，让我看一下。

（Patient extends tongue）

（患者伸出舌头）

Doctor：Your tongue has a reddish texture and a thin coating，which may be caused by excessive heart fire leading to insomnia. Let me take your pulse so that I can feel your physical condition.

你的舌头质地较红,舌苔较薄,可能是心火偏旺导致的失眠。让我给你把脉,感受一下你的身体状况。

(Doctor performs pulse diagnosis)

(医生进行脉诊)

Doctor：Your pulse is tight, which indicates that your heart qi is weak. Based on your symptoms and pulse, you may suffer from inflammation of heart fire and insufficient heart yin. I suggest you adjust your schedule, avoid strenuous activities at night, and try to maintain a relaxed mood. You can consider some traditional Chinese medicines that nourish yin and clear heat, such as yejiaoteng and huangjing, to harmonize the yin and yang of the heart and improve the symptoms of insomnia.

你的脉象较紧,说明心气较虚。根据你的症状和脉象,你可能患有心火上炎、心阴不足的情况。建议你调整作息,晚上避免剧烈活动,尽量保持心情舒畅。可以考虑一些滋阴清热的中药,如夜交藤、黄精等,以调和心阴阳,改善失眠的症状。

2. Dialogue 2 对话 2

Doctor：Hello, may I ask if there is any discomfort that requires medical attention?

你好,请问有什么不适需要就诊吗?

Patient：I have been feeling very tired lately and often feel like sleeping during the day, even though I have plenty of rest at night.

最近总是感觉很疲倦,白天常常想睡觉,尽管晚上休息充足。

Doctor：How long did this situation last?

这种情况持续多久了?

Patient：It's been about two months now, and I've never been so sleepy before.

大概有两个月了,我以前可从没这么嗜睡过。

Doctor：Please extend your tongue for me to take a look.

请伸出你的舌头,让我看一下。

(Patient extends tongue)

(患者伸出舌头)

Doctor：There is a layer of white coating on your tongue, and the texture of the tongue is slightly light. The drowsiness may be due to weakness in the spleen and stomach. Let me take your pulse so that I can feel your physical condition.

你的舌头上有一层白苔,舌质稍淡,可能是脾胃虚弱导致的嗜睡。让我给你把脉,感受一下你的身体状况。

(Doctor performs pulse diagnosis)

(医生进行脉诊)

Doctor：Your pulse is relatively slow, indicating a slow flow of qi and blood in the body. Based on your symptoms and pulse, you may suffer from spleen and stomach weakness and insufficient qi and blood. I suggest you adjust your diet, add some easily digestible foods and avoid overwork. Consider some traditional Chinese medicines that can nourish qi and blood, such as Chinese angelica and huangjing, to nourish the spleen and stomach and improve symptoms of drowsiness.

你的脉象较缓,说明体内气血运行较慢。根据你的症状和脉象,你可能患有脾胃虚弱、气血不足的情况。建议你调整饮食,增加一些易于消化的食物,避免过度劳累。可以考虑一些益气养血的中药,如当归、黄精等,以滋养脾胃,改善嗜睡的症状。

3．Dialogue 3 对话 3

Doctor：Hello, may I ask if there is any discomfort that requires medical attention?

你好,请问有什么不适需要就诊吗?

Patient：Recently, I have noticed a significant decline in my memory and sometimes I suddenly forget important things, which makes me feel very troubled.

最近我发现自己的记忆力明显下降,有时候会突然忘记一些重要的事情,感觉很困扰。

Doctor：How long did this situation last?

这种情况持续多久了？

Patient：It's been about six months now, and I'm starting to feel that this is not just ordinary forgetfulness.

大概有半年了，我开始觉得这不仅仅是普通的健忘。

Doctor：Please extend your tongue for me to take a look.

请伸出你的舌头，让我看一下。

(Patient extends tongue)

(患者伸出舌头)

Doctor：There are some pale cracks on your tongue, and the texture of the tongue is relatively light. It may be ammesia caused by a loss of kidney essence. Let me take your pulse so that I can feel your physical condition.

你的舌头上有一些淡白的裂纹，舌质较淡，可能是肾精亏损导致的遗忘症。让我给你把脉，感受一下你的身体状况。

(Doctor performs pulse diagnosis)

(医生进行脉诊)

Doctor：Your pulse is weak, indicating a deficiency of kidney essence. Based on your symptoms and pulse, you may suffer from a deficiency of kidney essence and disharmony between the heart and spleen. I suggest that you maintain a regular routine to avoid excessive fatigue. You can consider some traditional Chinese medicines that tonify the kidney and nourish the heart, such as goji berries and longan, to nourish kidney essence and improve symptoms of memory loss.

你的脉象较细弱，说明肾精亏虚。根据你的症状和脉象，你可能患有肾精亏损、心脾不交的情况。建议你保持规律的作息，避免过度疲劳。你可以考虑一些补肾养心的中药，如枸杞、龙眼等，以滋养肾精，改善失忆的症状。

Section 12　Abnormal Bowel and Urinary Functions

第 12 节　大小便异常

Ⅰ. Common Diseases 常见病症

1. Constipation 便秘

Constipation is a morbid condition due to abnormal conveyance function of the large intestine. It is characterized by undue hardening of the feces so that unusual straining is required to achieve defecation, or by lengthening the interval between bowel movements to three or four days or more.

便秘是一种由于大肠运输功能异常而引起的疾病。其特征是粪便过度硬化,需要异常用力才能排便,或将排便间隔延长至三四天或更长时间。

Generally, constipation can be classified into two categories: constipation of excess type and that of deficiency type. The former is most likely caused by either accumulated heat in the stomach and intestines that consumes the intestinal fluids, or stagnant qi that impedes the conveyance function of the large intestine. The latter can be encountered in any of the deficiency conditions of qi, blood, yin or yang, which lead to either deficiency of the intestinal fluids or reduced ability of conveyance.

一般来说,便秘可分为两类:过量型便秘和缺乏型便秘。前者最有可能是由胃肠内积聚的热量消耗肠液,或是滞气阻碍大肠的输送功能引起的。后者可出现在任何气、血、阴或阳不足的情况下,导致肠液不足或运输能力下降。

2. Diarrhea 腹泻

Diarrhea refers to abnormally frequent intestinal evacuations with more or less liquid stools. A variety of factors may cause diarrhea, including external contraction of wind, cold, summer-heat, heat or dampness, as well as internal injuries due to intake of improper food or emotional disorder. Dysentery, which is also accompanied by abnormally frequent fecal output, is mainly identified by bloody-and-purulent stools and tenesmus, and thus will not be discussed here.

　　腹泻是指异常频繁的肠道排空,伴有或多或少的液体粪便。多种因素可能导致腹泻,包括风、寒、暑、热或湿的外部收缩,以及因摄入不当食物或情绪障碍而造成的内伤。痢疾也伴随着异常频繁的粪便排出,主要通过血便、脓便和里急后重来识别,因此这里不再讨论。

　　Clinically, diarrhea is subdivided into two categories in accordance with its onset and duration, namely acute diarrhea and chronic diarrhea. The former term denotes diarrhea that has a sudden onset and short course, while the latter is marked by long duration or frequent recurrence. In most cases, acute diarrhea is caused by cold-dampness, dampness-heat or improper food, and chronic diarrhea is mainly due to spleen deficiency. One major cause that leads to chronic diarrhea is emotional disorder. This may induce liver qi stagnation, which restricts the spleen function. Another major cause is kidney yang deficiency, which leads to insufficient warmth of the spleen. Diarrhea of this type usually occurs early in the morning, and is sometimes called fifth watch diarrhea, or diarrhea before dawn.

　　临床上,腹泻根据发病和持续时间可分为两类,即急性腹泻和慢性腹泻。前者表示突然发作、病程短的腹泻,而后者则以持续时间长或频繁复发为特征。多数情况下,急性腹泻是由寒湿、湿热或饮食不当引起的,慢性腹泻主要是由脾虚引起的。导致慢性腹泻的一个主要原因是情绪障碍。这可能会导致肝气郁结,从而限制脾脏功能。另一个主要原因是肾阳虚,导致脾温不足。这种类型的腹泻通常发生在清晨,有时被称为五更腹泻,或黎明前腹泻。

3. Frequent Urination (Urinary Frequency) 尿频

　　Frequent urination or urinary frequency means voiding urine at abnormally brief intervals. Patients with such symptom may urinate for up to dozens of times a day. Frequent urination may be subdivided into deficiency and excess patterns. Among the deficiency patterns, yang deficiency is predominant, and is manifested as long voiding of unclear urine. Dampness-heat is always the leading cause of urinary frequency of the excess pattern. In this case, urgent and/or painful urination, as well as other discomfort during urination, are accompanying symptoms.

　　尿频是指以不正常的短暂间隔排尿。有这种症状的患者每天可能会小便数十次。尿频可分为虚证和实证。在虚证中,阳虚占主导地位,表现为长时间小便不清。湿热一直是导致实证型尿频的主要原因。在这种情况下,伴随症状包括尿急和/或尿痛,以及排尿过程中的其他不适。

The body fluids are controlled by the lung, the spleen and the kidney, disorders of any of which may lead to frequent urination.

体液由肺、脾和肾控制,其中任何一个器官的功能紊乱都可能导致尿频。

4. Nocturia 夜尿症

Nocturia refers to excessive urination at night in terms of both frequency and amount. Patients with such symptom urinate at a normal level during the daytime, but need to wake up for urination during the night more than two or three times, and the amount of urine discharged at night is more than one fourth of the total amount of urine discharged during a day and night. In some extreme cases, the total amount of the urine released in the night is close to or even more than that in the day.

夜尿症是指夜间尿频和尿量过多。有这种症状的患者白天排尿正常,但夜间需要醒来排尿两三次以上,夜间排出的尿液量超过昼夜排出总量的四分之一。在某些极端情况下,夜间释放的尿液总量接近甚至超过白天。

Nocturia is an immediate consequence of disorders of the kidney and bladder. Since daytime is yang, and night-time is yin, night-time is considered to be a period in which the yin ovetakes the yang. Nocturia is generally attributed to kidney yang deficiency. In some cases, however, deficiency of the spleen yang, which fails to replenish the kidney yang, may lead to yang deficiency of both the spleen and the kidney. And when this happens, nocturia may also ensue. The major difference in symptoms between patients with kidney yang deficiency and those with spleen-kidney yang deficiency lies in that the latter usually have low body weight, poor appetite and loose stools, in addition to the common symptoms of kidney deficiency such as sore lower back and tinnitus.

夜尿症是肾脏和膀胱出现问题的直接后果。由于白天是阳,夜晚是阴,因此夜间被认为是阴取阳的时期。夜尿症通常被认为是肾阳虚。然而,在某些情况下,脾阳不补肾阳,可能导致脾肾两虚。当这种情况发生时,夜尿症也可能随之而来。肾阳虚患者与脾肾阳虚患者在症状上的主要区别在于,脾肾阳虚患者除常见的腰酸背痛、耳鸣等肾虚症状外,通常还伴有体重低、食欲差、大便稀等症状。

5. Incontinence of Urine 尿失禁

Although both incontinence of urine and enuresis denote involuntary discharge of urine, there is a fundamental difference between them. While enuresis occurs only during sleep, incontinence of urine takes place even when awake. Post-micturition dribble is a term that describes the involuntary discharge of residual urine after urination. In this case, the process of urination is still under the patient's control. So the concept of incontinence of urine includes neither enuresis nor dribbling after urination.

尽管尿失禁和遗尿都表示不自主排出尿液,但它们之间有根本的区别。遗尿只发生在睡眠中,而尿失禁即使在清醒的时候也会发生。尿后滴沥是一个术语,描述了排尿后残余尿液的不自主排出。在这种情况下,排尿过程仍在患者的控制之下。因此,尿失禁的概念既不包括遗尿,也不包括尿后滴沥。

Incontinence of urine of the deficiency pattern is most commonly encountered in clinical practice. Deficiency-cold of kidney qi, qi deficiency of the lung and spleen, and deficiency of liver-kidney yin can all disturb qi transformation of the bladder and disable its function in containment of urine. Incontinence of urine can also occur due to dampness-heat of the bladder, which is an excess pattern. In this case, dampness-heat runs down to the bladder and disables its functions.

虚证尿失禁是临床上最常见的尿失禁。肾气虚寒、肺脾气虚、肝肾阴亏虚,都会干扰膀胱的气化,使膀胱的阻尿功能失效。小便失禁也可能是由于膀胱湿热引起的,这是一种实证。在这种情况下,湿热会转移到膀胱,使其功能失效。

6. Post-Micturition Dribble 尿后滴沥

Post-micturition dribble refers to involuntary discharge of residual urine after urination. Patients who are physically weak due to a chronic disease may have such a symptom. In those cases, kidney deficiency may lead to bladder cold, which impairs the function of qi transformation in the bladder, and eventually lead to post-micturition dribble. Improper food intake and fatigue may weaken the middle qi, resulting in a reduction in its lifting power. Without sufficient lifting power, the residual fluids may run downward, leading to post-micturition dribble. Acute post-micturition dribble, accompanied by a painful sensation and difficulty in urination, is usually due to dampness-heat in the bladder.

尿后滴沥是指排尿后残余尿液的不自主排出。由于慢性疾病而身体虚弱的患者可能会出现这种症状。在这些情况下,肾虚可能导致膀胱寒证,从而损害膀胱的气化功能,并最终导致尿后滴沥。不适当的食物摄入和疲劳可能会削弱中气,导致其升力下降。如果没有足够的升力,残留的液体可能会向下流动,导致尿后滴沥。急性尿后滴沥伴有疼痛感和排尿困难,通常是由于膀胱湿热引起的。

Ⅱ. Key Sentences 核心语句

(1) I know it is embarrassing to verbalize the conditions of your bowel movements, but it is important if I am to solve your problem.
我知道描述大便的情况不雅,但对于解决你的问题却至关重要。

(2) How long have you been suffering from constipation?
你患便秘有多久了?

(3) How frequent are your bowel movements? Once a day, once every two or three days?
几天大便一次? 每天一次还是两三天一次?

(4) (If the interval between bowel movements is over three days) Is it because you do not have an urge to empty your bowels, or you have the urge but cannot do so? (Is it because you do not have any sense of rectal fullness or you have such a sense but cannot empty your bowels?)
(如果三天以上才排便一次)是根本没有便意,还是有便意但排不出来?

(5) Can you explain why you have difficulty in defecation? Are your stools too dry and hard, or are they not hard but you do not have the strength to pass them out?
能不能解释一下为什么排便困难? 是因为大便干燥坚硬,排不出来,还是大便不硬,却没有力量排出来?

(6) Do you feel relief or fatigue after a bowel movement?
大便之后感到舒畅还是感到全身乏力?

(7) If there is no bowel movement for several days, do you experience any rumbling in the stomach (bowel sound), breaking wind, abdominal distention (fullness sensation), or abdominal pain?
几天不排便时有没有肠鸣矢气,腹胀腹痛等不适?

(8) Does constipation affect your appetite?
便秘对你的食欲有影响吗?

(9) Are you aware of dryness in your mouth and throat?

有没有感到口干咽干？

(10) Have you or people near you sensed foul breath from you?

你自己能感觉到口臭或者别人能闻到你口臭吗？

(11) Do you prefer hot or cold drinks?

你喜欢喝热饮还是冷饮？

(12) Are your limbs often cold? Have you ever felt coldness or pain in the stomach?

平时四肢发凉吗？腹中感到发冷或疼痛吗？

(13) How is the quality of your sleep? Besides constipation, do you also have problems sleeping?

你的睡眠怎么样？除便秘之外，你的睡眠也有障碍吗？

(14) Do you have any other discomfort?

你还有什么其他不适？

(15) How long have you been suffering from diarrhea? Is it a sudden and acute case, or has it been like this for a long time?

你腹泻几天了？是突发的急病还是已经患病很久了？

(16) (To acute diarrhea patients) Do you happen to know the reason for your diarrhea? Did you eat food that might have been spoiled? Did you catch a cold? Or did you overeat?

（对于急性腹泻者）你自己知道这次腹泻的原因吗？有没有吃不干净的东西？有没有受寒？或者有没有暴饮暴食？

(17) Did you catch a cold, accompanied by symptoms like chills, fever and headache?

有没有受凉感冒，伴有恶寒、发热、头痛的症状？

(18) Do you have abdominal pain?

肚子痛吗？

(19) Is your abdominal pain alleviated when you press your abdomen or warm it with a hot-water bag?

用手按压或者用热水袋焐，能使肚子痛减轻吗？

(20) Do your stools give off an unusual odor? Do they smell worse than usual or even give an extremely fetid smell like rotten eggs?

大便的臭味有什么异常吗？比平时的大便要臭，甚至像臭鸡蛋那样臭味浓重吗？

(21) Do you have painful and burning sensation in the anus when you empty your bowels?

排便时肛门感到灼热疼痛吗？

(22) (To chronic diarrhea patients) Has your diarrhea been off and on, or has it lasted continuously?

(对于慢性腹泻者)你的腹泻是时好时坏,还是一直不好？

(23) Is there any particular reason for each attack of diarrhea or aggravation of it? Does it have anything to do with improper food, emotions, or any other abnormal factors that you can think of? Or is there simply no reason?

每次腹泻发作或加重有什么原因吗？与不当的饮食、情绪,或其他你能想到的异常的因素有关吗？还是没有任何原因？

(24) Do you have diarrhea at any particular time during the day? For example, do you have diarrhea at dawn every day and feel comfortable afterwards?

每天腹泻有没有固定时间？比如是不是清晨天未亮时必然腹痛腹泻,泻完就舒服了？

(25) Are there a lot of food dregs in the stools?

排出的大便中有很多未消化的食物吗？

(26) Are you more intolerant of coldness than others? Are your hands and feet always cold or warm?

你平时比别人怕冷吗？手脚是凉的还是热的？

(27) Has chronic diarrhea had any impact on your health? For example, do you have chronic fatigue or a sore lower back and limp knees?

长期腹泻对身体有什么影响吗？比如感到身体疲倦乏力,或者腰膝酸软吗？

(28) You say that you have to urinate too many times a day. Can you please tell me how many?

你说每天排尿次数太多,一天要排尿多少次？

(29) How long have you been suffering from frequent urination?

你尿频的症状多久了？

(30) (To those with acute onset) Do you have any discomfort when you urinate? Do you feel any pain? When you have the urge to urinate, can you control the process?

（对于新近发病者）排尿时有什么不适的感觉吗？感到疼痛吗？有尿意时能憋得住吗？

（31）Did you have any discomfort in your lower abdomen before you started to have the urination problem?

排尿次数增多前,你排尿时小腹处有什么不舒服吗？

（32）Have you had a fever recently?

最近发过烧吗？

（33）Are there any changes in the appearance of the urine? For example, has it become turbid?

尿液有什么变化吗？比如变浑浊了吗？

（34）(In chronic cases) Is there any change in the urine amount on each voiding? Is it (the urine amount on each voiding) less than before?

（对于发病已久者）每泡尿量与以往排尿正常时比较有变化吗？是不是减少了？

（35）Have you ever lost control of your bladder?

有没有发生过憋不住尿以致失禁的情况？

（36）Do you have a burning sensation in the palms of your hands and soles of your feet? Or do you feel cold in your hands and feet?

你感到手脚心发热还是手脚发凉？

（37）Are you less tolerant of coldness than before?

全身有没有比以前怕冷？

（38）Do you have dizziness and tinnitus as well?

有没有同时出现头晕耳鸣的症状？

（39）Is your appetite reduced? Are you less energetic than before? Have you been getting tired more easily?

食量有没有减少？精神是不是比以前差了？有没有感到愈来愈容易疲倦？

（40）Do you often cough? Do you bring up mucus when you cough? Do you feel shortness of breath?

你平时咳嗽吗？咯痰吗？有没有感到气短？

（41）When did you start to notice that you were waking at night frequently to urinate?

你从什么时候开始注意到夜尿增多？

（42）During the daytime, do you dribble urine right after you urinate?

你白天小便有没有尿后余沥点滴不尽的现象？

（43）Is there any change in your hearing ability?

听力有什么变化吗？

（44）Do you have tinnitus?

有没有出现耳鸣的症状？

（45）Have you had a good appetite in recent years? Have you lost weight?

你近年来胃口一直很好吗？身体有没有比以前消瘦？

（46）Have your stools turned loose?

大便有没有变稀？

（47）How long have you been suffering from involuntary discharge of urine?

你患小便失禁的毛病有多久了？

（48）Did it start suddenly or gradually?

是突然发生的还是逐渐发生的？

（49）Do you leak urine all the time, or only under certain circumstances, for example, when you cough or sneeze?

是随时都有尿液流出，还是在一定情况下才有尿液流出，比如在咳嗽时或者打喷嚏时？

（50）Did you catch any respiratory illness such as persistent coughing before you perceived the urination problem?

发生小便失禁之前，你有没有得过诸如长时间的咳嗽等呼吸系统的疾病？

（51）Do you have a burning or stinging pain when urine comes out of the urethra (the canal that carries the urine out of the body)?

尿液流出时尿道有灼热刺痛之类的症状吗？

（52）Do you urinate more frequently than before?

排尿的次数有没有增多？

（53）Is the amount of urine on each voiding increased or decreased?

每次的尿量比没有小便失禁时是增多了还是减少了？

（54）Do you have a sore lower back and limp legs?

有没有腰酸腿软之类的症状？

（55）Do you feel colder in your hands and feet compared with the past? Or do you feel warmer? Is there a burning sensation in the palms of your hands and soles of your feet? Do you have night sweats?

你感到手脚比以前凉了还是热了？有没有手脚心发热，夜间盗汗的情况？

(56) Since you first had the urination problem, have you noticed any other changes in your health, such as your energy and appetite?

自从小便失禁以来你的身体状况有什么其他变化吗，比如体力和食欲方面？

(57) How long have you been dribbling after urination? Did it occur recently or some time ago?

你患有尿后点滴不尽的病症有多久了？是新近发生的还是由来已久了？

(58) (In acute cases) Besides dribbling after urination，do you have difficulty in urination and a burning sensation in the urethra?

（对于新病患者）除尿后点滴不尽外，有没有排尿困难和尿道灼痛？

(59) Is your urine clear or cloudy?

你排出的尿液一般是清亮的还是浑浊的？

(60) (In chronic cases) Do you dribble every time or only sometimes after urination?

（对于久病患者）是每次排尿后都有余沥不尽，还是有时有，有时没有？

(61) Besides the dribbling，do you have a sore lower back or cold limbs?

除尿后点滴不尽外，你有没有腰背酸软、四肢发凉等不适？

(62) Is your appetite not as good as before? Do you have loose stools?

有没有食量减少，大便稀溏的症状？

Ⅲ. Dialogues 情景对话

1. Dialogue 1 对话 1

Doctor：Hello, may I ask if you have any discomfort or need medical attention?

你好，请问你有什么不适需要就诊吗？

Patient：Recently, I often feel my stomach is swollen and my bowel movements are not smooth. Sometimes it takes several days to go to the bathroom.

最近经常感觉肚子很胀,而且排便不畅,有时候好几天才能上一次厕所。

Doctor：How long did this situation last?

这种情况持续多久了?

Patient：It has been about two months now，and I have tried some laxatives，but the effect is not very good.

大概有两个月了,我尝试了一些通便的药物,但效果不是很好。

Doctor：Please extend your tongue for me to take a look.

请伸出你的舌头,让我看一下。

(Patient extends tongue)

(患者伸出舌头)

Doctor：Your tongue has a thick coating and slightly red texture，which may be caused by intestinal dryness and constipation. Let me take your pulse so that I can feel your physical condition.

你的舌苔较厚,舌质稍红,可能是肠燥便秘导致的。让我给你把脉,感受一下你的身体状况。

(Doctor performs pulse diagnosis)

(医生进行脉诊)

Doctor：Your pulse is tight，indicating intestinal qi stagnation. Based on your symptoms and pulse，you may suffer from intestinal dryness and constipation. It is recommended that you drink more water and consume foods rich in fiber. You can consider some Chinese herbal medicines that can moisten the intestines and relieve constipation，such as rhubarb root and rhizome，mirabilite，to improve the symptoms of constipation.

你的脉象较紧,说明肠道气滞。根据你的症状和脉象,你可能患有肠燥便秘的情况。建议你多饮水、多摄入富含纤维的食物,可以考虑一些润肠通便的中药,如大黄、芒硝等,以改善便秘的症状。

2. Dialogue 2 对话 2

Doctor：Hello，may I ask if there is any discomfort that requires medical attention?

你好，请问有什么不适需要就诊吗？

Patient：In recent days，my stomach has been constantly hurting and I have frequent diarrhea，which makes me feel very uncomfortable.

最近几天肚子总是疼，而且频繁拉肚子，感觉很不舒服。

Doctor：How long did this situation last?

这种情况持续多久了？

Patient：It has been about a week now，and I have had diarrhea quite frequently，sometimes several times a day.

大概有一周了，拉肚子的次数比较多，有时候一天好几次。

Doctor：Please extend your tongue for me to take a look.

请伸出你的舌头，让我看一下。

(Patient extends tongue)

(患者伸出舌头)

Doctor：Your tongue has a thin coating and a slightly light texture，which may be caused by diarrhea due to spleen deficiency and dampness. Let me take your pulse so that I can feel your physical condition.

你的舌苔较薄，舌质稍淡，可能是脾虚湿盛导致的腹泻。让我来给你把脉，感受一下你的身体状况。

(Doctor performs pulse diagnosis)

(医生进行脉诊)

Doctor：Your pulse is moist，indicating a heavy dampness. Based on your symptoms and pulse，you may suffer from diarrhea due to spleen deficiency and dampness. It is recommended that you pay attention to dietary hygiene and avoid raw，cold，and greasy foods. You can consider some traditional Chinese medicines that can strengthen the spleen and remove dampness，such as dried tangerine peel and pinellia tuber，to regulate the spleen and stomach and improve the symptoms of diarrhea.

你的脉象较濡,说明湿邪较重。根据你的症状和脉象,你可能患有脾虚湿盛的情况。建议你注意饮食卫生,避免生冷油腻的食物,可以考虑一些健脾化湿的中药,如陈皮、半夏等,以调理脾胃,改善腹泻的症状。

3. Dialogue 3 对话3

Doctor:Hello, may I ask if there is any discomfort that requires medical attention?

你好,请问有什么不适需要就诊吗?

Patient:I have been feeling urgent to urinate in the past few days, and the number of times I use the restroom has significantly increased. Sometimes, just after using it, I feel like going to the restroom again.

最近几天总觉得尿急,上厕所的次数明显增多,有时候刚刚上完就又想上。

Doctor:How long did this situation last?

这种情况持续多久了?

Patient:It's been about a week now, and it's been like this day and night.

大概有一个星期了,白天晚上都这样。

Doctor:Please extend your tongue for me to take a look.

请伸出你的舌头,让我看一下。

(Patient extends tongue)

(患者伸出舌头)

Doctor:Your tongue has a thin coating and a slightly red texture, which may be due to frequent urination caused by damp heat in the bladder. Let me take your pulse so that I can feel your physical condition.

你的舌苔较薄,舌质稍红,可能是膀胱湿热导致的尿频。让我给你把脉,感受一下你的身体状况。

(Doctor performs pulse diagnosis)

(医生进行脉诊)

Doctor：Your pulse is slightly smooth, indicating a high level of dampness and heat. Based on your symptoms and pulse, you may suffer from bladder damp heat. I suggest you drink plenty of water, pay attention to a light diet, and consider some traditional Chinese medicines that can clear heat and remove dampness, such as dyers woad leaf and yinchenhao decoction, to regulate the bladder and improve symptoms of frequent urination.

你的脉象较滑，说明湿热较盛。根据你的症状和脉象，你可能患有膀胱湿热的情况。建议你多喝水，注意饮食清淡，可以考虑一些清热利湿的中药，如大青叶、茵陈蒿汤等，以调理膀胱，改善尿频的症状。

4. Dialogue 4 对话 4

Doctor：Hello, may I ask if there is any discomfort that requires medical attention?

你好，请问有什么不适需要就诊吗？

Patient：In the past few months, I have to wake up several times every night to use the restroom, which has affected the quality of my sleep.

最近几个月每天晚上都要起床好几次上厕所，影响了我的睡眠质量。

Doctor：How long did this situation last?

这种情况持续多久了？

Patient：It's been about three months now, and sometimes I can't fall asleep anymore after waking up and going to the bathroom at night.

大概有三个月了，而且有时候夜间起床上厕所后再也无法入睡。

Doctor：Please extend your tongue for me to take a look.

请伸出你的舌头，让我看一下。

(Patient extends tongue)

（患者伸出舌头）

Doctor：Your tongue has a thin coating and a slightly red texture, which may be due to nocturia caused by weak kidney yang. Let me take your pulse so that I can feel your physical condition.

你的舌苔较薄,舌质稍红,可能是肾阳虚弱导致的夜尿。让我给你把脉,感受一下你的身体状况。

(Doctor performs pulse diagnosis)

(医生进行脉诊)

Doctor：Your pulse is relatively weak, indicating a deficiency in kidney yang. Based on your symptoms and pulse, you may have nocturia due to kidney yang deficiency. It is recommended that you keep warm and avoid cold stimulation. You can consider some traditional Chinese medicines that can warm and tonify kidney yang, such as guifu dihuang wan, to regulate kidney yang and improve the symptoms of nocturia.

你的脉象较弱,说明肾阳较虚。根据你的症状和脉象,你可能患有肾阳虚夜尿的情况。建议你保持温暖,避免寒冷刺激,可考虑一些温补肾阳的中药,如桂附地黄丸等,以调理肾阳,改善夜尿的症状。

5. Dialogue 5 对话5

Doctor：Hello, may I ask if there is any discomfort that requires medical attention?

你好,请问有什么不适需要就诊吗?

Patient：I have been experiencing urinary incontinence lately, constantly wetting my pants and feeling very embarrassed.

我最近老是尿失禁,动不动就尿湿裤子,感觉很尴尬。

Doctor：How long did this situation last?

这种情况持续多久了?

Patient：It's been about a month now, and I was fine before.

大概有一个月了,之前还好好的。

Doctor：Please extend your tongue for me to take a look.

请伸出你的舌头,让我看一下。

(Patient extends tongue)

(患者伸出舌头)

Doctor：Your tongue has a thick coating and slightly dark texture, which may be due to urinary incontinence caused by bladder qi deficiency. Let me take your pulse so that I can feel your physical condition.

你的舌苔较厚，舌质稍暗，可能是膀胱气虚导致的尿失禁。让我给你把脉，感受一下你的身体状况。

(Doctor performs pulse diagnosis)

（医生进行脉诊）

Doctor：Your pulse is weak, indicating significant bladder qi deficiency. Based on your symptoms and pulse, you may have urinary incontinence due to bladder qi deficiency. I suggest you adjust your diet to avoid spicy and stimulating foods. You can consider some traditional Chinese medicines that can strengthen the spleen and nourish qi, such as liujunzi decoction, to regulate the bladder and improve symptoms of urinary incontinence.

你的脉象较弱，说明膀胱气虚较明显。根据你的症状和脉象，你可能患有膀胱气虚尿失禁的情况。建议你调整饮食结构，避免辛辣刺激的食物，可以考虑一些健脾益气的中药，如六君子汤等，以调理膀胱，改善尿失禁的症状。

6. Dialogue 6 对话 6

Doctor：Hello, may I ask if there is any discomfort that requires medical attention?

你好，请问有什么不适需要就诊吗？

Patient：After using the restroom, I always feel that my urethra is not fully satisfied and there may be dripping after urination.

每次上完厕所后总觉得尿道没有尽兴，还会有尿后滴沥的情况。

Doctor：How long did this situation last?

这种情况持续多久了？

Patient：It's been about two months now and I feel quite troubled.

大概有两个月了，感觉挺困扰的。

Doctor：Please extend your tongue for me to take a look.

请伸出你的舌头，让我看一下。

(Patient extends tongue)

（患者伸出舌头）

Doctor：Your tongue has a thin coating and a slightly light texture, which may be due to dripping after urination caused by damp heat in the bladder. Let me take your pulse so that I can feel your physical condition.

你的舌苔较薄,舌质稍淡,可能是膀胱湿热导致的尿后滴沥。让我给你把脉,感受一下你的身体状况。

(Doctor performs pulse diagnosis)

（医生进行脉诊）

Doctor：Your pulse is smooth，indicating a high level of damp heat. Based on your symptoms and pulse，you may have dribbling after urination due to bladder damp heat. I suggest you drink plenty of water to avoid spicy and stimulating foods. You can consider some traditional Chinese medicines that can clear heat and remove dampness，such as yinchenhao decoction，to regulate the bladder and improve symptoms of dripping after urination.

你的脉象较滑,说明湿热较盛。根据你的症状和脉象,你可能患有膀胱湿热尿后滴沥的情况。建议你多喝水,避免辛辣刺激的食物,可以考虑一些清热利湿的中药,如茵陈蒿汤等,以调理膀胱,改善尿后滴沥的症状。

Section 13　Gynecological Complaints
第 13 节　妇科疾病

Ⅰ. Common Diseases 常见病症

1. Advanced Menstruation（Advanced Periods）经期提前

The term advanced menstruation or advanced periods denotes occurrence of menstruation one to two weeks ahead of due time. Menstruation that occurs in advance occasionally or only three to five days before the due time does not belong to the category of advanced periods. Clinically, there are two major types of advanced periods, namely qi deficiency and blood heat. Qi deficiency can be subdivided into spleen qi deficiency and kidney qi deficiency, while blood heat can be subdivided into yang exuberance blood heat, yin deficiency blood heat and heat due to liver depression.

月经提前指月经时间提前一到两周的情况。偶尔提前或仅提前三到五天的月经不属于此类情况。临床上，有两种主要类型，即气虚和血热。气虚可细分为脾气虚和肾气虚，而血热可细分为阳盛血热、阴虚血热和肝郁热。

2. Infrequent Menstruation (Late Periods) 经期延后

The term late periods refers to menstruation occurring more than seven days after the due date, with normal duration of menstruation. Since the frequency of menstruation is lowered, for example, once every three to five months in extreme cases, the term late periods may be substituted by infrequent menstruation. The main mechanism involves disruption of the rhythmic ebb and flow of the blood due to insufficient blood level. The insufficiency may be caused by either deficiency of essence and blood or pathogenic-qi-induced stagnation. The former results from kidney deficiency or blood deficiency, while the latter, from blood-cold, stagnant qi or phlegm-dampness.

经期延后指月经时间拖后七天或以上，月经持续时间正常的情况。由于月经频率较低，例如，在极端情况下，每三到五个月来一次月经，因此月经延后一词可能会被月经不频繁取代。主要机制包括由于血液水平不足而破坏血液的节律性涨落。血液水平不足由精血不足或邪气郁结所致。前者由肾虚或血虚引起，后者由血寒、气滞或痰湿引起。

3. Irregular Menstrual Cycle (Irregular Periods) 月经周期不规律（月经不规律）

The term irregular menstrual cycle or irregular periods denotes a condition in which menstrual periods come at unpredictable times, usually over seven days ahead of or after the due date. The main mechanism of the disorder lies in the disharmony of the qi and blood in the thoroughfare and conception vessels followed by irregular ebb and flow of the blood level. Three syndrome patterns are commonly encountered in clinical practice: kidney deficiency, spleen deficiency and liver depression.

月经周期不规律或月经不规律是指月经周期出现在不可预测的时间，通常在预测经期之前或之后超过七天。其发病机制主要表现为冲任二脉气血不调和,血液水平不规则起伏。临床常见三种证型:肾虚、脾虚、肝郁。

4. Hypomenorrhea (Scanty Periods) 月经过少

Hypomenorrhea, also called scanty periods, refers to menstrual discharge of apparently less than normal amount or extremely sparse like a drip occurring at regular intervals, or shortened duration of the menstrual period with the bleeding lasting fewer than two days. Generally speaking, hypomenorrhea is either due to deficiency of essence-blood that leads to inadequacy of qi and blood in the thoroughfare and conception vessels or due to presence of congealing cold that impedes the flow of qi and blood in those vessels. Four patterns are commonly encountered in clinical practice: kidney deficiency, blood deficiency, blood cold and blood stasis.

月经过少是指月经量明显低于正常水平,或极为稀少,如每隔一段时间滴一滴,或月经周期缩短,出血持续时间少于两天。一般来说,月经过少要么是由于精血不足,导致冲任二脉气血不足,要么是由于寒凝,阻碍了这些经脉中的气血流动。临床上常见四种类型:肾虚、血虚、血寒、血瘀。

5. Amenorrhea 闭经

Amenorrhea refers to failure of menarche by age 18, or absence of menstruation for six months for women with previous periodic menses. The former is categorized as primary, and the latter as secondary. Absence of menstruation during pregnancy or lactation, and after the menopausal period is a normal physiological activity, and does not fulfill the criteria of amenorrhea.

闭经是指18岁时未经初潮,或者有月经周期的女性月经六个月不来。前者被归类为原发性,后者被归类为继发性。妊娠期或哺乳期以及绝经后无月经是一种正常的生理活动,不符合闭经的标准。

6. Metrorrhagia and Metrostaxis (Abnormal Uterine Bleeding) 子宫出血和子宫滴血(子宫异常出血)

Metrorrhagia and metrostaxis refer to abnormally profuse bleeding and slight but persistent bleeding from the vagina during intermenstrual periods, respectively. Both metrorrhagia and metrostaxis follow the same mechanism, which involves the loss of control of the uterine blood due to damage to the thoroughfare and conception vessels. In clinical practice, syndrome patterns such as kidney deficiency, spleen deficiency, blood heat and blood stasis are most commonly encountered.

子宫出血和子宫滴血分别是指月经间隙阴道异常大量出血和轻微但持续的出血。子宫出血和子宫滴血遵循相同的机制，即由于冲任二脉损伤而导致子宫血液失去控制。在临床上，肾虚、脾虚、血热和血瘀等证型最为常见。

Kidney deficiency is usually due to premature sexual activity, repeated childbirths, and excessive sexual activities, as well as decline of kidney qi during menopause. In patients with kidney yin deficiency, exuberant internal heat due to yin deficiency may affect the thoroughfare and conception vessels and push the blood to flow in unwanted directions. In patients with kidney yang deficiency, abnormal uterine bleeding occurs due to loss of the kidney's storage power, impairing the control of the qi and blood in the thoroughfare and conception vessels.

肾虚通常是由于性活动过早、重复生育、性活动过度以及更年期肾气下降引起的。肾阴虚患者，阴虚引起的内热旺盛可能会影响冲任二脉，使血液朝着无用的方向流动。肾阳虚的患者，由于肾的储存能力丧失，影响了对冲任二脉气血的控制，导致子宫异常出血。

Spleen qi damaging factors, such as anxiety, improper diet and fatigue, may lead to spleen deficiency. When the spleen loses control over the blood flow, bleeding from the vagina may occur at times other than menstrual periods.

焦虑、饮食不当、疲劳等脾气损害因素可能导致脾虚。当脾脏失去对血流的控制时，阴道出血可能发生在月经期以外的时间。

Patients with blood heat may also be prone to metrorrhagia or metrostaxis. The blood heat in those patients may be attributed to constitutional exuberance of yang, fire transformed from liver depression due to emotional disorders, external pathogens or exuberant internal heat due to excessive intake of hot and spicy food. All those factors may induce exuberant internal heat or fire, and damage the thoroughfare and conception vessels, pushing the blood to flow in unwanted directions.

血热患者也可能容易出现子宫出血或子宫滴血。这些患者的血热可能是由于体质阳盛、情绪障碍引起的肝郁转化为火、外感病原体或过多摄入辛辣食物引起的内热旺盛。所有这些因素都可能引发旺盛的内热或内火，破坏冲任二脉，促使血液朝着无用的方向流动。

Blood stasis due to emotion-induced internal injury may lead to obstruction of the thoroughfare and conception vessels, forcing the blood to bypass the vessels.

情绪内伤导致的瘀血可能会导致冲任二脉堵塞,迫使血液绕过经脉。

7. Dysmenorrhea (Painful Periods) 痛经(经期疼痛)

Dysmenorrhea or painful periods refers (refer) to the symptom in which lower abdominal pain occurs just prior to, during or right after menstruation. There are two major mechanisms that may induce pain during or around periods: One is obstruction in the flow of qi and blood. A Chinese medical maxim is, "Wherever there is obstruction, there is pain." The other is insufficient supply of qi and blood. Another proverb is, "Wherever there is undernourishment, there is pain."

痛经或经期疼痛是指在月经前、月经中或月经后出现下腹疼痛的症状。在经期或经期前后引起疼痛的主要机制有两种:一种是气血流动受阻。中国医学的一句格言是:"哪里有梗阻,哪里就有疼痛。"另一种是气血不足。另一句谚语是:"哪里有营养不良,哪里就有疼痛。"

The syndrome patterns commonly encountered in the cases of dysmenorrhea include kidney qi deficiency, deficiency-cold of spleen and stomach, qi stagnation and blood stasis, cold congealment and blood stasis, and dampness-heat accumulation.

痛经常见的证型有肾气虚、脾胃虚寒、气滞血瘀、寒凝血瘀、湿热瘀阻。

8. Menopausal Syndrome (Climacteric Syndrome) 更年期综合征

Menopausal syndrome or climacteric syndrome refers to the symptoms occurring around and during menopause, including hot flushes, sweating, irritability, tinnitus, palpitations, insomnia, amnesia, dizziness and irregular menstruation. These symptoms are associated with the physiological changes happening around and during menopause. In women at the age of menopause, the kidney qi starts declining. Predisposition towards exuberance or decline of yin or yang is likely to cause imbalance of yin and yang, and hence the syndrome. So kidney deficiency is the fundamental causal factor of menopausal syndrome, which can be subdivided into kidney yin deficiency, kidney yang deficiency, and deficiency of both kidney yin and kidney yang.

更年期综合征是指发生在更年期前后和更年期期间的症状,包括潮热、出汗、易怒、耳鸣、心悸、失眠、健忘、头晕和月经不调。这些症状与更年期前后发生的生理变化有关。在更年期的女性中,肾脏气开始下降。倾向于阴阳盛衰,易引起阴阳失衡,从而引起证候。肾虚是更年期综合征的根本病因,可分为肾阴虚、肾阳虚、肾阴肾阳两虚。

II. Key Sentences 核心语句

(1) How many days before the due date did your periods come recently?

你近来提前几天来例假?

(2) For how many months have you been like this?

已经连续这样几个月了?

(3) Is the bleeding heavy or light?

经量是增多了还是减少了?

(4) Is there any change in the color of the blood?

经血的颜色有什么变化吗?

(5) What is the color of the blood now? Is it pale red, deep red or red purple?

经血现在是什么颜色的? 是淡红的,深红的,还是紫红的?

(6) Has the change of your periods had any impact on your general health? For example, do you feel sluggish and tired? Do you have soreness in the lower back and weakness in the legs, or dizziness and tinnitus?

经期的变化对全身有什么影响吗? 比如有精神不好,四肢疲倦,或者腰酸腿软,头晕耳鸣的症状吗?

(7) Do you feel upset or have a sensation of oppression in the chest during menstruation?

行经期间有没有心烦胸闷的感觉?

(8) Do you feel fullness, pain or tenderness in your breasts, rib areas and lower abdomen before menstruation?

经期之前有没有感到乳房、两胁和小腹部胀痛?

(9) Do you sleep well at night?

夜里睡得好吗?

(10) Do you have to wake up to urinate at night?

起夜吗?

(11) How many times a night do you need to get up?

一晚上要起夜几次?

(12) Do you frequently have a dry sensation in the mouth and throat? Do you have a heat sensation in the palms of your hands and soles of your feet?

平时有没有咽干口燥、手脚心发热的感觉?

(13) Are you chronically thirsty? Do you prefer cold or hot drinks?

经常口渴吗? 喜欢喝冷饮还是热饮?

(14) How about your bowel movements? Are you constipated?

大便的情况怎么样? 便秘吗?

(15) How about your urination? Do you have short voidings of dark urine?

小便的情况怎么样? 有没有每次量少,尿色加深的现象?

(16) How many days late do your periods come? How frequently do they come?

你的例假错后多少天? 多久来一次?

(17) How long has this situation lasted?

这种情况已经有多久了?

(18) Is your menstrual blood sticky (viscous) or watery? Is it pale red or dark red in color? Are there any clots in it?

经血是黏稠的还是清稀的? 颜色是淡红的还是暗红的? 有没有血块?

(19) Do you have lower abdominal pain?

小腹疼痛吗?

(20) Is it a dull, bloating or hollow pain?

是隐隐作痛,胀痛,还是空痛?

(21) Can it (your lower abdominal pain) be alleviated or aggravated when you press your abdomen?

小腹疼痛时按压能减轻还是加重?

(22) How about warming it with a hot-water bag?

用热水袋焐焐管用吗?

(23) Do you have a larger amount of vaginal discharge than usual?

白带比以前增多了吗?

(24) Is it watery or sticky (viscous)?

是清稀的还是黏稠的?

(25) Do you have dizziness with blurred vision, palpitations or shortness of breath?

有没有头晕眼花,心悸气短之类的症状?

(26) Have you noticed any changes in your emotional or mental conditions?

自己感觉到有精神、情绪方面的变化吗?

(27) Do you have a tight feeling in the chest?

有胸闷的感觉吗?

(28) Do you have a sensation of upper abdominal fullness? Do you feel nauseous?

有上腹部胀闷恶心的感觉吗?

(29) Please describe in detail your irregular periods. Do the periods come ahead of or behind the due time for more than one week?

请你描述一下月经来潮不规律的具体情况。时而提前时而错后都在一周以上,是吗?

(30) Are your periods heavier or lighter than normal?

每次来潮的经血量比平常多还是少?

(31) How about the color?

颜色呢?

(32) Are there clots in the blood?

经血中有血块吗?

(33) Do you have dizziness, tinnitus, a sore lower back and limp legs?

有没有头晕耳鸣、腰酸腿软的症状?

(34) Do you have upper abdominal distension (fullness sensation)? Do you have a good appetie? Have you ever not felt like eating?

上腹部感到胀满吗?胃口好吗?有没有食欲不振,不想吃饭?

(35) During the periods, do you have distending pain (pain with a sensation of fullness) in the ribs, breasts and lower abdomen?

经期有没有胸胁乳房和下腹部胀痛的症状?

(36) Have you felt any emotional changes during your periods, such as depression and frequent sighing for no reason?

经期有没有精神上的变化,比如郁闷不舒,时常想要叹气?

(37) When did you start to have less bleeding during the period?

你从什么时候开始月经量减少了?

(38) How many days does each period last? By how much is the blood reduced?

你现在每次行经持续几天？经量减少了多少？

(39) Is the blood pale red or dark red? Or is it red purple?

经血的颜色是淡红的，暗红的，还是紫红的？

(40) Are there clots in it?

经血中混有血块吗？

(41) Have you had an induced abortion?

以前做过人工流产的手术吗？

(42) Is there any reason that you can think of for the lighter bleeding? For example, did you catch cold during a period or right after you bore a baby? Did anything seriously unpleasant happen to you during a period?

经量减少有什么明显的原因吗？比如是不是曾在经期或产后受寒，或者在经期发生过不愉快的事情严重影响了情绪？

(43) Do you suffer from a sore lower back and limp legs, dizziness or tinnitus?

平时有腰酸腿软、头晕耳鸣的症状吗？

(44) Do you often feel cold in the lower abdomen? How about the rest of your body, especially your limbs?

小腹发凉吗？身上和四肢发凉吗？

(45) Do you feel any pain in the lower abdomen during your periods?

行经期间小腹疼痛吗？

(46) (To a sufferer from lower abdominal pain) What does your pain feel like? Is it dull or stinging?

(对于小腹疼痛者)怎么个疼法？隐痛还是刺痛？

(47) Have you ever tried to relieve it with a hot-water bag? Was it helpful?

有没有用热水袋焐焐？能减轻吗？

(48) (To patients who suffer from primary amenorrhea) Do you have any discomfort, such as dizziness, tinnitus, soreness in the lower back and weakness in the legs?

(对原发性闭经患者)你有没有什么不舒服，比如头晕耳鸣、腰酸腿软？

（49）Are you intolerant of a cold or hot environment?

你平素怕冷还是怕热？

（50）Are your hands and feet always cold or warm? Do you have a burning sensation in the palms of your hands and soles of your feet? Do you feel better when you touch something cold with your palms?

手脚是经常凉的还是热的？手脚心有没有发热的感觉？是不是摸凉的东西感觉舒服？

（51）Do you have night sweats?

夜间有没有盗汗的现象？

（52）Do you wake up to urinate many times a night?

夜间起床小便的次数多吗？

（53）（To patients who suffer from secondary amenorrhea）Were your periods normal before? How long is it since you last had a period?

（对继发性闭经患者）你以前的例假正常吗？这次有多久没来例假了？

（54）Have you had a large amount of vaginal discharge? What is the color? Is it watery or viscous（sticky）?

白带多吗？什么颜色的？稀的还是稠的？

（55）Do you have a poor appetite, abdominal fullness or loose stools?

你有没有食欲不振、脘腹胀闷、大便溏薄等不适？

（56）Have you experienced dizziness with blurred vision or palpitations?

你有没有头晕眼花、心悸怔忡等不适？

（57）Have you had lower abdominal pain?

小腹疼吗？

（58）（If abdominal pain exists）What kind of pain is it? Is the pain dull or sharp? Is it accompanied by distension（fullness sensation）or by a coldness sensation? Do you feel better or worse when you press your abdomen? Is the pain alleviated when you warm it with a hot-water bag?

（如有小腹痛）怎么个疼法？是隐隐作痛还是剧痛？是胀痛还是冷痛？用手按时，是加重还是减轻？用热水袋焐能够减轻吗？

（59）Has there been any change in your emotions or temperament? For example, do you get depressed often, or do you get upset or even furious more easily?

你的性情和脾气有变化吗？比如说，精神上压抑郁闷,容易不耐烦或者生气发怒吗？

(60) I have noticed that you have sighed several times while sitting here. Is it because you feel fullness or tightness in the chest and feel relief when you sigh?

我看你坐在这里叹了好几回气,你是不是胸胁发胀、发满,长出口气会感到舒服些？

(61) How has your health been recently? Are you as energetic as before? Have you ever felt too tired to talk?

你近来身体怎么样？精力和以前一样吗？有没有感到疲乏无力,懒得说话？

(62) At normal times do you feel thirsty and want to drink cold water or other cold beverages? Are your stools hard and dry? And is your urine dark in color? How about during the periods?

平时有没有口渴想喝冷饮,大便干结,小便色深的情况？行经期间呢？

(63) When did you have your last period? It is not the due time now, is it?

你上次是什么时候来的例假？现在不该是经期,对吗？

(64) Is there any obvious reason behind the accidental vaginal bleeding?

这次突然阴道出血,有什么明显的原因吗？

(65) Is the blood pale red, bright red, dark red or dark purple? Are there any clots in it?

血色是淡红的,鲜红的,暗红的,还是暗紫的？夹杂血块吗？

(66) Is the blood watery or viscous (sticky)?

血的质地是稀的还是稠的？

(67) Do you have lower abdominal pain?

小腹疼不疼？

(68) Do you feel better or worse when you press the painful area?

用手按压疼的地方感觉好一些还是更疼了？

(69) Do you have dizziness, tinnitus, a sore lower back and limp knees, or a burning sensation in the palms of your hands and soles of your feet?

有没有头晕耳鸣,腰膝酸软,手足心热的症状?

(70) Do you have such symptoms as intolerance of coldness in general，with cold hands and feet in particular?

有没有全身怕冷,手脚发凉的症状?

(71) Do you often feel tired，and have a poor appetite?

有没有身体疲倦,不想吃饭的症状?

(72) Do you often feel thirsty，and crave a cold drink?

有没有口渴,想喝冷饮的症状?

(73) Are your bowel movements normal?（If not）Are your stools dry and hard or loose?

大便正常吗?(如不正常)是干结还是稀溏?

(74) Have you noticed any change of temperament? Are you feeling more irritable，or are you getting upset more easily?

性情方面有变化吗? 比如是否变得急躁不耐烦或容易生气发脾气?

(75) Do you feel bitterness and dryness in your mouth and throat? Are you constipated? Have you found your urine turning dark with short voidings recently?

有没有口苦咽干、大便秘结、小便短赤的现象?

(76) How long have you been suffering from painful periods?

你痛经多久了?

(77) Is there any reason that you can think of for the painful periods? For example, any illness, catching a cold after childbirth, anger, taking too much cold or uncooked food during a menstrual period?

你的痛经有什么原因吗? 比如生过什么病以后出现痛经,产后受凉,愤怒生气,经期吃了很多生冷的东西,等等。

(78) Can you describe your lower abdominal pain? Is it dull or sharp? Do you also have a burning sensation or a cold sensation in the painful area?

来例假时小腹怎么个痛法? 隐痛还是剧痛? 灼痛还是冷痛?

(79) Do you feel better when you press your lower abdomen? Or do you feel worse?

按压小腹是使疼痛减轻还是加重?

(80) Do you feel better when you warm your lower abdomen with a hot-water bag?

用热水袋焐能使小腹疼痛减轻吗？

(81) Do you have pain in the lower abdomen only, or does it travel to the rear?

痛经只限于小腹疼痛,还是连腰骶部都感到疼痛？

(82) Do you also have pain and distension in the chest and breasts?

胸胁和乳房是不是也感到胀痛？

(83) Is the amount of your periods increased or decreased compared with that of the past?

月经血量与过去不痛经时比较是增多了,还是减少了？

(84) How does the blood look? Is it paler or darker? More watery or more viscous?

经血的颜色和质地呢？变淡了还是发暗了？变稀了还是变稠了？

(85) Are there any blood clots in it? Are there a lot?

经血中有血块吗？血块多吗？

(86) Do you have a normal vaginal discharge? Is the amount increased? Is it watery or viscous? Is it white or yellow?

白带正常吗？比平常多吗？稀的还是稠的？白色的还是黄色的？

(87) Do you have dizziness and tinnitus, or a sore lower back and limp knees?

平时有没有头晕耳鸣、腰膝酸软的症状？

(88) You say that you are at the age of menopause, and have experienced discomfort related to it. Please update me on the conditions of your periods for the past few months: Have your periods come on time? Have your periods become heavy or scanty? Or did your periods stop several months ago?

你认为可能是更年期,现在有很多不舒服,请先说一下近几个月的月经情况:经期准不准？经量多了还是少了？还是已经有几个月没来例假了？

(89) Do you feel waves of chilliness or hot flushes?

身上感到一阵阵发冷还是烘热？

(90) Do you sweat for no reason?

无缘无故地出汗吗？

(91) Are you more intolerant of heat or cold than before?

你比以前怕冷还是比以前怕热？

(92) Do you feel chilly and hot alternately?

有没有一会儿怕冷一会儿怕热的情况？

(93) Do you have a burning sensation in the palms of your hands and soles of your feet?

有没有手脚心发热的感觉？

(94) Can you sleep well at night? Have you experienced sleeplessness recently?

夜间睡眠好吗？近来有没有失眠？

(95) Are there any changes in your emotions? Do you get upset easily? Can you control your emotions? Do you cry easily?

情绪方面有什么变化吗？有没有感到烦躁，容易生气，或者控制不住自己，容易哭泣？

(96) Have you found any changes in your mental state? Do you feel sluggish and even reluctant to talk with others?

精神方面有什么变化吗？有没有感到萎靡不振，连话都懒得说？

(97) Are you as energetic as before? Do you have a sore lower back and limp legs?

体力和以前一样吗？有没有腰酸腿软之类的症状？

Ⅲ. Dialogues 情景对话

1. Dialogue 1 对话 1

Patient：Doctor, my menstrual cycle has been abnormal recently and I have been experiencing severe pain during my period. Can you help me see what's going on?

医生，最近我月经周期不太正常，而且经期疼痛得很厉害，你能帮我看看是怎么回事吗？

Doctor：Hello, after learning about your situation，I would like to know if your menstrual cycle has changed，and what is the color and texture of menstrual blood? What is the specific feeling of pain?

你好，了解到你的情况后，我想了解一下你的月经周期是否有变化，经血的颜色和质地如何？疼痛的具体感觉是什么样的？

Patient：Yes，the menstrual cycle has become quite irregular recently，sometimes early and sometimes late. The color of menstrual blood is darker，the texture is thicker，and the pain feels like a throbbing pain，sometimes accompanied by lower back pain.

是的,最近月经周期变得比较不规律,有时提前,有时推迟。经血颜色较深,质地也较厚,而且疼痛感觉像是一阵阵的抽痛,有时还伴随着腰酸背痛。

Doctor：Thank you for your description. These symptoms may involve poor circulation of qi and blood，leading to the aggregation of menstrual blood into clumps. I will carefully check your tongue and pulse to confirm the diagnosis. May I ask if your daily routine and dietary habits have changed？

谢谢你的描述。这些症状可能涉及气血运行不畅,导致经血凝聚而成块。我会仔细检查一下你的舌头和脉搏,以确认诊断。请问你平时的作息和饮食习惯有没有变化?

Patient：Recently，I have been quite busy with work，and my schedule is indeed irregular. Perhaps I am not particular about food.

最近工作比较忙,作息时间确实有些不规律,可能饮食上也没有很讲究。

Doctor：I understand. These factors may have a certain impact on the circulation of qi and blood in the body. I will prescribe some traditional Chinese medicine to regulate menstruation and promote blood circulation for you. At the same time, I suggest that you pay attention to the regulation of your daily routine and diet，and maintain good lifestyle habits.

了解了。这些因素可能对体内的气血运行产生一定的影响。我会给你开一些调经活血的中药,同时建议你注意作息和饮食的调理,保持良好的生活习惯。

2. Dialogue 2 对话2

Patient：Doctor，I have been feeling bloating and pain in my lower abdomen recently，and I often urinate frequently. What do you think is the problem？

医生,我最近感觉下腹部胀痛,而且经常尿频,你觉得这是什么问题呢?

Doctor：Hello, after understanding your symptoms, I would like to have a detailed understanding of your specific feeling of lower abdominal distension and pain. Does it appear at a specific time or persist? Is frequent urination persistent?

你好,了解到你的症状后,我想详细了解一下你的下腹部胀痛的具体感觉。是在特定的时间出现还是一直存在? 尿频是持续性的吗?

Patient：The distention and pain in the lower abdomen feels like a heavy sensation, sometimes more pronounced before and after menstruation. Urinary frequency is relatively persistent, occurring both day and night, and the urine output is not very high.

这个下腹部胀痛感觉像是一种沉重的感觉,有时候在经期前后会更加明显。尿频是比较持续的,白天晚上都有,而且尿量并不是很多。

Doctor：Thank you for your description. These symptoms may be related to qi stagnation, blood stasis, damp heat, etc. I will check your tongue and pulse to better understand the condition. May I ask if you have been experiencing any discomfort with your daily routine or diet recently?

谢谢你的描述。这些症状可能与气滞血瘀、湿热等有关。我会检查一下你的舌头和脉搏,以便更好地了解病情。请问你最近有没有生活作息或饮食方面的不适?

Patient：Recently, I have been under a lot of work pressure and may have irregular sleep patterns. I also haven't paid much attention to my diet.

最近工作压力比较大,可能作息不太规律,饮食上也没有很注意。

Doctor：Understood. These factors may affect the circulation of qi and blood in the body. I will prescribe some traditional Chinese medicine that can soothe the liver, regulate qi, regulate menstruation and promote blood circulation for you. At the same time, I suggest that you adjust your daily routine, pay attention to keeping warm, and avoid getting cold. If you have any other discomfort, feel free to let me know.

了解了。这些因素可能影响到体内的气血运行。我会给你开一些疏肝理气、调经活血的中药,同时建议你调整作息,注意保暖,避免受凉。如果有其他不适,随时告诉我。

3. Dialogues 3 对话 3

Doctor: Hello, may I ask if there is any discomfort?

你好,请问有什么不适?

Patient: Recently, the menstrual cycle has been irregular, sometimes early and sometimes delayed, and the volume is also unstable.

最近月经周期不规律,有时提前,有时推迟,而且量也不稳定。

Doctor: I understand. Menstrual abnormalities may be related to poor circulation of qi and blood in the body. Do you have any recent stress or emotional fluctuations in your life?

了解。月经异常可能与体内气血运行不畅有关。最近你有没有生活上的压力或情绪波动?

Patient: I have been under a lot of work pressure recently and I am also prone to fatigue.

最近确实有点工作压力大,也容易疲劳。

Doctor: Okay, I will check your pulse and tongue coating to gain a more comprehensive understanding of your physical condition.

好的,我会检查一下你的脉象和舌苔,以更全面地了解你的身体状况。

(Doctor's examination completed)

(医生检查完毕)

Doctor: Your pulse is slightly weak and the tongue coating is slightly white, which may be caused by insufficient qi and blood. I will prescribe a traditional Chinese medicine formula to harmonize qi and blood for you, and I suggest that you pay attention to adjusting your life to avoid excessive fatigue.

你的脉象稍弱,舌苔稍白,可能是气血不足引起的。我会给你开一服调和气血的中药方,并建议你注意调整生活,避免过度疲劳。

Patient：How do I take traditional Chinese medicine?

中药需要怎么服用?

Doctor：I will provide a detailed explanation of the medication method. Please take it on time and in the appropriate amount. In addition, adjusting one's daily routine and exercising moderately can also help regulate menstruation.

我会详细说明用药方法,请按时按量服用。此外,调整作息、适度锻炼对月经调理也有帮助。

Patient：Okay, I will follow the doctor's advice. Thank you, doctor.

好的,我会按医生的建议去做。谢谢医生。

Doctor：You're welcome. I hope your menstrual cycle can gradually become regular. If you have any other questions, feel free to contact me.

不客气,希望你的月经周期能够逐渐规律起来。如果有其他问题,随时联系我。

4．Dialogues 4 对话 4

Doctor：Hello, may I ask if there is any discomfort?

你好,请问有什么不适?

Patient：I haven't had my period in the past few months and I feel very worried.

我最近几个月都没有来月经了,感觉很担心。

Doctor：Understood. Amenorrhea may have multiple reasons, including insufficient qi and blood in the body, unstable emotions, etc. Have you been experiencing any stress or emotional fluctuations in your life recently?

了解。闭经可能有多种原因,包括体内的气血不足、情绪不稳定等。你最近有没有生活上的压力或情绪波动?

Patient：I have been under some pressure recently and also feeling a bit down.

最近确实有一些压力,也有点情绪低落。

Doctor：Okay, I will check your pulse and tongue coating to gain a more comprehensive understanding of your physical condition.

好的,我会检查一下你的脉象和舌苔,以更全面地了解你的身体状况。

(Doctor's examination completed)

(医生检查完毕)

Doctor：Your pulse is slender and the tongue coating is thin and white, which may be caused by poor circulation of qi and blood. I will prescribe a traditional Chinese medicine formula to harmonize qi and blood for you, and I suggest that you pay attention to emotional regulation to avoid excessive stress.

你的脉象弦细,舌苔薄白,可能是气血运行不畅引起的。我会给你开一服调和气血的中药方,并建议你注意情绪调理,避免过度压力。

Patient：How do I take traditional Chinese medicine?

中药需要怎么服用?

Doctor：I will provide a detailed explanation of the medication method. Please take it on time and in the appropriate amount. At the same time, maintaining a good mindset and avoiding emotional fluctuations is also important for relieving amenorrhea.

我会详细说明用药方法,请按时按量服用。同时,保持良好的心态、避免情绪波动对闭经的缓解也很重要。

Patient：Okay, I will follow the doctor's advice. Thank you, doctor.

好的,我会按医生的建议去做。谢谢医生。

Doctor：You're welcome. I hope your menstrual cycle can return to normal as soon as possible. If you have any other questions, feel free to contact me.

不客气,希望你的月经周期能够尽快恢复正常。如果有其他问题,随时联系我。

5. Dialogues 5 对话 5

Doctor：Hello, may I ask if there is any discomfort?

你好,请问有什么不适?

Patient：Recently, I have noticed some abnormalities. The menstrual interval is very short and the amount is quite large, sometimes with some continuous bleeding.

最近发现有点异常，月经间隔很短，而且量比较多，有时候还会持续出血。

Doctor：Understood. Uterine bleeding may involve poor circulation of qi and blood in the uterus. Do you have any recent stress or other symptoms in your life?

了解。子宫出血可能涉及子宫的气血运行不畅。最近你有没有生活上的压力或其他症状？

Patient：Recently, I have been busy with work and a bit tired.

最近工作比较忙，而且有点疲劳。

Doctor：Okay, I will check your pulse and tongue coating to gain a more comprehensive understanding of your physical condition.

好的，我会检查一下你的脉象和舌苔，以更全面地了解你的身体状况。

(Doctor's examination completed)

(医生检查完毕)

Doctor：Your pulse is slightly smooth and your tongue coating is slightly yellow, which may be caused by the accumulation of dampness and heat. I will prescribe a traditional Chinese medicine formula for clearing heat and removing dampness for you, and I suggest that you adjust your lifestyle to avoid excessive fatigue.

你的脉象稍滑，舌苔稍黄，可能是湿热内蕴引起的。我会给你开一服清热利湿的中药方，并建议你调整生活，避免过度疲劳。

Patient：How do I take traditional Chinese medicine?

中药需要怎么服用？

Doctor：I will provide a detailed explanation of the medication method. Please take it on time and in the appropriate amount. In addition, maintaining good lifestyle habits is also crucial for alleviating uterine bleeding.

我会详细说明用药方法，请按时按量服用。另外，保持良好的生活习惯对于子宫出血的缓解也很关键。

Patient：Okay, I will follow the doctor's advice. Thank you, doctor.

好的，我会按医生的建议去做。谢谢医生。

Doctor：You're welcome. I hope your symptoms can be relieved. If you have any other questions, feel free to contact me.

不客气,希望你的症状能够得到缓解。如果有其他问题,随时联系我。

6. Dialogues 6 对话6

Doctor：Hello, may I ask if there is any discomfort?

你好,请问有什么不适?

Patient：I have been feeling a surge of heat lately and my emotions are also quite unstable. I am a bit worried if it is a symptom of menopause.

最近总是感觉热潮涌上来,情绪也比较不稳定,有点担心是不是更年期的症状。

Doctor：I understand. Menopause is often accompanied by symptoms of yin-yang imbalance. Do you have any other discomforts besides hot flashes and emotional fluctuations, such as insomnia and headaches?

了解。更年期常常伴随着阴阳失衡的症状。除了潮热和情绪波动,你还有其他的不适吗,比如失眠、头痛等?

Patient：Sometimes insomnia occurs, and there are also more headaches.

有时候失眠,而且头痛的情况也比较多。

Doctor：Okay, I will check your pulse and tongue coating to gain a more comprehensive understanding of your physical condition.

好的,我会检查一下你的脉象和舌苔,以更全面地了解你的身体状况。

(Doctor's examination completed)

(医生检查完毕)

Doctor：Your pulse is slightly curved and your tongue coating is slightly yellow, which does show some signs of imbalance between yin and yang. I will prescribe a traditional Chinese medicine formula to harmonize yin and yang for you, and I suggest that you pay attention to adjusting your lifestyle and maintaining good sleep and dietary habits.

你的脉象稍弦,舌苔稍黄,确实显示了一些阴阳失衡的迹象。我会给你开一服调和阴阳的中药方,并建议你注意调整生活,保持良好的作息和饮食习惯。

Patient：How do I take traditional Chinese medicine?

中药需要怎么服用?

Doctor：I will provide a detailed explanation of the medication method. Take it on time and in the appropriate amount. In addition, paying attention to emotional regulation can help alleviate symptoms through deep breathing, relaxation techniques, and other methods.

我会详细说明用药方法,请按时按量服用。此外,注意情绪调理,可以通过深呼吸、放松技巧等方式来帮助缓解症状。

Patient：Okay, I will follow the doctor's advice. Thank you, doctor.

好的,我会按医生的建议去做。谢谢医生。

Doctor：You're welcome. Menopausal period is a natural physiological process, and through the regulation of traditional Chinese medicine, your symptoms should be able to be relieved. If you have any other questions, feel free to contact me.

不客气,更年期是一个自然的生理过程,通过中医的调理,你的症状应该能够得到缓解。如果有其他问题,随时联系我。

Section 14　Pediatric Complaints
第 14 节　小儿病症

Ⅰ. Common Diseases 常见病症

1. Hyperkinetic Disorder in Children〔Attention Deficit Hyperactivity Disorder (ADHD)〕儿童多动障碍(注意力缺陷多动障碍或多动症)

Hyperkinetic disorder, also called attention deficit hyperactivity disorder (ADHD), is a behavioral abnormality characterized by hyperactivity, inattention and impulsiveness. It commonly occurs among school-age children, resulting in poor school performance. In most cases, ADHD is due to insufficiency of natural endowment. However, postnatal physical weakness and incomplete recovery from certain diseases may also be important factors. The main mechanism involves disharmony of yin and yang, yin deficiency with exuberant yang, or upward floating of asthenic yang. In clinical practice, heart deficiency, kidney deficiency with hyperactive liver, and heart-spleen deficiency are the most commonly encountered syndrome patterns. Doctors need to differentiate the children with hyperkinetic disorder from those who are simply energetic or naughty. Naughty children may also exhibit occasional inattention and get addicted to little tricks in class. However, they are able to exhibit normal school performance and refrain from improper behavior after correction from teachers.

多动障碍,也称为注意力缺陷多动障碍(ADHD),是一种以多动、注意力不集中和冲动为特征的行为异常,常见于学龄儿童,导致其学校表现不佳。在大多数情况下,多动症是由于天生禀赋不足。然而,产后身体虚弱和某些疾病的不完全康复也可能是重要因素。其主要机制为阴阳不调和、阴虚阳盛、虚阳上浮。在临床上,心虚、肾虚肝亢、心脾虚是最常见的证型。医生需要将患有多动障碍的儿童与那些精力充沛或顽皮的儿童区分开来。顽皮的孩子也可能偶尔表现出注意力不集中,在课堂上沉迷于小把戏。然而,经过老师的纠正,他们能够有正常的学校表现,并避免不当行为。

2. Parorexia (Pica) 食欲倒错(异食癖)

Parorexia or pica refers to disordered appetite with a craving for unusual foods or substances, such as uncooked rice, mud or paper. It may occur among children who are infested with parasites and those who suffer from malnutrition or mental disorders.

食欲倒错或异食癖是指食欲紊乱,渴望不寻常的食物或物质,如生米、泥或纸。它可能发生在感染寄生虫的儿童和营养不良或精神障碍的儿童中。

3. Enuresis (Bed-Wetting) 遗尿症(尿床)

Enuresis or bed-wetting refers to the involuntary passage of urine during sleep at night. Enuresis is normal in infants because their urinary control ability has not yet been established. Nor is it abnormal that a school-age child occasionally urinates in bed during a sound sleep. However, children beyond the age of three who still wet the bed every night are considered to be enuretic. Enuresis is often encountered in syndrome patterns of kidney qi insecurity, spleen-lung qi deficiency, and stagnant heat in the liver meridian.

遗尿或尿床是指夜间睡眠时尿液不自主排出。婴儿遗尿是正常的，因为他们的尿液控制能力尚未建立。学龄儿童在酣睡时偶尔会在床上小便，这也不奇怪。然而，三岁以上的儿童如果每晚仍尿床，则被认为是遗尿症。遗尿多见于肾气不安、脾肺气虚、肝经郁热等证型。

Ⅱ. Key Sentences 核心语句

To the parents：问家长：

(1) How old is your child? What grade is he (she) in?

你的孩子多大了？现在在上几年级？

(2) You say that your child cannot focus on listening but constantly plays little tricks in class. Does he (she) stop doing that after correction by his (her) teacher?

你说你的孩子上课不能专心听课，喜欢做小动作，老师制止后能够停止吗？

(3) Does your child have trouble sitting still during meals, while at school or doing homework? Is he (she) always fidgeting and squirming?

你的孩子吃饭、上课和在家里做作业时坐得住吗？总是在座位上动来动去不能安静吗？

(4) How is his (her) school performance? Can he (she) cope with his (her) homework?

你的孩子学习成绩怎么样？能够完成作业吗？

(5) How is his (her) temperament? Does he (she) get upset easily?

他(她)的脾气怎么样？脾气暴躁，容易激动吗？

(6) Does he (she) often wet the bed?

他(她)经常尿床吗？

(7) Does he (she) have night sweats?

他(她)有夜间睡觉出汗的毛病吗？

(8) How is his (her) diet? Does he (she) have a good appetite? Does he (she) prefer one type of food over others?

他(她)平时的饮食情况怎么样？吃饭香吗？有没有偏食的情况？

To the child：问患儿：

(9) Do you find it difficult to follow the teacher's instructions?

你觉得听老师讲课难不难？

(10) Do you find school interesting or boring?

你觉得上学有趣还是无聊？

(11) Do you feel tired in class?

你觉得上课累不累？

(12) Do you have vivid dreams while you sleep?

你夜里睡觉时做梦多吗？

To the parents：问家长：

(13) What kind of unusual things or foods does your child like to eat?

你的孩子都喜欢吃哪些异物？

(14) Do you tell him（her）that those things are not edible? Does he（she）listen to you，and do as you tell him（her）?

你有没有告诉他（她）这些东西不能吃？ 他（她）听你的话，照做吗？

(15) How long has he（she）been doing this?

他（她）有这个毛病多久了？

(16) Does it affect his（her）normal meals?

对日常饮食有影响吗？

(17) Did he（she）vomit or expel in stools any parasites like roundworms?

他（她）吐过或随大便排出过蛔虫之类的寄生虫吗？

(18) Have you found anything abnormal in his（her）psychological make-up?

他（她）的精神和情绪有没有异常的情况？

(19) What grade is your child in? How is his（her）school performance?

你的孩子上几年级了？ 学习成绩怎么样？

(20) Is your child liable to perspire? Is it easy for him（her）to catch a cold?

孩子平时容易出汗吗？ 容易感冒吗？

(21) Does he（she）eat more than other children of the same age，or less?

饭量与同龄孩子比较是多是少？

(22) How about his（her）temperament? Is he（she）a grumpy child?

孩子的脾气好吗？性情急躁吗？

（23）Does he（she）talk in his（her）sleep？

孩子夜里睡眠时说梦话吗？

（24）（If yes）Very often or occasionally？

（如果说梦话）经常说还是偶尔说？

（25）Does he（she）often grind his（her）teeth during sleep？

睡眠中常有磨牙的情况吗？

III. Dialogues 情景对话

1. Dialogue 1 对话 1

Patient's parents：Doctor, my baby has been coughing and losing appetite recently. Can you help me see what's going on?

医生，我家宝宝最近总是咳嗽，而且食欲不振，你能帮忙看看是怎么回事吗？

Doctor：Hello, it seems that your baby may have been affected by wind and cold. I need to know his specific symptoms. For example, what is the sound of coughing like? Is there any nasal congestion or runny nose? Are there any other discomforts?

你好，看来你的宝宝可能受到了风寒侵袭。我需要了解一下他的具体症状。比如，咳嗽的声音是什么样的？是否有鼻塞、流鼻涕的情况？还有其他不适的地方吗？

Patient's parents：Well, he has a dry cough and sometimes has a slight nasal congestion，but there is not much runny nose. He has been feeling a little feverish lately.

嗯，他咳嗽声音比较干燥，有时候会有点儿鼻塞，但没怎么流鼻涕。最近也有点儿发热。

Doctor：Thank you for your description. These symptoms are consistent with the characteristics of wind-cold common cold. I will check his tongue and pulse in detail to see if there are any other signs. Besides, what is his mental state? How is the quality of sleep?

谢谢你的描述。这些症状符合风寒感冒的特征。我会详细检查一下他的舌头和脉搏,看看是否有其他体征。除此之外,他的精神状态如何? 睡眠质量怎么样?

Patient's parents: His mental state has been average recently, and sometimes his sleep is affected by coughing.

他最近精神状态一般,有时候会因为咳嗽而影响睡眠。

Doctor: Understood. I will further observe his tongue coating and pulse, and then provide a targeted treatment plan. Meanwhile, it is recommended that you pay attention to keeping him warm and avoid cold outdoor air.

了解了。我会进一步观察他的舌苔、脉象,然后给出一个针对性的治疗方案。同时,建议你注意给孩子保暖,抵御室外寒冷的空气。

2. Dialogue 2 对话 2

Patient's parents: Doctor, my baby has been suffering from diarrhea and losing appetite recently. He also has a fever. Can you help me see what's going on?

医生,我家小孩最近总是拉肚子,而且食欲很差,有点发热,怎么回事啊?

Doctor: Hello, I'm sorry to hear that the child is not feeling well. How often is the diarrhea? How do the stools look? Are there any other discomforts?

你好,很抱歉听到小孩不舒服。请问拉肚子的次数是多久一次? 大便的颜色和质地如何? 有没有其他不适的症状?

Patient's parents: About three or four times a day. It is mushy, sometimes a little yellow. And he is always rubbing his eyes, looking a little tired.

大概一天拉三四次,大便呈现稀糊状,有时候带一点儿黄色。他还总是揉眼睛,看起来有点儿疲倦。

Doctor: Thank you for your description. These symptoms are consistent with the characteristics of stomach upset caused by damp heat. I will check his tongue and pulse in detail to confirm the diagnosis. Besides, Is there anything irregular about his diet?

谢谢你的描述。这些症状可能与湿热引起的肠胃不适有关。我会检查一下他的舌头和脉搏,以确认诊断。请问他平时饮食有什么不规律的地方吗?

Patient's parents：Maybe. Lately he's been eating ice cream and something cold.

可能是。最近他吃了一些冰淇淋和凉的东西。

Doctor：Understood. These foods may lead to the increase of cold dampness in the body. I will prescribe some traditional Chinese medicines to clear heat and remove dampness for him. It is recomended to adjust his diet, avoid cold foods and eat more mild and digestible foods.

了解了。这些食物可能导致体内寒凉湿气增加。我会给他开一些清热化湿的中药,并建议你调整他的饮食,避免寒凉食物,多吃一些温和易消化的食物。

3. Dialogue 3 对话 3

Doctor：Hello, may I ask if you have any questions to consult?

你好,请问有什么问题需要咨询?

Parent：I bring my child to see a doctor and recently I've found that he is particularly active and lacks concentration. The teacher also reported that he has difficulty calming down at school, and I am a bit worried about whether it is ADHD.

我带着我的孩子来看病,最近发现他特别活跃,注意力不集中。老师也反映说他在学校难以安静下来,我有点担心是不是多动症。

Doctor：Understood. From the perspective of traditional Chinese medicine, ADHD can be understood as spleen deficiency with poor circulation or excessive liver fire. I will first carefully inquire about the child's lifestyle and dietary habits, and then perform pulse and tongue examinations for him.

了解。多动症在中医角度可以理解为脾虚不运或肝火偏亢。我会先仔细询问一下孩子的生活习惯和饮食情况,然后为他进行脉诊和舌诊。

(Doctor performs corresponding examinations)

(医生进行相应的检查)

Doctor：Through examination, I found that his pulse is slightly weak and his tongue coating is slightly yellow. This may be caused by spleen deficiency. I will prescribe a traditional Chinese medicine for him to invigorate the spleen and qi, and I suggest that you pay attention to giving him some easily digestible foods to avoid stimulating foods.

通过检查,我发现他的脉象稍弱,舌苔有些黄。这可能是脾虚引起的。我会给他开一服健脾益气的中药方,并建议你在饮食上注意给他一些易消化的食物,避免刺激性食物。

Parent：Okay, I will follow the doctor's advice. Thank you, doctor.

好的,我会按照医生的建议去做,谢谢医生。

Doctor：You're welcome. Please have regular follow-up visits, and we will adjust the treatment plan based on his specific situation.

不客气,请定期复诊,我们会根据他的具体情况来调整治疗方案。

4. Dialogue 4 对话 4

Doctor：Hello, may I ask if you have any questions to consult?

你好,请问有什么问题需要咨询?

Parents：I bring my child to see a doctor. He has already passed the first grade of elementary school, but he has been bedwetting recently. I don't know if there is any problem.

我带着孩子来看病,他已经过了小学一年级,但最近还在尿床,我不知道是不是有什么问题。

Doctor：I understand. Bedwetting may be related to kidney deficiency in traditional Chinese medicine. I will first understand his diet and sleep situation, and then perform corresponding pulse and tongue examinations.

了解。尿床在中医中可能与肾虚有关。我会先了解一下他的饮食和睡眠情况,然后进行相应的脉诊和舌诊。

(Doctor performs corresponding examinations)

（医生进行相应的检查）

Doctor：Through examination, I found that his pulse is relatively weak and his tongue coating is thin. This may be related to kidney deficiency. I will prescribe a traditional Chinese medicine formula to nourish kidney qi for him, and I suggest that you control his water intake at night and avoid consuming stimulating foods.

通过检查,我发现他的脉象相对较弱,舌苔较薄。这可能与肾虚有关。我会给他开一服滋补肾气的中药方,并建议晚上控制饮水量,避免食用刺激性食物。

Parent：Okay, I will follow the doctor's advice. Thank you, doctor.

好的,我会按照医生的建议去做,谢谢医生。

Doctor：You're welcome. Please have regular follow-up visits, and we will adjust the treatment plan based on his specific situation. Feel free to contact me if you have any other questions.

不客气,请定期复诊,我们会根据他的具体情况来调整治疗方案。如果有其他问题,随时联系我。

Section 15　Traditional Chinese Medicine (TCM) and Medical Herbs

第 15 节　中医和中药

Ⅰ. Dialogues 情景对话

1. Learning about Chinese Medicine 了解中医

Patient：Doctor, I want to try Chinese Medicine, but truly speaking, I really don't know its effectiveness. Would you please explain it simply for me?

医生,我想尝试着用中医治疗,可是说实话,我不太了解中医,不知道中医治疗到底有没有效。你能简单给我解释一下吗?

Doctor：OK. The medical management of traditional Chinese medicine includes the four diagnostics and differential diagnostication. That is to say, the treatment just bases on the syndrome differentiated through an overall analysis of the data being collected by means of observation(inspection), ausculation and smelling（ausculation and olfaction）, interrogation, pulse feeling and palpation.

好吧。中医诊断疾病的方法包括四诊和辨证两个环节。也就是说,中医的治疗是基于望(诊)、闻(诊)、问(诊)、切(诊)等方法,把收集到的病人信息通过全面分析,综合成不同的证候群,再进行辨证施治的。

Patient：But what does a syndrome mean, doctor?

医生,那什么又叫证候群呢?

Doctor：A syndrome, simply speaking, is a group of symptoms and signs which have a common pathophysiological basis and often appear together during the course of illness.

简单地说,证候群就是人们在发病过程中同时出现的一组症状和体征,而且它们(这些症状和体征)都具有共同的病理生理基础。

Patient：Oh, it sounds so complicated and mysterious.

啊呀,听起来好难理解呢。

2. Acute Coryza 急性鼻炎

Patient：Doctor, my nose is blocked and I feel chilly and feverish since I went outdoors and became soaking wet in a downpour last night.

医生,昨晚我出门时,被大雨浇淋之后,鼻子就感觉堵了,并且还感到浑身发冷发热的。

Doctor：It's a case of common flu. It may take you two to three days' bed rest to recover. There is an epidemic of influenza in the city these days. Did you run a high fever?

你这是感冒了,可能需要卧床休息两到三天才能恢复。这几天流感特厉害,你发高烧了吗?

Patient：Yes. I had a high fever accompanied by severe joint pain and general malaise, but it has subsided now. It started with a running nose. At first the secretion was watery, but the following days it turned into a yellow and sticky substance.

是的。我发高烧了,有时我还感觉关节疼得很、浑身无力,但是现在已经退烧了。开始时就流鼻涕,先流的是清鼻涕,可几天后就变成黄色黏稠的鼻涕了。

Doctor：Please put on a flu mask when you go out. I advise you to drink plenty of warm water and to do some hot steam inhalation.

你出门时最好戴上口罩。我劝你要多喝热水,还要做些热蒸汽吸入的治疗。

Patient：These nose drops don't work very well. Could you please change to some more effective ones for me, doctor?

医生,这滴鼻药不太管用,能不能请你给我开些效果好的药呀?

Doctor：Steam inhalation with a big basin is very easy to do at home. A powdered mixture of Chinese herbs called "influenza decoction" is also quite effective for a common cold.

在家里自己用大盆做蒸汽吸入的治疗也很方便。还有一种叫作"感冒冲剂"的中草药对治疗流行性感冒的效果相当好。

3. Deficiency of Vital Energy of Spleen and Stomach 脾胃两虚

Patient：I have no idea, doctor, why I have experienced a feeling of general malaise for quite a long time.

医生,我也不知道为什么,好长一段时间以来,我总是感到全身无力。

Doctor：Since when?

大概从什么时候开始的?

Patient：For nearly one sharp year.

几乎一整年了。

Doctor：How is your appetite?

你的胃口怎样?

Patient：Honestly speaking, I have no appetite at all.

老实说,我根本就没什么胃口。

Doctor：Have you lost any weight?

你的体重减轻了吗?

Patient：Yes, I really have lost sixteen pounds since last year.

是的,从去年到现在减了十六磅。

Doctor：Any discomfort in your abdomen? And how about your bowel movement?

你腹部有什么不适吗? 还有,你的大便正常吗?

Patient：Yes, I always have a feeling of fullness in the upper abdomen. And I have been suffering from loose bowel movements for three months.

是的,我总是觉得上腹部有胀满的感觉。还有,我腹泻也有三个月了。

Doctor：How many times a day?

一天拉几次呢?

Patient：Two or three, doctor. And the first motion is usually urgent. As soon as I get up in the morning I have to go to the toilet immediately.

两三次吧。一般第一次都是很急的,只要我一起床,就得赶紧上厕所。

Doctor：Have you had any swelling around your eyes or in the legs and feet?

你的眼、腿和脚肿吗?

Patient：Yes, doctor. I have puffiness of face usually in the morning and swelling of the ankles in the afternoon. I really feel my legs are very heavy.

是的,我早晨起来脸是肿的,下午脚踝肿,而且我总是觉得腿沉沉的。

Doctor：And have you noticed any bleeding from the gums?

你的牙龈也出血吗?

Patient：Yes.

是的。

Doctor：OK，let me feel your pulse. Lay your wrist on the little pillow. Put your right wrist on the pillow with the palm facing upward. That's right，please give me the other hand.

好,把手腕放在脉枕上,让我看看你的脉象。把右手腕放在脉枕上，手心朝上。好，换另一只手吧。

Patient：How is my pulse, doctor? Is it all right?

我的脉象怎样，医生？ 正常吗？

Doctor：Your pulse is deep and thready.

你的脉象沉而细。

Patient：What does it mean, doctor?

医生，这是什么意思啊？

Doctor：It means there is a deficiency of vital energy. Now show me your tongue, pull it out a little bit, please.

你的气虚。现在让我看看你的舌头，请往外伸一点。

Patient：How is my tongue, doctor?

医生，我的舌头怎样啊？

Doctor：Your tongue appears swollen and is coated with a thin layer of a white fur.

你的舌头肿大，还有一层薄薄的白苔。

Patient：What is a swollen tongue?

舌头肿又说明了什么？

Doctor：Your tongue as well as your pulse together with the symptoms all denote a deficiency of the vital energy of spleen and stomach.

你的舌征和脉象及你的症状表现都说明你脾胃两虚。

4. How to Take the Herb Medicine 如何服中药

Patient：How do I take (make) the herb medicine, doctor ?

医生，我该怎样服（煎、熬）中药呢？

Doctor：Put the herbs into a sand (grit) pot, then add about 500cc of cold water to soak them for 30 minutes. After the water boils, please simmer gently for another 20 minutes. Then drain the solution, and the amount left is about 40-50cc. This is the first dose, but don't throw (cast) the herbs away. Do (perform) the same as the former, then get the second dose. Take the first dose in the morning, the second dose in the evening. Or you just mix two doses together, drink one part in the morning and another part in the evening.

把草药放入砂锅中,加入冷水 500 毫升,浸泡 30 分钟,待大火煮沸后,文火再煮 20 分钟,将药水滤出约 40－50 毫升。这是头煎,不要将药渣倒掉。按照煎头遍的方法再煎一次,这是二煎。头煎早上服,二煎晚上服。也可以把头煎、二煎混匀了,分早晚两次服用。

Patient：Oh, it's hard to remember, let me write it down.

噢,我记不住,还是让我写下来吧。

Doctor：Oh, madame. We can make the solution for you for five days. Take one bottle daily, half in the morning, and half in the evening. Please remember to put them in the refrigerator (in a very cool place). Don't take the medicine while it is cold.

噢,夫人。我们可以把五天的药都给你煎好。你只需每天服一瓶就行,早上半瓶,晚上半瓶。其他的药要存放在冰箱里冷藏(凉爽的地方)。不要喝冷的药。

Patient：Must I boil it before I take it?

请问,我每次服药都要将它煮开吗?

Doctor：No. Just put it in a glass and warm it in a bowl of hot water.

不用。还放在瓶中,你只需把它放在一碗热水中温热喝就行了。

Ⅱ. Sentences 替换句型

(1) It's not a big deal, just a common cold. Here is some Chinese traditional medicine, which is very effective for treating colds. You will be fine in a few days.

没什么大事儿(不要紧的),只不过是普通感冒而已。吃点中药,治感冒很有效的。用不了几天你就会好的。

(2) Hello, doctor. My child has had a cough and a poor appetite for two weeks. I have brought him to the clinic three times and given him the medicine prescribed, but he isn't getting better. That's why I bring him to see Chinese Medicine.

医生,我的孩子咳嗽和胃口不好已经两星期了。我已经带他到门诊去过三次,也按时服完了药,但是他一直不见好,我想今天来看看中医。

(3) His poor appetite is most likely related to his liver troubles. The

Chinese traditional medicine might help him. Would you like to try it and see?

他胃口不好很可能是由于肝病引起的。我想中药会对他的病有些帮助的。你愿意让他试试看吗？

(4) Here is the prescription，madame. Take it to the pharmacy. The medicine has to be specially prepared. Come back tomorrow morning for it. Two bottles for four days. Give him half a bottle each day divided into two to four portions. Put the bottle in a small basin of warm water to heat the medicine a little. Add a little sugar if you wish. Give it to him two to three hours after food to avoid vomiting.

这是处方,夫人。拿到药房去吧。这药必须特殊配制。明天早晨你来取药。一共两瓶的药四天的量。每天让他喝半瓶,最好分成二到四份。把瓶子放到一碗温水里将药稍稍加热。也可以稍加些糖。饭后二到三个小时就可以服药了,这样可以避免引起呕吐。

(5) I'll give you some Chinese traditional medicine pills. Apply a hot water pad over the knees. You can also have short-wave diathermy.

我给你开一点中药丸。你可以在膝关节上做热敷,还可以同时用超短波透热疗法。

(6) Have you ever had any swelling or pain in your other small joints such as your wrist，fingers，or toes?

其他小关节如腕、指、趾关节也疼,也肿吗?

(7) Is it worse when the weather changes?

天气变化时疼得厉害吗?

(8) Some Chinese herbs have an excellent therapeutic effect for tonsillitis,especially in its acute stage. One of the advantages of Chinese herbs is that there is less chance of drug allergy and side reactions.

有些中药对扁桃体炎,特别是在急性发作期有很好的疗效。中药的优点之一在于它引起药物过敏和副作用的概率较小。

Ⅲ. Words and Expressions 单词和短语

cold as an exogenous pathogenic factor dwelling in the liver channel 寒凝肝脉

common cold due to wind and cold 风寒感冒

common syndromes frequently met with in the clinic 临床常见的证候群

deficiency of vital energy of heart and spleen 心脾两虚

deficiency of vital energy of spleen and stomach 脾胃虚弱

deficiency of yang (the function) of spleen and kidney 脾肾阳虚

deficiency of Yin （body fluid and essence of secretion）of lung and kidney 肺肾阴虚

diseases caused by cold or retardation of functional metabolism 寒证

diseases caused by heat or over-exuberance of functional metabolism 热证

diseases of serious infection or hypermetabolism 实证

diseases of the exterior 表证　　diseases of the interior 里证

diseases of weakness or exhaustion 虚证

emotional evil effects 内伤

excess of yang （the function）occurs as a result of deficiency of yin （body fluid and essence of secretion）阴虚阳亢

external infection 外感

five organs；five viscera （heart，liver，lungs，spleen and kidneys）五脏（心、肝、肺、脾、肾）

five primary elements （metal，wood，water，fire and earth）五行（金、木、水、火、土）

floating pulse 浮脉　　collapsing pulse 沉脉

full pulse 洪脉　　paradoxical pulse 逆脉

intrusion of damp and heat into the lower part of the body cavity 下焦湿热

large and vertical channels 经　　small and horizontal channels 络

medical herbs 中药　　patent medicine 成药

medical tea；herbal broths；potions brewed from herbs；decoction 汤药

negative elements；yin 阴　　positive elements；yang 阳

philosophy of the pulse 脉理

principal channels （for circulation of vital energy, blood and nutriment）经络（用于促进气血与营养的循环）

running pulse 数脉　　slow pulse 迟脉

seven passions （joy, anger, grief, meditation, sorrow, terror and fright）七情（喜、怒、忧、思、悲、恐、惊）

six entrails （gall bladder, stomach, small intestime, large intestine, bladder and triple energizer) 六腑(胆、胃、小肠、大肠、膀胱、三焦)

six evils (wind, cold, heat, wetness, dryness and fire) 六淫(风、寒、暑、湿、燥、火)

stagnancy of liver qi (vital energy through the liver channel) 肝气郁滞

to feel the pulse; palpation 把脉

triple energizer (upper energizer, middle energizer and lower energizer) 三焦(上焦、中焦、下焦)

vigour /vɪgə/; functional power; qi 气　　saliva /səˈlaɪvə/; body fluid 津液

vital energy; jing 精　　nutriment and blood 营血

weak pulse 弱脉　　stagnant pulse 涩脉

wood generates fire 木生火　　earth destroys water 土克水

Section 16　Acupuncture and Recovery

第16节　针灸和康复

Ⅰ. Dialogues 情景对话

1. Moxibustion and Massage 艾灸和按摩

Doctor：When did your pain start?

你的疼痛是从什么时候开始的？

Patient：Three days ago.

三天前。

Doctor：Can you move as usual? Is there any swelling?

影响活动吗？肿不肿呢？

Patient：My motions are limited, but there is no swelling.

不肿，就是活动受限制。

Doctor：Let's try acupuncture to see if any effects are produced (made).

Take it easy, do you feel numb now?

那我给你扎扎针灸吧。放松，告诉我你感到麻了吗？

Patient：Yes, but I also feel dizzy.

麻了,可是我感到也有点头晕呀。

Doctor：In that case, I will do some moxibustion instead of using needles for you. Please let me know if it's so (too) hot.

要是这样的话,我再给你试试艾灸吧,感觉热的时候,告诉我。

Patient：OK … Doctor, I think moxibustion is more suitable for me, now I feel relaxed after the treatment.

好的……医生,我觉得艾灸对我更合适些,做完治疗后,我感到轻松(舒服)多了。

Doctor：Mr. Smith, I would like to give you some massage which may be much better (helpful) to you.

史密斯先生,我给你再增加一些按摩,效果可能会更好点儿。

Patient：Thanks a lot, doctor.

多谢了,医生。

2. Femur Fracture 股骨骨折

Doctor：Hello, I'm an orthopedic surgeon. What happened to your leg?

你好,我是骨科医生。你的腿怎么了?

Patient：I fell down the stairs. Immediately, I felt a bad pain in my left hip and I couldn't stand at all.

我从楼梯上摔了下来,马上感到左髋疼得厉害,我简直站不起来了。

Doctor：When did it happen?

什么时候发生的?

Patient：Two hours ago.

两小时以前。

Doctor：Have you taken any pain-killers?

你用过什么止疼药吗?

Patient：No, I came directly here.

没有,我直接就来了。

Doctor：Please lie on the bed, loosen your belt. And point to the spot where you feel the most pain.

请躺下,松开你的腰带,请你指出最疼的部位。

Patient：It's here, around the left hip.

就在这里,左髋关节周围。

Doctor：I'm afraid your femur is broken. We'd better X-ray it, just to be sure. Take this paper to the office, and the nurse will show you the X-ray department.

你的股骨恐怕断了。得去照几张 X 光片来确定一下。拿这张申请单到办公室去,护士会带你到放射科去。

Patient：Doctor, will it heal properly?

医生,能治好吗?

Doctor：Of course, it will, don't worry. I think you should be admitted to hospital. You need an operation to fix it.

当然能治好,不要着急。我想你得住院做复位固定手术。

3. Lumbago 腰疼

Patient：Doctor, the lower part of my back hurts so much that I'm not able to move.

医生,我腰疼得都不能活动了。

Doctor：How did it happen?

怎样引起的?

Patient：When I tried to get something off a high shelf, I suddenly felt a pain in my back.

我从高处拿东西时,突然觉得腰疼。

Doctor：Is the pain localized to just that spot?

疼就固定在那一块儿吗?

Patient：Yes, only there. (No, I feel it go down my leg when I cough.)

是的,就在那个地方。(不,我咳嗽时,疼痛就往腿上窜。)

Doctor：Is the pain worse when straightening up (stooping down)?

你伸腰(弯腰)时疼痛加重吗?

Patient：Yes, it's worse while straightening up (stooping down).

是的,尤其是伸腰(弯腰)时。

Doctor：Does anything help it?

怎么样就好些呢?

Patient：It's better after resting, but when I try to walk again it hurts so much, and I have to stop.

休息后好些,但是我只要再走一点道儿,就疼得不得不再停下。

Doctor：Please stand up. Let me examine your back. Please bend forward and backward. That's fine. Please turn to the right and left. All right. Please lie on your back. If I hurt you let me know. Please raise your left leg with the knee straight. Please lie on your abdomen. Do you feel pain when I press here?

站起来我给你检查一下背部。请向前弯、向后仰,好。向左右侧弯,对。请仰卧。如果感到疼你就告诉我。抬起你的左腿,伸直。再俯卧,好。我按的部位你觉得疼吗?

Patient：Yes, right here. Anything serious, doctor?

是的,就这儿疼。医生,病得重吗?

Doctor：Nothing serious, it's just a strained back. Acupuncture is the most effective treatment for this kind of backache. You have a protrusion of intervertebral disc.

不严重,只是扭伤了腰。针灸治这种腰疼最有效了。你得了椎间盘突出症。

Patient：Can it be cured?

能治好吗?

Doctor：Certainly, only it takes time. I'll prescribe some medicine for you. You should have acupuncture every other day. Sleep on a hard bed and rest well. You'll be all right within two or three weeks.

当然能治好,只是得花时间。我给你开点药。此外你要每隔一天来针灸一次。最好睡硬板床,还要好好休息。二三周后你就会痊愈的。

II. Sentences 替换句型

(1) How long have you been suffering from rheumatism? Look, the joints are all swelling.

你患风湿病多久了? 瞧瞧,这些关节都肿了。

(2) Which of your joints, for example, the knees, are affected?

你的哪些关节受到了影响,比如说膝关节?

(3) When does your pain become more intensive? Is it unbearable on

motions or in (during) rainy days?

你什么时候感觉最疼？活动的时候或者下雨天感觉疼痛难忍吗？

(4) Doctor，besides(in addition to) aching，I also feel stiffening and fatigue，typically in the late afternoon.

医生，除了疼，我还感到身体僵硬和疲倦，特别是在傍晚的时候。

(5) I have heard(it's said) that acupuncture may help people to stop (quit；give up) smoking. Is that true?

我听说(据说)针灸能帮人戒烟，是真的吗？

(6) Yes，it's true. The acupuncture is so effective to help you stop smoking，but in addition you must have the determination and a strong will，and also cooperate well with your doctor in order to obtain the desired result.

是真的，针灸能帮人戒烟。不过戒烟者本人必须要有决心、有毅力与医生配合好才能达到很好的戒烟效果。

(7) OK，I'll put these silver needles into some points on your body. So please lie down in the bed and keep still. Then take it easy. I'll start，does it (acupuncture) hurt?

好的，我就准备用这些针给你针灸了。轻放松，躺在床上别动，我就要扎了，疼吗？

(8) Acupuncture may cause just a little pain，but it also brings (causes) a certain feeling of numbness and distension. We will try it every day for seven days，will that be all right?

针灸只有些轻微的疼痛，还会有些麻麻、胀胀的感觉。给你每天针灸一次，连续七天，你看好吗？

(9) And when I lifted a heavy box，I felt a pain in my back.

当我抬起一个重箱子时，我觉得腰疼。

(10) It's just (exactly) like what you said. It feels a little distention and numbness，but I haven't neither faintness nor nausea.

就像你所说的那样，有一种胀麻感，不过我一点都不感到头晕恶心。

(11) I would like to affix a few small hard needs (wangbuliuxing) on the skin of your ears which will be kept in places by a piece of adhesive tape. And please press and knead that particular spot between your thumb and index finger until you feel painful and warm. Repeat this three times a day (the more you repeat it，the better).

我用胶布往你的耳朵穴位上贴一些王不留行籽儿,你用拇指和食指揉捏贴处,感觉微微发疼发热就行了。每天三次(捏的次数越多越好)。

(12) While you are getting acupuncture your nose may feel sore and your eyes may also fill with tears. That's a good sign showing the treatment is effective. Don't worry about it.

针灸时你会感觉到鼻子发酸,而且还流眼泪,这说明针灸治疗有效果了,用不着担心害怕。

(13) Deafness due to nervous factors is difficult to cure. Acupuncture may have some effect, but a prolonged treatment is needed.

神经性耳聋不太容易治好,针灸可能有些效果,但是需要长期治疗。

(14) Acupuncture may be helpful for short-sightedness (near-eyesight), but a rather prolonged treatment is needed. However, in some cases, it's useless. If you want to have a try, please go to the eye clinic to have a new check-up first.

针灸治疗近视眼可能有效,但需要很长的治疗时间。可是,对某些近视患者,针灸毫无效果。如果你想尝试治疗的话,请再去眼科重新检验一次吧。

(15) Doctor, I come here to seek help for my son. He has been stone deaf since birth. Can you cure him with acupuncture?

请给我儿子看看病吧,医生,他生下来就一点也听不见。针刺能治好他的病吗?

(16) I am sorry, acupuncture is not always helpful for deaf-muteness. It is only effective in cases of early and mild deafness.

很抱歉,针刺只对早期轻微耳聋有效,对聋哑症的针刺效果似乎不怎么好。

III. Words and Expressions 单词和短语

abalone shell 石决明

acupuncture anesthesia 针刺麻醉

acupuncture /ˈækjupʌŋktʃə/;
  stylostixis /ˌstaɪləʊˈstɪksɪs/;
  needling /ˈniːdlɪŋ/ n. 针刺

agrimony /ˈæɡrɪməni/ n. 仙鹤草

ailanthus /eɪˈlænθəs/ n. 臭椿

alisma /əˈlɪzmə/ n. 泽泻

allium /ˈæliəm/ n. 薤白

allium odorum 胡韭子

almond /'ɑːmənd/ n. 杏仁

alum /'æləm/ n. 明矾

ambergris /'æmbəˌgriːs/ n. 龙涎香

amber /'æmbə/ n. 琥珀

American ginseng 西洋参

anemone /ə'neməni/ n. 白头翁

angelica decursiva 前湖

angelica /æn'dʒelɪkə/ n. 当归

angelica sinensis 当归

aniseed /'ænəsiːd/ n. 八角

antler /'æntlə/; tine /taɪn/ n. 鹿茸

areca /'ærɪkə/ n. 槟榔

aristolochia /ˌærɪstəu'ləukɪə/ n. 马兜铃

arrowroot /'ærəuˌruːt/ n. 竹芋

arsenic white 砒霜

artemisia /ˌɑːtɪ'mɪːziə/ n. 蒿属植物

asafoetida /ˌæsə'fetɪdə/ n. 阿魏

asparagus /ə'spærəgəs/ n. 天门冬

aster /'æstə/ n. 紫菀

atractylic lancea 白术

atractylodes n. 苍术

balsam /'bɔːlsəm/ n. 凤仙花

bamboo endodermis 竹茹

bark of eucommia 杜仲

bark of magnolia 厚朴

betony /'betəni/ n. 藿香

borneol /'bɔːnɪˌɒl/ n. 冰片

broomrape /'bruːmˌreɪp/ n. 列当

buddleia /'bʌdlɪə/ n. 密蒙花

bufotoxin /bʌfəu'tɒksɪn/ n. 蟾蜍毒

buplever /bjuː'plevə/ n. 柴胡

burdock /'bɜːdɒk/ n. 牛蒡子

calabash /'kæləbæʃ/ n. 葫芦

calamus root；sweetflag root 芦根

calcite /'kælsaɪt/ n. 方解石

calendula /kə'lendjulə/ n. 金盏花

camphor /'kæmfə/ n. 樟脑

cannabis /'kænəbɪs/ n. 大麻

carapace /'kærəˌpeɪs/ n. 龟壳

cardamon /'kɑːdəmən/ n. 豆蔻

carnation /kɑː'neɪʃn/ n. 香石竹；康乃馨

cassia /'kæsɪə/ n.（肉）桂皮；决明

castor bean 蓖麻子

catalpa /kə'tælpə/ n. 梓实

catechu /'kætɪˌtʃuː/ n. 儿茶

celandine /'selənˌdaɪn/ n. 白屈菜

chamois horn 羚羊角

chinese celery 水芹

chrysanthemum /krɪ'sænθəməm/ n. 菊花

cibotium barometz 狗脊

cinnabar /'sɪnəˌbɑː/ n. 朱砂

cinnamon /'sɪnəmən/ n. 桂皮

clam shell 蛤壳

clematis /'klemətɪs/ n. 铁线莲

coltsfoot /'kəultsˌfut/ n. 款冬

common bletilla rubber（*Bletilla striata*）白及

conch shell 海螺壳

convolvulus /kən'vɒlvjələs/ n. 旋复花

corydalis /kə'rɪdəlɪs/ n. 紫堇

cow bezoar 牛黄

crab apple 山楂

croton /'krəutn/ n. 巴豆

cumin /'kʌmɪn/；fennel /'fenl/ n. 茴香

curcuma /'kɜːkjumə/ n. 姜黄

cuttlebone /'kʌtlˌbəun/ n. 海螵蛸

danshen root（*Salvia mitiorrhiza*）丹参

daphne /'dæfni/ n. 瑞香

datura /dəˈtjʊərə/ n. 曼陀罗

diospyros lotus 酸枣

dodder /ˈdɒdə/ n. 菟丝子

domain of taboo 禁区

duckweed /ˈdʌkwiːd/ n. 浮萍

ear-acupuncture therapy 耳针疗法

earth worm 地龙

endodermis of chicken gizzard 鸡内金

ephedra /ɪˈfedrə/ n. 麻黄

equisetum /ˌekwɪˈsiːtəm/ n. 木贼

ergot /ˈɜːɡət/ n. 麦角

eupatorium /ˌjuːpəˈtɔːriəm/ n. 西洋兰

exuviae of cicada 蝉蜕

exuviae of snake 蛇蜕

fig /fɪɡ/ n. 无花果

flax seed 亚麻子

footstalk of musk melon 苦丁香(蒂)

forsythia /fɔːˈsaɪθiə/ n. 连翘

foxglove /ˈfɒksˌɡlʌv/ n. 毛地黄

fritillary /frɪˈtɪləri/ (Fritillaria) n. 贝母

fruit of glossy privet 女贞子

galangal /ɡəˈlæŋɡəl/ n. 良姜

gamboge /ɡæmˈbuːʒ/ n. 藤黄

gelatin /ˈdʒelətɪn/ n. 明胶

gentian /ˈdʒenʃən/ n. 龙胆草

gingko /ˈɡɪŋkəʊ/ n. 白果

ginseng /ˈdʒɪnseŋ/ (Panax ginseng) n. 人参

golden thread 黄连

gypsum /ˈdʒɪpsəm/ n. 石膏

haematic iron ore 赭石

hedgehog skin 刺猬

hellebore /ˈheliˌbɔː/ (Veratrum nigrum) n. 藜芦

hemerocallis /ˌheməraʊˈkælɪs/ n. 萱草

hemp seed 火麻仁

hibiscus /hɪˈbɪskəs/ n. 木槿

honeysuckle /ˈhʌnisʌkl/ n. 金银花;忍冬

hornet-hive 蜂房

insertion /ɪnˈsɜːʃn/ n. 进针

Japanese ampelopsis root (Ampelopsis japonica) 白蔹

Job's-tears 薏苡

Judas tree 南欧紫荆

jujube /ˈdʒuːdʒuːb/ n. 枣

jujube kernel 枣仁

juncus /ˈdʒʌŋkəs/ n. 灯心

kneading /ˈniːdɪŋ/ n. 推

leech /liːtʃ/ n. 水蛭

lily /ˈlɪli/ n. 百合

lily of the valley 铃兰

liquidambar /ˌlɪkwɪdˈæmbə/ n. 枫香

liquorice /ˈlɪkərɪs/ (Glycyrrhiza uralensis) n. 甘草

lobelia /ləʊˈbiːliə/ n. 山梗菜

locust bean 槐角

loquat /ˈləʊkwɒt/ n. 枇杷

lotus leaf 荷叶

lotus seed-case 莲房

lotus seed 莲子

lysium chinense 枸杞子

madder /ˈmædə/ n. 茜草

magnolia /mæɡˈnəʊliə/ n. 木兰

mallow /ˈmæləʊ/ n. 锦葵

massage /ˈmæsɑːʒ/ n. 推拿;按摩

medicated wine 药酒

meretrix shell 蛤壳

milkvetch root 黄芪

mole cricket 蝼蛄

morning glory 牵牛

motherwort /ˈmʌðəˌwɜːt/ *n*. 益母草

moxa punk 艾绒

moxibustion /ˌmɒksɪˈbʌstʃən/；

　cauterization /ˌkɔːtəraɪˈzeɪʃən/ *n*. 艾灼

mulberry branch 桑枝

mulberry root-bark 桑白皮

musk /mʌsk/ *n*. 麝香

mustard /ˈmʌstəd/ *n*. 白芥子

myrrh /mɜː/ *n*. 没药

nutgall /ˈnʌtˌgɔːl/ *n*. 五倍子

nutmeg /ˈnʌtmeg/ *n*. 肉豆蔻

olibanum gum 乳香

opium /ˈəupiəm/ *n*. 鸦片

orange peel 橘皮

orpiment /ˈɔːpɪmənt/ *n*. 雌黄

osmanthus /ɒsˈmænθəs/ *n*. 桂花

oxalis /ˈɒksəlɪs/ *n*. 酢浆草

oyster /ˈɔɪstə/ *n*. 牡蛎

papaya /pəˈpaɪə/ *n*. 木瓜

peach kernel 桃仁

persimmon sugar 柿霜

pine leaves 松针

pinellia tuber (*Pinellia ternata*) 半夏

pine pollen 松花粉

plantain /ˈplæntɪn/ *n*. 车前草

platy codon 桔梗

point /pɔɪnt/；sinus /ˈsaɪnəs/ *n*. 穴；穴道

polygala /pəˈlɪgələ/ *n*. 远志

polygonum /pəˈlɪgənəm/ *n*. 蓼属

portulaca /ˌpɔːtjʊˈlækə/ *n*. 马齿苋

prune /pruːn/ *n*. 乌梅

pseudo-ginseng 三七

psoralea /səˈreɪlɪə/ *n*. 补骨脂

pumpkin seed 南瓜子

realgar /rɪˈælgə/ *n*. 雄黄

red kaoline 赤石脂

red peony 赤芍

rhinoceros horn 犀角

rhizome of Chinese monkshood
　(*Aconitum carmichaelii*) n. 乌头

rhizome of chuanxiong 川芎

rhododendron /ˈrəudəˈdendrən/ *n*. 满山红

rhubarb /ˈruːbaːb/ *n*. 大黄

root-bark of tree peony 牡丹皮

root of Beijing euphorbia (*Euphorbia
　kansui*) n. 甘遂

rose /rəuz/ *n*. 刺玫

royal jelly 蜂王浆

rub /rʌb/ *v*. 搓

rue /ruː/ *n*. 芸香

safflower /ˈsæflauə/ *n*.；saffron(藏)红花

sandalwood /ˈsændlwud/ *n*. 檀香

schisandra /skiˈzændrə/ *n*. 五味子

scorpion /ˈskɔːpiən/ *n*. 蝎子

sea tangle n. 海带

sea-tortoises shell 玳瑁

seaweed /ˈsiːwiːd/ *n*. 海藻

sedative point 镇静穴

selfheal /ˈselfˌhiːl/ *n*. 夏枯草

sesame /ˈsesəmi/ *n*. 芝麻

skull cap 黄芩

smilax /ˈsmaɪlæks/ *n*. 叶门冬

snail /sneɪl/ *n*. 蜗牛

snakegourd fruit (*Trichosanthes
　kirilowii*) n. 栝楼

soap-pod 皂荚

soft rush 通草

spearmint /'spɪəmɪnt/；peppermint /'pepəmɪnt/ *n*. 薄荷

spinal pinching 捏背

straight ladybell root（*Adenophora stricta*）*n*. 沙参

storax /'stɔːræks/ *n*. 苏合香

syringa /sɪ'rɪŋgə/ *n*. (amurensis) 山梅花

tamarisk /'tæmərɪsk/ *n*. 柽柳

tap /tæp/ *v*. 拍打

taraxacum /tə'ræksəkəm/ *n*. 蒲公英

tendon-pinching 捏筋

the datura flower 洋金花

thistle /'θɪsl/ *n*. 大蓟

thyme /taɪm/ *n*. 百里香

tinder agaric 灵芝

tonic point 补穴

tuberose /'tjuːbəˌrəʊs/ *n*. 夜来香

tuckahoe /'tʌkəˌhəʊ/ *n*. 茯苓

tulip /'tjuːlɪp/ *n*. 郁金香

turmeric /'tɜːmərɪk/ *n*. 郁金

turnip seed 莱菔子

twirl /twɜːl/ *v*. 行针

urtica /'ɜːtɪkə/ *n*. 荨麻

valerian /və'lɪərɪən/ *n*. 缬草

veronica /və'rɒnɪkə/ *n*. 婆婆纳

virgina creeper 爬山虎；刺南蛇藤

walnut /'wɔːlnʌt/ *n*. 核桃

water lily 睡莲

white agaric 银耳

wild poppy 野罂粟

yam /jæm/ *n*. 山药

zingiber /'zɪndʒɪbə/；ginger /'dʒɪndʒə/ *n*. 姜

Section 17　Main Collateral Channels and Physiotherapy in TCM
第 17 节　中医经络及物理治疗

Ⅰ. Dialogues 情景对话

1. Lumbar Pain and Sciatica 腰疼和坐骨神经疼

Doctor：Mr.（Mrs.）Smith. Can you tell me in which area of your back you feel much pain? Only in the middle，or on the sides also? 史密斯先生(夫人)，你能告诉我你觉得你背部哪个地方疼吗？是只在中间疼，还是两边都疼？

Patient：Only in the middle part.

只是中间这地方疼。

Doctor：Does the pain radiate（react）to the leg?

你觉得疼往腿上窜吗？

Patient：Yes，and sometimes it radiates straight（directly）down to my heel.

是的，有时一直往下窜到脚后跟。

Doctor：Can you move as usual?

你能正常活动吗？

Patient：I can move a little，but my motions are quite limited. I feel pain when bending down. And it hurts when I stand up after sitting for a long period of time.

我能活动那么一点点，但动作受限，一弯腰就疼。还有稍坐久一点，一站起来也疼。

Doctor：Have you ever twisted your lumbar region?

请问你的腰扭伤过吗？

Patient：A week ago，I carried a heavy piece of luggage，and I think maybe（perhaps）I twisted my back at that time.

一个星期前，我提重物时，我想可能是把腰给扭了。

Doctor：Then have you ever had any other illness，for instance（such as）nephritis，gall-stones（or any gynecological diseases）?

那你还得过其他病吗，比如说，肾炎、胆结石（或什么妇科病）？

Patient：Yes，I had nephritis，but that was five years ago.

是的，我得过肾炎，不过那是五年前的事了。

Doctor：Do you feel any pain when I press here?

我用手压的这个地方疼吗？

Patient：No，I don't.

不疼。

Doctor：I'm going to give you a shot of vitamin B_{12} and Chinese angelica solution into certain acupuncture points to relieve your sharp pain.

我准备把维生素 B_{12} 和当归提取液给你注入到针刺的穴位内，这样可以很好地缓解疼痛。

Patient：Is it painful?

疼吗？

Doctor：It's just like an injection and it only causes a slight (light, less) pain.

只是像打针一样,只稍微有点疼。

Patient：OK,I see. Thank you very much.

好,我知道了,谢谢你。

2. Spur 骨刺

Doctor： I would like to arrange for you to have three sessions of physiotherapy. Is it convenient for you to come everyday?

我打算给你安排三次理疗。你是每天都能来吗?

Patient：I'm rather busy, but I'll try to come.

我很忙,但是我尽量抽时间来吧。

Doctor： How long has your leg (shoulder, lumbar region, hip) been hurting?

你的腿(肩、腰、髋)疼了有多久了?

Patient： Already for half a year now.

已经疼了有半年了。

Doctor：Does the pain at the back of your shoulder move along your arms? Does it feel numb?

你肩膀后面的疼痛往胳膊上窜吗? 有麻木的感觉吗?

Patient：If I turn my neck, the back of my shoulder feels heavy, painful and numb. It moves along my right arm. I feel numb all the way to the tips of my fingers. The lumbar pain goes to the outside and back of my left leg. Can you tell me what is wrong with me, doctor?

我一扭脖子,肩膀后面就感到发沉,发疼,发麻。而且这种感觉还往我的右胳膊窜,我甚至觉得一直都麻到指头尖了。腰部的疼痛是往我左腿外侧和后面窜。医生我这是得了什么病呀?

Doctor： According to your symptoms and X-ray report, you are suffering from spur of cervical vertebrae (lumbar spine, knee joint).

根据你的症状描述和 X 光片的报告显示,你的颈椎(腰椎、膝关节)长有骨刺了。

Patient：Is there any danger? What can I do to relieve the pain?

有危险吗？怎么样才能减轻这样的疼痛呢？

Doctor：Generally speaking, spur is degeneration of the skeletal system. It's a chronic disease associated with aging. There is no danger at all. You'd better avoid too much exercises. Physiotherapy might relieve your symptoms.

一般来说，骨刺是骨骼的退行性改变，它是一种跟年龄增长有关的慢性病，虽然没什么危险性，不过最好还是避免过量的活动。理疗可能会缓解你的症状。

Patient：What kind of treatment are you going to give me?

你准备怎么给我治疗呢？

Doctor：I would like to give you two kinds of treatments. One is an acetic acid ion transfer. It may reduce your pain and numbness. Another treatment is a traction of your neck. It may widen the narrowing of the vertebrae and reduce the irritation on the nerves, muscles and other tissues to alleviate the pain.

我准备给你做两种形式的治疗。一种是醋酸离子导入疗法，它主要是减轻你的疼痛和麻木。另一种是颈部牵引，它可以把椎间隙拉宽，从而缓解椎骨因神经、肌肉以及其他组织的刺激所引起的疼痛。

Patient：Does it hurt?

疼吗？

Doctor：No, only a slight prickling sensation. There may be some itchy skin after treatment. You can apply alcohol or glycerin to it, but try not to scratch it. Remember，there mustn't be any skin trauma, or the treatment can't continue.

不疼，只有轻微的针刺感。治疗后局部皮肤可能会有些痒，你可以在上面涂些酒精或甘油，但尽量不要抓挠它。记着皮肤不能有创伤，否则就不能继续进行治疗了。

Patient：Why?

为什么呢？

Doctor：Even a very small lesion will cause a severe pain. The current will be concentrated on the lesion.

因为哪怕很小的一点创伤，治疗时电流就会集中在伤口上，这样反而会引起更剧烈的疼痛。

Patient：I see，by the way，how many times should I come?

我明白了，那我需要来多少次呢?

Doctor：This treatment will last for ten to fifteen sessions. You can repeat it in two weeks if it is effective.

这种治疗要持续做十到十五次。如果有效的话，两周后再重复做一个疗程。

Ⅱ. Sentences 替换句型

(1) Does traction cause any discomfort，doctor?

医生，做牵引有什么不舒服吗?

(2) Don't worry. The weight we use is ten to twenty pounds each time for twenty minutes. We start at twelve pounds. We can do it ten to fifteen times or more. If you feel no palpitation，dizziness or fatigue，we can increase the weight gradually. If you don't feel well，we can reduce it.

你不要有什么顾虑。治疗时用的重量仅仅只有 10 至 20 磅，每次做 20 分钟。我们先从 12 磅开始，这样做 10 至 15 次或更多次。假如你没有心跳、头晕或疲劳的感觉，还可以逐渐增加重量。如果你感觉不舒服，我们也可以减少重量。

(3) How long has your finger been swollen and red?

你的手指红肿多久了?

(4) It has been hurting for about one week already，and has been red and swollen for two days. I did not bump (sprain，bruise) it.

已经疼了将近一个星期，红肿已两天了。我并没有碰伤（扭伤、挫伤）它。

(5) It seems that the inflammation is localized and that there is some pus. Please register and see the surgeon.

你的这个局部的炎症看来已经很厉害了，而且里面已经有脓了。请你挂号看看外科吧。

(6) Is the pain getting less severe?

疼痛减轻些了吗?

(7) Much less. (There is no change at all. It remains swollen and

painful.）

轻得多了。（完全没有什么变化,还是又肿又疼。）

（8）I would like to give you the treatment four to six times. You can come everyday or every other day. What time do you prefer? How about half past eight in the morning?

我给你做4至6次治疗。你每天来或隔天来都行。你愿意在什么时间来? 你看,对你来说早晨八点半来合适吗?

（9）I can't come in the morning. May I come in the afternoon?

我上午来不了。你看我下午来行吗?

（10）You may. Our clinic starts at half past two. We have no clinic on Wednesday and Saturday so please don't come on those days.

可以的。我们的门诊治疗下午两点半开始。周三和周六没有门诊,所以请你来治疗时错开这两天。

（11）How long have you been coughing? Do you bring up any sputum? Are you running a temperature? Is your nose blocked? Is there any abnormal discharge?

你咳嗽多久了? 有痰吗? 你发烧吗? 你的鼻子堵吗? 有没有异常分泌物?

（12）The discharge from my nose（ear）is yellowish and contains some pus.

从我鼻子里（耳朵里）流出来的东西都是黄的,而且里面还有脓。

（13）Please raise（extend）your arm. And put your arm behind your back.

请抬起（伸出）你的胳膊。把你的胳膊向背后伸。

（14）It is not necessary to take off all your clothing. Only expose the part where you feel pain.

不需要脱衣服了,只露出疼痛的部位就行了。

（15）After the treatment please raise your limbs for a while to improve your circulation.

做完治疗后请把胳膊腿抬起一会儿,这样可以更好地改进血液循环。

（16）We'll use an electric current for treatment. There will be a slight pricking sensation. Please let me know if you feel any pain. I'll reduce the current.

现在要用一种电流给你做治疗,可能会有一点轻微的针刺感。你要是感觉疼痛就告诉我,我可以降低一点电流量。

(17) I'll treat you with ultraviolet rays. It may diminish the inflammation and reduce the pain. Because the light is so strong that I have to cover up your eyes to protect them. The treatment only lasts a few seconds. After that your skin may become red and tanned a little bit as if you had been sunbathing. It will fade away in a few days.

现在给你用紫外线做几秒钟的治疗,它可以消炎止疼。不过这光线有点强,为了保护眼睛,需要把眼睛盖上。治疗后皮肤可能变得就像晒过太阳似的,不用担心,几天后就会褪去的。

(18) I'll treat you with visible light and a kind of electric current. Visible light gives you a warm sensation. The electric current has three types of waves that produce different feelings. The first wave gives you a feeling of numbness. The second wave gives you a feeling of being lightly hammered. The third wave renders the part numbness from time to time.

我要用太阳灯结合一种电流给你做治疗。太阳灯会让你有一种温热的感觉。电流会产生三种不同的波形让你有不同的感觉。第一种是麻的感觉,第二种有如小锤敲打的感觉,第三种是一阵阵麻的感觉。

(19) I'll treat you with ultrashort wave (diathermy). It might improve the blood and lymph circulation so as to reduce the pain. You'll feel nothing during the treatment. Please don't apply any hot compress locally. During your monthly period the treatment should be stopped.

我用超短波(透热疗法)给你治疗。它可以促进血液和淋巴循环,从而达到减轻疼痛的目的。治疗时没有什么特别的感觉。治疗后不需要在局部再做热敷了。月经期间不适合做这种治疗。

(20) We'll treat you with ultrasonic waves. It is helpful in absorbing scar formation and hard lumps. You will feel vibrations and warmth.

我要用超声波给你治疗。它有助于吸收瘢痕和硬结。治疗中稍有震颤和温热的感觉。

(21) We'll use whirlpool bath for your treatment. Put your arm (leg) into the water. The bubbles in the water are a form of massage.

The warm water will improve your circulation.

我要用漩水浴给你治疗。请将你的胳膊(腿)放入水里,汩汩冒起的水泡可以起到按摩的作用,温热的水还可以促进你的血液循环。

（22）We'll give you laser treatment. Don't worry. You won't feel anything during the treatment. Please don't look at it directly. Put on these dark glasses.

我用激光给你治疗。请不要怕。治疗中你不会有什么特别的感觉。注意眼睛不要直接看着它。请你戴上墨镜。

（23）We'd better use interference current therapy in your case. You'll feel numbness, trembling and chafing. Please tell me if you think it is too strong. I'll adjust the amount of current.

你的情况最好用干扰电流治疗。治疗中你会有麻、震和按摩的感觉。假如你感觉电流太强,请告诉我,我会给你调节一下电流量的。

（24）I'll use a kind of electric current therapy in your case. It can help stop itching, act as a pain-killer, and improve the circulation and metabolism. Take off everything made of metal that you are wearing. There is only a pricking sensation. After the treatment you will feel quite comfortable.

我用的这种电流治疗有止痒、镇痛、促进血液循环及营养代谢的作用。请你把身上戴的所有金属制品摘下来。不要怕,只有一种针刺感,治疗后你会感到很舒服的。

（25）I'll treat you with paraffin therapy. Please don't move during the treatment. Don't hesitate to tell me if you feel too hot.

我用石蜡给你做治疗。治疗时不要动,若感到太热就马上告诉我。

（26）This is your card for physiotherapy. Please take this to the cashier where you pay. Whenever you come please show us this card.

这是你的理疗卡片。请拿着它到收费处交费。每次来治疗时记得要出示你的卡片。

Ⅲ. Words and Expressions 单词和短语

1. The Lung Channel of Hand-Taiyin and its Acupuncture Points 手太阴肺经及其相关经穴

chize 尺泽

jingqu 经渠

kongzui 孔最

lieque 列缺

shaoshang 少商

taiyuan 太渊

tianfu 天府

xiabai 侠白

yuji 鱼际

yunmen 云门

zhongfu 中府

2. The Large Intestine Channel of Hand-Yangming and its Acupuncture Points 手阳明大肠经及其相关经穴

binao 臂臑

erjian 二间

futu 扶突

hegu 合谷

heliao 禾髎

jianyu 肩髃

jugu 巨骨

pianli 偏历

quchi 曲池

sanjian 三间

shanglian 上廉

shangyang 商阳

shousanli 手三里

shouwuli 手五里

tianding 天鼎

wenliu 温溜

xialian 下廉

yangxi 阳溪

yingxiang 迎香

zhouliao 肘髎

3. The Stomach Channel of Foot-Yangming and its Acupuncture Points 足阳明胃经及其相关经穴

biguan 髀关

burong 不容

chengman 承满

chengqi 承泣

chongyang 冲阳

daju 大巨

daying 大迎

dicang 地仓

dubi 犊鼻

fenglong 丰隆

futu 伏兔

guanmen 关门

guilai 归来

huaroumen 滑肉门

jiache 颊车

jiexi 解溪

juliao 巨髎

kufang 库房

liangmen 梁门

liangqiu 梁丘

lidui 厉兑

qichong 气冲

qihu 气户

qishe 气舍

quepen 缺盆

renying 人迎

rugen 乳根

ruzhong 乳中

shangjuxu 上巨虚

shuidao 水道

shuitu 水突

sibai 四白

taiyi 太乙

tianshu 天枢

tiaokou 条口

touwei 头维

wailing 外陵

wuyi 屋翳

xiaguan 下关

xiajuxu 下巨虚

xiangu 陷谷

yingchuang 膺窗

yinshi 阴市

zusanli 足三里

4. The Spleen Channel of Foot-Taiyin and its Acupuncture Points 足太阴脾经及其相关经穴

chongmen 冲门

dabao 大包

dadu 大都

daheng 大横

diji 地机

fuai 腹哀

fujie 腹结

fushe 府舍

gongsun 公孙

jimen 箕门

lougu 漏谷

sanyinjiao 三阴交

shangqiu 商丘

shidou 食窦

taibai 太白

tianxi 天溪

xiongxiang 胸乡

xuehai 血海

yinbai 隐白

yinlingquan 阴陵泉

zhourong 周荣

5. The Heart Channel of Hand-Shaoyin and its Acupuncture Points 手少阴心经及其相关经穴

jiquan 极泉

lingdao 灵道

qingling 青灵

shaochong 少冲

shaofu 少府

shaohai 少海

shenmen 神门

tongli 通里

yinxi 阴郄

6. The Small Intestine Channel of Hand-Taiyang and its Acupuncture Points 手太阳小肠经及其相关经穴

bingfeng 秉风

houxi 后溪

jianwaishu 肩外俞

jianzhen 肩贞

jianzhongshu 肩中俞

naoshu 臑俞

qiangu 前谷

quyuan 曲垣

shaoze 少泽

tianchuang 天窗

tianrong 天容

tianzong 天宗

tinggong 听宫

wangu 腕骨

xiaohai 小海

yanggu 阳谷

yanglao 养老

zhizheng 支正

7. The Urinary Bladder Channel of Foot-Taiyang and its Acupuncture Points 足太阳膀胱经及其相关经穴

baihuanshu 白环俞

baomang 胞肓

chengfu 承扶

chengguang 承光

chengjin 承筋

chengshan 承山

ciliao 次髎

cuanzhu 攒竹

dachangshu 大肠俞

danshu 胆俞

dashu 大杼

dushu 督俞

feishu 肺俞

feiyang 飞扬

fengmen 风门

fufen 附分

fuxi 浮郄

fuyang 跗阳

ganshu 肝俞

gaohuangshu 膏肓俞

geguan 膈关

geshu 膈俞

guanyuanshu 关元俞

heyang 合阳

huangmen 肓门

huiyang 会阳

hunmen 魂门

jinggu 京骨

jinmen 金门

jueyinshu 厥阴俞

kunlun 昆仑

luoque 络却

meichong 眉冲

pangguangshu 膀胱俞

pishu 脾俞

pohu 魄户

pucan 仆参

qihaishu 气海俞

qingming 晴明

qucha 曲差

sanjiaoshu 三脚俞

shangliao 上髎

shenmai 申脉

shenshu 肾俞

shentang 神堂

shugu 束骨

tianzhu 天柱

tongtian 通天

weicang 胃仓

weishu 胃俞

weiyang 委阳

weizhong 委中

wuchu 五处

xialiao 下髎

xiaochangshu 小肠俞

xinshu 心俞

yanggang 阳纲

yinmen 殷门

yishe 意舍

yixi 譩嘻

yuzhen 玉枕

zhibian 秩边

zhishi 志室

zhiyin 至阴

zhongliao 中髎

zhonglvshu 中膂俞

zutonggu 足通骨

8. The Kidney Channel of Foot-Shaoyin and its Acupuncture Points 足少阴肾经及其相关经穴

bulang 步廊

dahe 大赫

dazhong 大钟

fuliu 复溜

futonggu 腹通谷

henggu 横骨

huangshu 肓俞

jiaoxin 交信

lingxu 灵墟

qixue 气穴

rangu 然谷

shangqu 商曲

shencang 神藏

shenfeng 神封

shiguan 石关

shufu 俞府

shuiquan 水泉

siman 四满

taixi 太溪

yindu 阴都

yingu 阴谷

yongquan 涌泉

youmen 幽门

yuzhong 彧中

zhaohai 照海

zhongzhu 中注

zhubin 筑宾

9. The Pericardium Channel of Hand-Jueyin and its Acupuncture Points 手厥阴心包经及其相关经穴

daling 大陵

jianshi 间使

laogong 劳宫

neiguan 内关

quze 曲泽

tianchi 天池

tianquan 天泉

ximen 郄门

zhongchong 中冲

10. The Sanjiao Channel of Hand-Shaoyang and its Acupuncture Points 手少阳三焦经及其相关经穴

ermen 耳门

guanchong 关冲

heliao 和髎

huizong 会宗

jianliao 肩髎

jiaosun 角孙

luxi 颅息

naohui 臑会

qimai 契脉

qinglengyuan 清冷渊

sanyangluo 三阳络

sidu 四渎

sizhukong 丝竹空

tianjing 天井

tianliao 天髎

tianyou 天牖

waiguan 外关

xiaoluo 消泺

yangchi 阳池

yemen 液门

yifeng 翳风

zhigou 支沟

zhongzhu 中渚

11. The Gall Bladder Channel of Foot-Shaoyang and its Acupuncture Points 足少阳胆经及其相关经穴

benshen 本神

chengling 承灵

daimai 带脉

diwuhui 地五会

fengchi 风池

fengshi 风市

fubai 浮白

guangming 光明

hanyan 颔厌

huantiao 环跳

jianjing 肩井

jingmen 京门

juliao 居髎

muchuang 目窗

naokong 脑空

qiuxu 丘墟

qubin 曲鬓

riyue 日月

shangguan 上关

shuaigu 率谷

tianchong 天冲

tinghui 听会

tongziliao 瞳子髎

toulinqi 头临泣

touqiaoyin 头窍阴

waiqiu 外丘

wangu 完骨

weidao 维道

wushu 五枢

xiaxi 侠溪

xiyangguan 膝阳关

xuanli 悬厘

xuanlu 悬颅

xuanzhong 悬钟

yangbai 阳白

yangfu 阳辅

yangjiao 阳交

yanglingquan 阳陵泉

yuanye 渊腋

zhejin 辄筋

zhengying 正营

zhongdu 中渎

zulinqi 足临泣

zuqiaoyin 足窍阴

12. The Liver Channel of Foot-Jueyin and its Acupuncture Points 足厥阴肝经及其相关经穴

dadun 大敦

jimai 急脉

ligou 蠡沟

qimen 期门

ququan 曲泉

taichong 太冲

xiguan 膝关

xingjian 行间

yinbao 阴包

yinlian 阴廉

zhangmen 章门

zhongdu 中都

zhongfeng 中封

zuwuli 足五里

13. The Front Midline Channel and its Acupuncture Points 任脉及其相关经穴

chengjiang 承浆

danzhong 膻中

guanyuan 关元

huagai 华盖

huiyin 会阴

jianli 建里

jiuwei 鸠尾

juque 巨阙

lianquan 廉泉

qihai 气海

qugu 曲骨

shangwan 上脘

shenque 神阙

shimen 石门

shuifen 水分

tiantu 天突

xiawan 下脘

xuanji 璇玑

yinjiao 阴交

yutang 玉堂

zhongji 中极

zhongting 中庭

zhongwan 中脘

zigong 紫宫

14. The Back Midline Channel and its Acupuncture Points 督脉及其相关经穴

anmian 安眠

bafeng 八风

baichongwo 百虫窝

baihui 百会

bailao 百劳

baxie 八邪

cephalo-cerical points 头颈部

changqiang 长强

chonggu 崇骨

dagukong 大骨空

dannangxue 胆囊穴

dazhui 大椎

dingchuan 定喘

duiduan 兑端

duoming 夺命

duyin 独阴

erbai 二白

erjian 耳尖

fengfu 风府

heding 鹤顶

houding 后顶

hukou 虎口

jiachengjiang 夹承浆

jiaji 夹肌

jiali 颊里

jianqian 肩前

jieji 接脊

jingbi 颈臂

jingling 精灵

jinjin 金津

jinsuo 筋缩

jizhong 脊中

juquan 聚泉

juqueshu 巨阙俞

lanweixue 阑尾穴

lineiting 里内庭

linghou 陵后

lingtai 灵台

liniaoxue 利尿穴

mingmen 命门

naohu 脑户

neiyingxiang 内迎香

nüxi 女膝

pigen 痞根

points of limbs 四肢部

qianding 前顶

qiangjian 强间

qianzheng 牵正

qiduan 气端

qimen 气门

qiuhou 球后

qizhongsibian 脐中四边

quanjian 拳尖

sanjiaojiu 三角灸

shanglianquan 上廉泉

shangxing 上星

shangyingxiang 上迎香

shencong 神聪

shendao 神道

shenting 神庭

shenzhu 身柱

shiqizhuixue 十七椎穴

shixuan 十宣

shounizhu 手逆注

shuigou 水沟

sifengxue 四缝穴

suliao 素髎

taiyang 太阳

taodao 陶道

tituo 提托

truncal Points 躯干部

wailaogong 外劳宫

weiguanxiashu 胃管下俞

weiling 威灵

weishang 胃上

wuhu 五虎

xiajishu 下极俞

xiaogukong 小骨空

xinhui 囟会

xinshe 新设

xiyan 膝眼

xuanshu 悬枢

xueyadian 血压点

yamen 哑门

yaoqi 腰奇

yaoshu 腰俞

yaoyangguan 腰阳关

yaoyan 腰眼

yiming 翳明

yinjiao 龈交

yintang 印堂

yuyao 鱼腰

yuye 玉液

zhiyang 至阳

zhongkui 中魁

zhongquan 中泉

zhongshu 中枢

zhoujian 肘尖

zhouzhui 肘椎

zigongxue 子宫穴

Section 18　The Chinese Medical Formulary

第 18 节　中医方药

Ⅰ. Key Concepts 核心概念

（1）Prescription：A composition of different quantities of several Chinese medicinal herbs, as therapeutically indicated in traditional Chinese medicine, in certain dosages and forms of preparation, so as to be definitely effective and fit for a comprehensive therapy.

方即方剂,它是把不同剂量的中药按中医医理法则组合而成一定的剂量、剂型,以便能使药物更好地适应病人的病情。

（2）Principles, associates, adjuvents, and messengers：They are the four regular components and basic rules of a prescription. The principles are the drugs with the therapeutic effects, also called primary drugs; the associates, those to assist or to enhance the effects of the principles, also called subsidiary drugs; the adjuvents, those to assist the principles to treat the complications or to suppress their toxicity and reduce their drastic activities; and the messengers, those to lead the effects of the above drugs to the diseased regions and to harmonize their effects.

君臣佐使(主辅佐使)是指方剂组成的四个部分,同时也是组成方剂的原则。君是在一个药方中起主要治疗作用的药物,又称主药;臣则是辅助君药起治疗作用或加强君药疗效的药物,又称辅药;佐也是协助君药治疗兼症或抑制药物毒性及缓和君药烈性的药物;使是指引导其他药物到达疾病所在部位和起调和其他药物性能的药物。

（3）Composing a prescription：To combine different drugs according to the needs of the disease and the therapeutic principle of traditional Chinese medicine.

方剂配伍是指根据病情需要,按照中医理法原则来组合药物的方法。

（4）Seven prescriptions：An ancient Chinese classification of prescriptions. There are seven classes：Grandiose prescriptions, minor prescriptions, mild prescriptions, urgent prescriptions, odd-numbered prescriptions, even-numbered prescriptions and composite prescriptions.

七方是中国古代对方剂的一种分类方法,共计七类,即大方、小方、缓方、急方、奇方、偶方、复方。

(5) Grandiose prescriptions: Those with drugs drastic in action, great in variety, and large in dosage.

大方是指药力猛、药味多、药量重的方剂。

(6) Minor prescriptions: Those with drugs not drastic in action, a few in variety, and small in dosage.

小方是指药物性能不峻烈、药味少、药量轻的方剂。

(7) Mild prescriptions: Those composed of drugs moderate in action.

缓方是指药物作用缓和的方剂。

(8) Urgent prescriptions: Those with drugs of rapid effect.

急方是指药物作用迅速的方剂。

(9) Odd-numbered prescriptions: Those composed of an odd number of drugs.

奇方是指药味和于奇数的方剂。

(10) Even-numbered prescriptions: Those composed of an even number of drugs.

偶方是指药味和于偶数的方剂。

(11) Composite prescriptions: Those formed by combination of more than one prescription.

复方是指两个以上合起来使用的方剂。

(12) Additional prescriptions: An odd-numbered prescription is first tried and if not effective, then, an even-numbered prescription is employed.

重方是指先用奇方治病未愈,再用偶方治疗的方剂。

(13) Light prescriptions: Using either the odd-numbered or the even-numbered prescription only.

轻方是单用奇方或偶方治病的方剂。

(14) Complex prescriptions: It is composed of drugs of differrent effects, and mainly used in complicated diseases.

兼方是将性能不同的药物,组合于一方之中。此方多用于病情较复杂的病征。

（15）Simple prescriptions：It is composed of a few drugs，easy to prepare and convenient to use.

单方是指药味简单，取之容易而又便用的方剂。

（16）Classical prescriptions：Generally speaking，the prescriptions are those as recorded in *Shanghan Zabing Lun* (*On Fevers and Other Diseases*). Secondly，it can also refer to empirical formulas.

经方一般是指《伤寒杂病论》中所记载的方剂。此外，它还可以特别指"经验方"。

（17）Current prescriptions：On one hand，the prescriptions are those introduced after the Tang and Song Dynasties. And on the other hand，they are all the prescriptions except those as recorded in *Shanghan Zabing Lun* (*On Fevers and Other Diseases*).

时方是指唐、宋以后出现的方剂。另外，它还指除《伤寒杂病论》所载方剂之外的方剂。

（18）Arcanum (arcane prescriptions)：The secret prescriptions.

禁方即秘方。

（19）The ten prescriptions：Prescriptions were classified by ancient practitioners according to the effects into ten kinds，namely，dispersing prescriptions，mobilizing prescriptions，tonics，purgatives，light prescriptions，heavy prescriptions，lubricants，astringents，desiccants and moistants.

十剂是指古代医家按照方剂的功效而分的十类药剂，即宣剂、通剂、补剂、泄剂、轻剂、重剂、滑剂、涩剂、燥剂、湿剂。

（20）The twelve prescriptions：The ten prescriptions plus cold and hot prescriptions or plus elevating and depressant prescriptions.

十二剂是十剂增加了寒剂和热剂，或是十剂增加了升剂和降剂的方剂的总称。

（21）Dispersing prescriptions：Those with the effects of dispersing stasis，reducing phlegm，and promoting emesis.

宣剂是指有宣散、化痰、催吐等作用的一类方剂。

（22）Mobilizing prescriptions：Those with the effects of relieving stasis and obstruction.

通剂是指有通利作用的一类方剂。

（23）Tonic prescriptions：Those with the effects of reinforcing the weakened body and building strong constitution.

补剂是指有补虚强壮作用的一类方剂。

（24）Purgative prescriptions：Those with purgative effect.

泄剂是指有泄下等作用的一类方剂。

（25）Light prescriptions：Those with the effects of diaphoresis and removing exterior syndromes.

轻剂是指有发汗、解除表证等作用的一类方剂。

（26）Heavy prescriptions：Those composed of the drugs heavy in weight and having the effects of checking the yang, sedation, and tranquilizing.

重剂是指药物质地厚重，而且有镇静、潜阳、安神等作用的一类方剂。

（27）Lubricating prescriptions：Those with diuretic drugs having the effects of discharging the calculus and relieving urethral discharges.

滑剂是指药物性质滑利，有利石通淋等作用的一类方剂。

（28）Astringent prescriptions：Those with astringent effect and often for hyperhidrosis, spermatorrhea, chronic diarrhea, etc.

涩剂是指有收敛作用的一类方剂。中医常用这类方剂来治疗多汗、遗精、久泻等病征。

（29）Desiccating prescriptions：Those with the effect of removing pathogenic dampness, often for such symptom complexes as edema, tanyin（phlegm and excessive fluid）.

燥剂是指有去湿作用的一类方剂。中医常用这类方剂治疗水肿、痰饮等病征。

（30）Moistening prescriptions：Those with the effects of producing the liquid essence, enriching the blood, moistening the tissues, etc.

湿剂是指有生津、养血、滋润等作用的一类方剂。

（31）Cold prescriptions：Those with drugs of cold nature and for the heat symptom complex.

寒剂是指性质寒凉，能治疗热证的一类方剂。

（32）Heat prescriptions：Those with drugs of damp and hot nature and for the cold symptom complex.

热剂是指性质湿热,能治疗寒证的一类方剂。

（33）Elevating prescriptions：Those with the elevating effect and for prolapse of the rectum and the uterus, etc.

升剂是指有升提作用,能治疗脱肛、子宫脱垂等病征的一类方剂。

（34）Depressant prescriptions：Those with the effect of counteracting the abnormal rise of the vital principles, and for such symptom complexes as cough, vomiting, etc.

降剂是指有降逆作用,能治疗咳嗽、呕吐等病征的一类方剂。

（35）Single effect：One of the "seven features" of drugs, i. e., treating diseases by means of the effects of a single drug.

单行是药物的"七情"之一。它是指单用一味药就可以发挥效能来治疗疾病。

（36）Potentiation：One of the "seven features" of drugs. It refers to the combined use of two drugs, similar in property, which can potentiate each other.

相须也是药物的"七情"之一。它是指两种性能相类的药物同用,互相增强作用的配伍方法。

（37）Enhancement：One of the "seven features" of drugs. It refers to the combined use of more than two drugs, of which one is the main drug and the other are the adjuvents to enhance its effects.

相使也是药物的"七情"之一。它是指两种以上的药物同用,一药为主,余药为辅用以提高主药疗效的配伍方法。

（38）Counteraction：One of the "seven features" of drugs. One drug counteracts the effects of another.

相畏也是药物的"七情"之一,是指药物的相互抑制作用。

（39）Antagonism：One of the"seven features" of drugs, the antagonistic actions among drugs.

相恶是药物的"七情"之一,是指一种药物能减轻另一种药物的性能。

（40）Suppression：One of the "seven features" of drugs. One drug can suppress the toxic reactions of the other.

相杀是药物的"七情"之一,是指一种药物能减弱另一种药物的中毒反应。

（41）Incompatibility：One of the "seven features" of drugs. Two drugs, when used in combination, will give rise to severe adverse side reactions.

相反是药物的"七情"之一,是指两种药物同用后会发生强烈的副作用。

(42) Eighteen incompatibilities: Ancient practitioners held that eighteen kinds (actually nineteen kinds) of drugs would be incompatible with some other; and, if used together, strong side effects would be aroused. *Glycyrrhiza uralensis* counteracts *Euphorbia kansui*, *Euphorbia pekinensis*, *Daphne genkwa*, seaweed. *Aconitum carmichaelii* counteracts *Fritillaria*, *Trichosanthes kirilowii*, *Pinellia ternata*, *Ampelopsis japonica*, *Bletilla striata*. *Veratrum nigrum* counteracts *Panax ginseng*, *Adenophora stricta*, *Salvia mitiorrhiza*, *Sophora flavescens*, *Asarum*, *Radix paeoniae alba*.

十八反是指古代医家认为的十八种(实际为十九种)药物,它们性能相反,两药同用会产生剧烈的副作用。即甘草反甘遂、大戟、芫花、海藻,乌头反贝母、栝楼、半夏、白蔹、白及,藜芦反人参、沙参、丹参、苦参、细辛、白芍。

(43) Nineteen antagnonisms: Ancient practitioners held that nineteen kinds of drugs had mutually antagonistic properties, and if the two of them were used simultaneously, they would antagonize each other, or even completely destroy their effects. Sulphur antagonizes mirabilite, mercury antagonizes *Arsenicum sublimatum*, *Radix euphorbia* antagonizes *Lithargyrum*, *Croton tiglium* antagonizes *Semen pharbitidis*, *Flos caryophylli* antagonizes *Curcuma aromatica*, *Dental nitrate* antagonizes *Rhizoma sparganii*, *Aconitum carmichaelii* and *Aconitum kusnezoffii* antagonize cornu rhinoceri asiatici, *Panax ginseng* antagonizes *Faeces trogopterori*, *Cinnamomum cassia* antagonizes *Bolus rubra*.

十九畏是古代医家认为有十九种药物性能"相畏",如两种同用会发生强烈的抑制作用,甚至会使药物完全丧失功效。即硫黄畏朴硝,水银畏砒霜,狼毒畏密陀僧,巴豆畏牵牛子,丁香畏郁金,牙硝畏三棱,川乌、草乌畏犀角,人参畏五灵脂,肉桂畏赤石脂。

（44）Drugs contraindicated during pregnancy：Drugs that can induce abortion or harm the mother or fetus are contraindicated during pregnancy.

妊娠药忌是指妇女在怀孕期间，可能会引起流产或损害母子的药物。一般为妊娠忌用药。

（45）Guiding drugs：Those which are able to guide other drugs to the affected part. Actually, they exert special effects on the affected areas.

引经报使是指某些药物好像向导一样，有带引其他药物到达病变部位的功能，实质上是指这些药物对人体某些病变部位所起的特殊作用。

（46）Diaphoresis-contraindicated cases：Diaphoresis is contraindicated in such diseases as internal heat due to yin deficiency, external cold due to yang deficiency, hemorrhages, etc.

发汗禁例是指那些不适宜运用汗法治疗的病证，如阴虚内热证、阳虚外寒证、出血性疾病等。

（47）Emesis-contraindicated cases：Emesis is contraindicated in such diseases as cold due to gastrosplenic deficiency, the aged, the infirm, blood loss, etc.

涌吐禁例是指那些不适宜用吐法治疗的病证，如脾胃虚寒证、年老、虚弱及失血等。

（48）Purgation-contraindicated cases：Purgatives are contraindicated in such diseases as anemia and constipation in primipara, the half-exterior-half-interior syndrome, constipation and anemia in the aged.

泻下禁例是指那些不适宜泻下治疗的病症，如初产妇的贫血和便秘、半表半里证、老年血虚便秘证等。

（49）Processed drugs：Various forms of processed drugs, such as boiled solution, decoction, drink, extracts, pellets, pills, powders, tablets, etc.

剂（剂型）即药物通过加工后制成的各种不同的形式，如汤剂、煎剂、饮剂、膏剂、丹剂、丸剂、散剂、片剂等。

（50）Boiled solution：The medicinal solution obtained by boiling the drugs with an appropriate amount of water for a fixed period of time.

汤液是指将中药放入罐内,加适量水,煎沸一定时间后所得的药液。

(51) Decoction：Firstly, it's the term of decocting the drugs in an appropriate amount of water. Secondly, it's also the name of boiled solution.

煎一是指将中药加适量水煎煮的方法,二则是中药汤液的别称。

(52) Drink：The decoction that must be taken cold.

饮是指需要冷服的药液。

(53) Medicinal wine：The liquid prepared by soaking the drugs in wine for a fixed period of time and, then, filtering out the residue.

酒剂是指药浸入酒内,经过一定时间的浸泡,滤去渣后所制备的液体,又称药酒。

(54) Pill：Prepared by grinding drugs into powder, mixing it with honey, water or other drug juices, and making round masses of various sizes.

丸剂是根据中药配方将若干药物研成粉末,再用蜜或水或其他药汁等拌和制成圆球形大小不等的药丸。

(55) Pulvis：It's divided into two types. Pulvis for internal administration-drugs are first ground into coarse granules and then, boiled with water or drugs ground into fine powder taken orally with water, rice soup or wine. Besides, pulvis for topical application-drugs are ground into fine powder, dusted topically to the surface of the wound, or applied locally to the affected part after being mixed with wine, vinegar, or honey.

散分为两种。内服散剂是指将药物研成粗末,加水煮服;或将药物研成细粉末,用水、米汤或酒冲服。外用散剂是指将药物研成细粉末,用来撒在体表部位的伤口或溃疡处;或用酒、醋、蜜等调敷患处。

(56) Draft（boiled preparation）：The drugs are ground into coarse granules, boiled with water for a fixed period of time and, then, only the liquid is administered orally.

煮散是指药物研成粗末,加水煮沸一定时间后去渣服药液的方药。

(57) Paste：It's divided into two types. Paste for oral administration is prepared by decocting the drug in water, discarding the residue,

adding honey or granulated sugar, and, then, concentrating it to a paste. It is mostly used to treat chronic diseases. Besides, paste for external application is prepared by adding bees wax to sesameseed oil, cotton-seed oil or peanut oil, melting it with heat and while hot, adding fine powder of the drugs to it and stirring it constantly. The desired paste is formed after cooling. It is commonly used for skin diseases or suppurative infections.

膏分两种。内服膏是将药加水煎熬去渣后,再加入蜂蜜、砂糖等,浓缩成糊状,多用以治疗慢性疾病。而外用膏是把蜂蜡加入芝麻油或棉子油或花生油中,加热熔化后趁热加入药粉,不断搅拌,待冷凝制备而成,一般用来治疗皮肤病或外科痈疽肿毒。

(58) Magic portions: It's divided into two types. Those for external use are the powder prepared by subliming or melting medicinal minerals containing mercury or sulphur by heat. It is mostly used for treating skin diseases and suppurative infections. Besides, those for oral administration are prepared with more efficacious, and costly pulvis, pill or troche that need special technique.

丹分为两种。外用丹是将含有贡、硫等的矿物药经过熔化加热升华和提炼而成的粉末状制剂,多用来治疗皮肤病或外科痈疽肿毒。而内服丹是指用某些较特殊的制作方法制备而成的,功效较大,价格较昂贵的内服药粉、药丸或锭剂。

(59) Troche: A drug is ground into very fine powder and an appropriate amount of excipient is added. Solid cones or rectangular preparations are made.

锭是把药物研成细粉末,加一定的赋形剂后,制备而成的状如圆锥或长方形的固体制剂。

(60) Gelatin: Decocting drugs with animal skin, bone, shell or horn in water until the material is condensed to a dry mass. It is usually used as tonics, such as donkey-skin gelatin, tiger-bone gelatin, tortoise-plastron gelatin, deer-horn gelatin, etc.

胶是将药用动物皮、骨、甲、角等加水反复煎熬,浓缩后制成的干燥固体块状物质。多为补养药,如驴皮胶、虎骨胶、龟板胶、鹿角胶等。

(61) Medicinal tea: A medicinal preparation made by breaking the drug into coarse granules and compressing it into lump. After it is

infused or decocted with boiling water, the liquid is drunk as tea.

茶是指将药物轧成粗末,制成块状,用沸水泡或煎汁,代茶服用的一种制剂。

(62) Fermented drug：Prepared by mixing drug powder with flour, forming a lump and fermenting it.

曲是指将药粉与面粉混合,制成块状,使之发酵的制剂。

(63) Tablet：Made by processing the drug.

片是指药物经过加工后制成的药片。

(64) Infusion：Prepared by making an extract of the drug into a paste, adding amounts of sugar and flavoring agent and rendering it into fine granules. It is administered after infusing it with boiling water.

冲服剂是指将中药提炼成稠浸膏,加适量糖粉、调味剂等,再制成细颗粒样的制剂,服用时加开水冲服即可。

(65) Mixture：Prepared by decocting two or more drugs in water, and condensing it to a certain volume, or by making an extract of drugs, and dissolving it in water to form a solution.

合剂是指两种或两种以上的中药经水煎煮后浓缩成一定容量的液体,或是指中药的提取物以水为溶剂而配成的液体制剂。

(66) Pharmacopeia：Firstly, it refers to the special works with material medica in ancient times. Secondly, it's just a general term for herbal medicines.

本草一是指古时记载药物的专书,二则是指中药的统称。

(67) Folk medicinal herbs：A collective term for those medicinal plants which have neither been recorded in medical books nor widely used by physicians, and they are not available commercially, and usually not processed and prepared, but very popular with the masses.

草药是在一般医药书中没有记载,或有记载也很少为广大医生所使用,且未被列为商品药,一般也不用以加工炮制,但却在民间广泛流传的药用植物的统称。

(68) Chinese herbal medicines：A collective term for traditional Chinese drugs which have been recorded in medical books and available in pharmacies, and the folk medicinal herbs popular with the masses.

中草药是一般医药书上有记载、药店里有出售的中药,与民间流传的草药的合称。

(69) Four properties of drugs：They are cold，hot，warm，and cool. The drugs for heat diseases are of cold or cool nature, and those for cold diseases are of warm or hot nature.

四气是指药物的寒、热、温、凉四种性能。那些能够治疗热证的药物,就属于寒性或凉性;而那些能够治疗寒证的药物,则属于温性或热性。

(70) Five tastes of drugs：Pungent，sweet，sour，bitter，and salty.

五味即是指辛、甘、酸、苦、咸五种药味。

(71) Properties and tastes of drugs：A collective term for the four properties and the five tastes of drugs.

气味是药物四性(四气)和五味的合称。

(72) Ascending, descending, floating, and sinking：The tendencies of drug action. Ascending and floating refer to the inward and outward effects of drugs such as their yang-elevating, chill-dispersing, diaphorcetic and exterior-relieving actions, while descending and sinking, to the downward and inward effects, such as their depressing, reversing, astringent and purgative actions.

升降浮沉是指药物在人体机体内发挥作用的趋向。升、浮是指药物的效应有向上、向外的特点,如药物的升阳、散寒、发汗解表等作用;降、沉是指药物的效应有下行、向内的特点,如药物的降逆、收敛、泻下等作用。

(73) Effects：It collectively refers to "four properties, five tastes, ascending, descending, floating, and sinking actions of drugs and their clinical effectiveness.

性能是指药物的四气、五味和升降浮沉的属性及其所表现的临床效应。

(74) Channel-tropism：The theory to relate the action of drugs to the viscera, channels, and various parts of the body so as to explain their specific actions to the viscera, the channels or the particular part of the body.

归经是指把药物的作用与脏腑、经络和不同部位联系起来,用以说明某种药物对某些脏腑、经络或某部位所起的特殊治疗作用的理论。

(75) Color-and-taste-tropism：A part of channel-tropism theory. Basing on the theory of the five elements, the ancient physicians related the five colors (green, red, yellow, white and black) and the five tastes (sour, bitter, sweet, pungent, salty) of drugs to the five elements, viscera and channels, in order to explain the effect of drugs on different channels and different viscera. For example, the green and sour drugs identified with wood of the five elements, and related to the liver (gall bladder) channel; the yellow and sweet drugs identified with earth and related to the spleen (stomach) channel; the white and pungent drugs identified with metal and related to the lung (large intestine) channel; the black and salty drugs identified with water and related to the kidney (urinary bladder) channel.

五色五味所入是中药归经理论的内容之一。这是古代医家按五行学说把药物的五色(青、赤、黄、白、黑)和五味(酸、苦、甘、辛、咸)分别归属于五行和脏腑经络，从而对药物的效应加以解释的一种理论。如色青、味酸的药，在五行属木，入肝(胆)经；色黄、味甘的药，在五行属土，入脾(胃)经；色白、味辛的药，在五行属金，入肺(大肠)经；色黑、味咸的药，在五行属水，入肾(膀胱)经。

(76) Properties and tastes as yin and yang：The four properties, the five tastes, and ascending, descending, floating, and sinking actions of drugs may be categorized according to yin and yang. Of the four properties, the drugs of hot or warm nature belong to the yang, the drugs of cold or cool nature to the yin. Of the five tastes, the pungent and the sweet belong to the yang; the sour, the bitter and the salty to the yin. The ascending and the floating effects belong to the yang, the descending and the sinking effects to the yin.

气味阴阳是指药性四气、五味和升降浮沉的阴阳属性。如四气中，具有热、温性质的药物属阳，寒、凉性质的药物属阴。五味中具有辛、甘味的药物属阳，酸、苦、咸属阴。具有升、浮性能的属阳，沉、降属阴。

(77) The pungent and the sweet with dissipating effects are yang：The pungent and sweet drugs having dissipating effects are yang in

nature.

辛甘发散为阳是指辛味、甘味药有发散功效者属阳。

（78）The sour and the bitter with emetic and purgative effects are yin：The sour and bitter drugs having emetic or purgative effects are yin in nature.

酸苦涌泻为阴是指酸味、苦味药有催吐、泻下作用者属阴。

（79）The salty with emetic and purgative effects are yin：The salty drugs having emetic or purgative effects are yin in nature.

咸味涌泻为阴是指咸味药能催吐、泄下者属阴。

（80）Light taste excreting, and diuretic drugs are yang：The drugs of light taste having dampness-excreting and diuretic effects are yang in nature.

淡味渗泄为阳是指淡味药有排泄水湿、通利小便功效者属阳。

（81）No ascent with the sour and the salty, no descent with the sweet and the pungent：The action of the sour and the salty drugs tend to be downward and inward rather than ascending, and the action of the sweet and the pungent drugs tend to be upward and outward rather than descending.

酸咸无升，甘辛无降是指酸、咸味的药性是向下、向内的，没有升的趋向；甘、辛味的药性是向上、向外的，没有降的趋向。

（82）No floating with the cold, no sinking with the hot：The drugs of cold nature tend to act inward and downward rather than floating, while those of hot nature tend to be outward and upward rather than sinking.

寒无浮，热无沉是指寒性药的作用是向里、向下的，其功效没有上浮的趋势；热性药的作用是向外、向上的，其功效没有下沉的趋势。

（83）Five trends：The trends of actions of the five tastes of drugs. A sour drug tends to act first on the liver (the tendons)；a bitter one, the heart (blood)；a sweet one, the spleen (the muscles)；a pungent one, the lung (the qi)；a salty one, the kidney (the bone).

五走是指五味的药性走向，如酸先走肝(筋)，苦先走心(血)，甘先走脾(肉)，辛先走肺(气)，咸先走肾(骨)。

（84）Five grains：Rice, peas, wheat, beans, and millet.

五谷一般指米、小豆、麦、大豆、黄黍(黄米)。

(85) Five appropriate diets: The diets indicated for the diseases of the five parenchymatous viscera. Ancient practitioners held that wheat, mutton, apricot, etc. are indicated for heart diseases; husked sorghum, beef, jujube, etc. for spleen diseases; dog meat, plum, fragrant-flowered garlic, etc. for liver diseases; soybean, pork, chestnut, etc. for kidney diseases; millet, chicken, peach, and onion, etc. for lung diseases.

五宜是指五脏病所适宜的食物。古代医家认为:心病宜食麦、羊肉、杏等,脾病宜食秫米饭、牛肉、枣等,肝病宜食犬肉、李、韭等,肾病宜食大豆、猪肉、栗子等,肺病宜食黄黍、鸡肉、桃、葱等。

(86) Dietary therapy: The use of foods to treat diseases or as tonics.

食治是指用食物治疗疾病或调补身体的方法。

(87) Three grades (upper, middle and lower grades): A method of grading drugs in ancient times. Drugs, which are nontoxic, can be used for a long time and taken in large doses without harmful effect, are graded as the upper grade. Those, which are nontoxic or toxic but can be taken carefully, and cure deficiencies, are graded as the middle grade. Those, which are toxic and can't be used for a long time, but can remove pathogenic cold and heat, are graded as the lower grade.

三品(上、中、下品)是指古代的一种药物分类法。那些被认为没有毒性,可以久服、多服而不会损害机体的药物,列为上品;那些被认为没有毒性,或有毒性须斟酌使用,又可以治病补虚的药,列为中品;而那些被认为有毒性而不能长期使用,却能退寒热、除邪气的药,列为下品。

(88) Attacking pathogenic factor with poision: To treat a disease with poisonous drugs. Here, "poison" refers to certain special effects of a drug or certain side reactions of a drug or certain toxic reactions of a drug.

毒药攻邪是指使用有毒的药物来治疗疾病。"毒"在这里的意思是指药物的某些功效特性,或药物的某些副作用,或药物的毒性反应。

(89) Drastic poison, moderate poison, slight poison, non-poisonous drug: The method of grading the toxicity and other features of the

drugs. Drastically toxic drugs are called drastic poison；drugs with less toxicity，moderate poison；those with still lesser toxicity，slight poison；those without toxicity，non-poisonous drugs.

大毒、常毒、小毒、无毒是指对药物的毒性和某些特性的分级归纳。药物毒性剧烈的，称大毒；毒性仅次于剧毒药的，称常毒；毒性次于常毒药的，称小毒；而那些没有毒性的药物则被称为无毒。

（90）Methods of decocting drugs：The appropriate method to decoct drugs includes quantity of water added，duration of decoction，prior decoction，post decoction，etc.

煎药法是指药物加水煎煮时所应采取的适宜方法。如煎煮时间的长短，加水量的多少，以及药物的先煎、后下等，则都属于煎药方法的范畴。

（91）Prior decoction：Some drugs must be decocted prior to the others for some time. For example，mineral drugs and shell drugs are added to the decoction earlier to ensure the full release of their effective components.

先煎是指煎药时，一些药应较另一些药先煎一段时间。如矿物药、介壳药，要先煎，才能使有效成分充分释出。

（92）Post decoction：Some drugs must be decocted later than the others for some time. For example，gambir plant nod，rhubarb root and rhizome，etc. are added to the decoction later to avoid destruction of their effective components.

后下是指煎药时一些药应较其他药迟一段时间投入煎煮。如钩藤、大黄等后下，其有效成分才不至于因长时间煎煮而被破坏。

（93）Melting：Drugs such as mirabilite，malt sugar，honey，donkey skin glue，are dissolved in the solution of decoction（after removal of the residue）with gentle heat.

熔化是指在煎好去渣的药物内，放进某些药（如芒硝、饴糖、蜂蜜、阿胶等）后，再加温熔化。

（94）Decoction in packets：Certain drugs should be wrapped in a piece of cloth before decoction.

包煎是指某些药物需要用布包裹后再进行煎煮。

（95）Taking medicine after infusion：It refers to taking powered medicine after mixing it with boiling water, and also to certain drugs, which are infused with boiling decoction for a while, and then administered.

冲服是指某些粉末药加开水冲服后服下。也可指某些药先放入碗内,将其他煎好的药液趁热冲入碗内片刻,再服用。

(96) Taking mixed medicine：Taking medicine after mixing it well with water or the solution of decoction.

调服是指某些粉末药加入水或药液调匀后服用。

(97) Dissoving in mouth：Certain drugs may be held in the mouth and then swallowed slowly after they are dissolved.

噙化是指把某些药物含在口内,待其溶化后缓缓吞下。

(98) Taking medicine with fluid：Taking pills, tablets, etc. with warm boiled water or medicinal liquids.

送服是指把丸剂、片剂等和温开水或药液一起吞下。

(99) Taking medicine between meals：Taking medicine long after a meal or before the next meal.

食远服是指在两次进食时间中间服药为宜。

(100) Taking medicine with empty stomach：Taking medicine before breakfast in the morning.

空腹服是指早晨未进食之前服药。

(101) Taking medicine before meals：Medicines, such as tonics, are usually recommended to be taken before meals.

饭前服(在进食之前服药)：一般而言,补益药要饭前服。

(102) Taking medicine after meals：Most of medicines should be administered after meals except tonics and anthelmintics.

饭后服(在进食之后服药)：除补益药、驱虫药外,多数药要饭后服。

(103) Taking medicine before an attack：Taking medicine before the attack of a certain disease to control its symptoms. For example, malaria must be treated by administering antimalarials at a certain time before the expected attack.

未发病前服是指在疾病症状未发现之前服药,用以控制症状的发生。如疟疾,必须在其发作之前适当的时候服药。

(104) Taking a dose all at once：Taking a large amount of the medicinal

fluid completely at one time.

顿服是指将药液多量一次服完。

（105）Taking medicine in multiple doses：Taking a medicinal fluid in several small doses.

频服是指将药液少量多次服下。

（106）Taking medicine warm：Taking the decocted medicine when it is warm.

温服是指将煎好的药液在不冷不热时服下。

（107）Taking medicine hot：Taking the decocted medicine when it is hot.

热服是指将煎好的药液趁热服下。

（108）Taking medicine cold：Taking the decocted medicine when it is cold.

冷服是指待煎好的药液冷却后服下。

（109）Prohibited foods：For therapeutic purposes，certain foods are prohibited when certain drugs are administered.

忌口是指在患病服药期间，由于治疗的需要，要求病人忌食某些食物。

（110）Processing the drugs：The various processing procedures that medicinal materials undergo before being made into various dosage forms，for example，washing the collected herbs to get rid of sand and mud，discarding the non-medicinal parts，cutting them into pieces，soaking them in water，drying them in the sun，steaming them，calcining them，frying them，etc.

炮制是指药材在制成各种剂型之前的不同加工处理过程，如把采集到的药材洗去泥沙、去除非药用部位、切片、浸泡、晒干、蒸、煅、炒等。

（111）Quick-frying and roasting：Firstly，it refers to two processes of preparing Chinese drugs，quick-frying and roasting；secondly，it generally refers to the processes of preparing Chinese drugs，which is the same as processing drugs.

炮炙一是指炮和炙两种不同的制药方法；二是指药材加工处理的总称，与炮制义同。

（112）Purifying and cutting：The process of removing non-medicinal parts, and slicing, grinding or smashing the material to make medicinal preparations.

治削是指先去除混在药材中的杂物和非药用部分,再将药材切片、碾碎、捣烂用以制备药物前的操作技术。

(113) Washing: Washing the crude drug so as to get rid of sand, mud, and dirt.

洗是指用水洗去药材表面的泥沙或其他不洁物。

(114) Bleaching: The process of soaking crude drugs with frequent changes of water to remove dirt and to minimize their toxicity and their bad odor.

漂是指某些药材用经常换水的方法浸泡,用以去除药物中的杂质和减轻药物的毒性、去除腥味的处理过程。

(115) Soaking: Soaking drugs in water. This makes it easier to peel certain drugs after soaking, or in other words, the texture of certain drugs becomes softer after soaking, making it easier for further processing.

泡(浸泡)是指用水浸泡药物。这样使得某些药物经过浸泡后便于去皮,或者说某些药物浸泡后质地变软而便于进一步加工处理。

(116) Refining drugs with water: To the drug-powder a considerable amount of water is added and stirring is carried out. Then the supernatant solution of the drug is decanted and the drug-powder is separated by sediment and dried.

水飞(飞)是指在碾成粉末的药粉中加入较多的水后,待充分搅拌后,再把含有药粉的水倒出使之沉淀、干燥。

(117) Calcining: Burning the crude drug red-hot direct in the fire or indirectly in a container to make it loose and brittle.

锻是指把药物放在火内直接烧红,或放入耐火容器中间接烧红,使药物质地松脆的一种药物加工方法。

(118) Quick-frying: Frying the drug in an iron pot with high temperature until it becomes dark-brown or cracked.

炮是指把药物放在高温铁锅内炒至四面焦黄或炸裂的一种药物加工方法。

(119) Roasting in ashes: The drugs are wrapped in moistened paper, paste or yellow mud and heated in hot cinder until the coating is

charred or cracked, so that the drugs inside the wrapping have achieved the high-temperature processing.

煨是指把药物用湿纸、面糊或黄泥包裹，放入热灰中，待湿纸、面糊焦黑，黄泥干枯为止，而使被包裹的药物达到高温处理的一种药物加工过程。

(120) Stir-frying: To process the crude drugs in a frying pan with constant stirring.

炒是指将药材放入锅内加热，并不断翻拌的药物加工过程。

(121) Dry-curing or baking: Drying crude drugs with slow fire, by putting them in an oven, which is dry-curing; or on a tile or in a pot without charring them, which is baking.

烘、焙是指用微火(细火)对药材进行加热并使之干燥的药物制备方法。"烘"是把药物放在烘房或烘柜内，使药物干燥而又不焦黑；"焙"是把药材放在静瓦片上或锅内焙燥，但又不使其烧焦。

(122) Frying with liquids: Mixing the drugs with some liquid and stir-frying. For example, drugs fried with wine are called wine-fried; with vinegar, vinegar-fried; with honey, honey-fried; and the like.

炙是指药材与液体辅料共炒，使辅料渗入药物的加工方法，也叫和炒。如药材与酒共炒叫酒炙，药材与米醋汁共炒叫醋炙，药材和蜂蜜共炒叫蜜炙，等等。

(123) Charring: Burning certain drugs in a slow charcoal fire until their outer part chars and inner part browns. This is a common method to partially char drugs.

烧存性是把某些药物放入木炭火中烧至外部焦黑、内部焦黄，以使药物部分炭化的加工方法。

(124) Removing fire toxin: The process of removing fire toxin in the medicinal plasters or drugs fried with liquids. It means newly prepared medicinal plasters or drugs fried with liquids are ready for use after having been placed in a cool place for several day, and also refers to soaking a newly prepared medicinal plaster in cold water before use.

去火毒是指除去膏药或炒灸药中火毒的加工方法。它既可以把熬好的膏药或炒灸药放在阴凉处待数日后再使用，也可以把熬好的膏药放在凉水中浸泡数日后再使用。

(125) Steaming：The process of thoroughly heating drugs with steam. There are two techniques. One is steaming drugs directly in a steamer；and the other is steaming drugs which are getting along with ginger juice，wine or other liquids covered and steamed in a sealed container.

蒸是指利用水蒸气蒸制药物,使之熟透的加工方法。有两种技术,一种是直接在蒸锅中对药物进行清蒸;另一种是药物拌蒸,即将药物拌入姜汁、酒或其他辅料,另用容器装好,放置加热的锅中隔水加盖蒸熟。

(126) Distillation：The process of preparing the drug liquid by distilling the drugs and collecting the distillate by condensation.

蒸露是指药物经过蒸馏法而制成蒸馏药液的加工过程。

(127) Boiling：Boiling drugs in water or other liquids.

煮是将某些药物与清水或其他液体辅料同煮的方法。

(128) Quenching：The process of heating certain drugs red-hot and putting them immediately into cold water or vinegar repeatedly for several times. It is usually used to process mineral drugs.

淬是反复多次先把某些药物用火烧红后,再立刻投入水中或醋液中。这种方法一般用来加工矿物药。

(129) Simmering：The process of boiling the drugs with several changes of water，collecting and filtering the supernatant and condensing and solidifying it into a gel，or adding other ingredients before making a gel. In addition，it refers to the process of thoroughly boiling drugs in water.

熬是将某些药物反复加清水煮多次,把每次煮取的药液过滤后汇集在一起,再浓缩成固体胶状,或加入某些辅料后,浓缩成半流汁膏状的加工方法。此外它还指把药物煮烂的过程。

(130) Degreasing oils：The process of removing the oils and fats of certain drugs to minimize drastic reactions，toxicity or adverse side effects.

去油是指去掉某些药物的油脂,以降低药物的烈性、毒性或副作用。

(131) Making frost：It refers to the following three techniques of

processing medicine. Firstly, removing the oils of certain medicinal seeds，then，grinding them into a fine powder. Secondly，crystallizing certain drugs. Thirdly，grinding the residue after making medicinal gel with certain animal bones，shells，or horns，into a fine powder.

制霜是指以下三种加工药物的方法：一是将某些种子类药去掉油脂后研成细粉末，二是将某些药物析出结晶，三是将某些药用动物的骨、壳或角熬胶后剩下的药渣研成细粉末。

(132) Making pulp：Smashing certain plant drugs into a pulp.

制绒是指把某些植物药捣成绒状。

(133) Pulverization：Grinding drugs in a motar into very fine powder.

乳细是指把药物放在乳钵内研成细粉末的过程。

(134) Splitting：Splitting some drugs before boiling them. Jujube is often broken up before being decocted.

掰是指把某些药物先用手破开，后煎煮的方法。如红枣常需要破开后再煎煮。

(135) Biting and masticating：Drugs were broken by biting and masticating in the mouth in ancient times.

㕮咀是指古代将药物咬成粗粒制备药物的方法。

(136) Tablet for drink：Drugs are processed into tablets，pieces，etc. and then decocted with water for drinking.

饮片（咀片）是指将药材加工处理成为片、块等形状后再加水煎汤饮服。

(137) Equal amounts：The amounts of the drugs in a prescription are the same.

等分是指将处方中各味药的剂量均等。

(138) Slow fire and quick fire：Mild and slow fire is called slow fire；while rotating and quick fire，quick fire.

文火、武火：火力小而缓的称为文火，而火力大而猛的称为武火。

(139) Rice-washed water：Water having been used to wash the rice.

米泔水是指淘洗大米的水。

(140) Splashed water：Taking water out of a basin with a ladle，and pouring it back into it repeatedly until there are numerous bubbles rolling to and fro on the water surface.

甘澜水(劳水)是把水放在盆内,用瓢将水扬起来倒下去,如此反复多次,这样便能看到水面上水珠滚来滚去。

(141) Yin-yang water：Boiled water mixed with unboiled water.

阴阳水(生熟水)是把未煮沸的水和已煮沸的水混合在一起。

(142) Limeless wine：The wine with no added lime as made in ancient times，which is usually used for processing medicines.

无灰酒是指古代的一种酿制不放石灰的酒,多供药用。

Ⅱ. Dialogues 情景对话

1. Dialogue 1 对话 1

Doctor：Hello，this is your herbal prescription. Follow the instructions to use it. What is the dosage taken each time and what is the frequency?

你好,这是你的草药方子,请按照说明使用。每次服用的剂量是多少,频率是怎样的?

Patient：The prescription states that it should be taken twice after each decoction，but I am not sure about the specific dosage.

方子上写的是每次煎煮后分两次服用,但我不太清楚具体的剂量。

Doctor：Taking it twice each time is to maintain the stability of the drug effect. You can divide the entire dose in half and take it once in the morning and once in the evening. This is more conducive to the absorption of drugs.

每次分两次服用是为了保持药效的稳定,你可以将整剂分成两半,早晚各服一次。这样更有助于药物的吸收。

2. Dialogue 2 对话 2

Patient：Doctor，should this herb be taken before or after meals?

医生,这个草药是要在饭前还是饭后服用?

Doctor：This prescription is relatively mild and can be taken half an hour before or one hour after meals, which helps with drug absorption. However, it is best to avoid consuming stimulating foods such as alcohol and coffee at the same time.

这个方子比较温和,可以在饭前半小时或饭后一小时服用,这样有助于药物的吸收。不过最好避免与酒、咖啡等刺激性食物同时摄入。

Patient: Doctor, I am not very familiar with the method of boiling herbs. What should I do?

医生,我不太熟悉煎煮草药的方法,应该怎么做呢?

Doctor: No problem, I will explain it to you. Firstly, put the herbs into a decoction pot and add an appropriate amount of water. Then slowly simmer over low to medium heat until half of the water is left, turn off the heat and filter out the medicine. Finally, divide the medication into two doses for administration.

没问题,我会为你解释一下。首先,将草药放入煎药锅中,加入适量的清水。其次用中小火慢慢煎煮,待水剩下一半时,即可关火,滤出药液。最后,将药液分成两次服用。

Patient: Doctor, what should I do if I feel unwell or experience other reactions during the medication process?

医生,如果在用药过程中感觉身体不适或出现其他反应,应该怎么办?

Doctor: If you experience any discomfort, such as dizziness, nausea, you should stop taking the medication immediately and inform me promptly. I will adjust the formula according to the specific situation. Meanwhile, if other drugs are used simultaneously, it is best to inform in advance to avoid adverse interactions.

如果出现任何不适反应,比如头晕、恶心等,应立即停药并及时告诉我。我会根据具体情况调整方子。同时,如果有其他药物同时使用,最好提前告知,以免发生不良相互作用。

3. Dialogue 3 对话3

Doctor: Hello, is there anything bothering you?

你好,有什么让你烦恼的事情吗?

Patient：Recently, I have been under a lot of work pressure, and I always find it difficult to fall asleep at night. Additionally, my mood is relatively low during the day.

最近工作压力大,晚上总是难以入睡,而且白天情绪也比较低落。

Doctor：This is a typical case of qi stagnation and blood stasis. I will prescribe guizhi fuling wan with modifications, which helps to clear qi and regulate emotions.

这是一种典型的气滞血瘀的情况。我会开一服桂枝茯苓丸加减,有助于疏通气机、调理情绪。

Patient：Is there anything special to note about this herb?

这个草药有没有什么需要特别注意的地方?

Doctor：Guizhi fuling wan is a mild herb and generally does not have too strong side effects. But it is still recommended that you use the prescribed dosage to avoid overdose.

桂枝茯苓丸属于温和的草药,一般来说不会有太强的副作用。但还是建议你按照开具的剂量使用,避免过量。

4. Dialogue 4 对话 4

Doctor：Hello, is there any discomfort that I can help you solve?

你好,有什么不适的地方需要我帮助你解决吗?

Patient：I have been feeling unwell in my stomach lately, and sometimes I feel bloated when eating.

我最近总觉得胃部不舒服,有时候吃东西会胀气。

Doctor：It seems that you may have some digestive problems. I suggest you try taking some traditional Chinese medicine that can regulate qi and promote digestion, such as liujunzi decoction. This formula helps to adjust your gastrointestinal function and reduce discomfort.

看起来你可能有一些消化不良的问题。我建议你尝试服用一些理气消食的中药,比如六君子汤。这个方剂有助于调整你的胃肠功能,减轻不适感。

Patient：Does this prescription need to be taken for a long time?

这个方子需要长期服用吗?

Doctor：Normally，it is recommended that you take it continuously for about a week to observe the improvement of symptoms. If necessary，we can make further adjustments.

通常情况下,建议你连续服用一周左右,观察症状的改善情况。如果有需要,我们可以进行进一步调整。

Section 19   Inquiries into Past Medical History
第 19 节   既往病史问诊

Ⅰ. Key Sentences 核心语句

(1) Please tell me about any hospitalizations and surgeries you have undergone.

请告诉我你过去生病住过院或做过手术吗?

(2) What illnesses have you had in the past? Any injuries?

你过去生过什么病? 受过伤吗?

(3) Do you have any allergies?

你对什么过敏吗?

For family history：家族病史：

(4) Has anyone else in your family ever had problems like yours?

你的家族中有没有人得过与你一样的疾病?

(5) Please tell me about any illnesses that may run in your family, for example，diabetes，cancer or stroke?

请告诉我你的家族中有没有多发的疾病,比如糖尿病、癌症或卒中?

For personal life history：个人生活习惯：

(6) Do you smoke and/or drink?

你抽烟喝酒吗?

(7) (If the patient smokes) How long have you been smoking?

(如病人抽烟)你抽烟有多久了?

(8) (ib.) How many cigarettes do you smoke every day?

(同上)每天平均抽多少支?

(9) (If the patient drinks) How long have you been drinking?

(如病人喝酒)你喝酒有多久了？

(10) (ib.)What kind of alcoholic beverages do you drink?

(同上)你平时喝什么酒？

(11) (ib.)How much do you drink ordinarily?

(同上)每天大概喝多少？

(12) Do you drink tea habitually?

你有喝茶的习惯吗？

(13) Do you eat greasy food frequently?

你经常吃油腻的食物吗？

(14) Do you eat fruit and vegetables every day?

你每天吃蔬菜和水果吗？

(15) When do you get up every day?

你平日几点起床？

(16) When do you usually go to bed?

你通常几点睡觉？

(17) Do you participate in physical exercises regularly?

你常进行体育锻炼吗？

For inspecting the patient's tongue and checking the patient's pulse：为患者进行舌诊和脉诊：

(18) Please open your mouth, and let me check your tongue.

请张开嘴，让我看一下舌头。

(19) Please curl your tongue upward, and let me examine the underside of it.

请把舌头向上卷起，我看看舌头底面。

(20) Please stick out your tongue.

请把舌头伸出来。

(21) Now I would like to check your pulse. Please put your hand on the cushion with the palm facing upward.

现在给你号脉，请把手放在脉枕上，手心向上。

Ⅱ. Dialogues 情景对话

1. Dialogue 1 对话 1

Doctor：Hello，may I ask if you have had any previous experiences with colds，coughs，or other respiratory diseases?

你好，请问你以前有没有感冒、咳嗽或者其他呼吸道疾病的经历?

Patient：I remember having a cold last winter. My throat hurt for a few days，and then I coughed. At that time，I went to see a family doctor who prescribed some medicine. It took me about a week to recover.

我记得上个冬天有一次感冒，嗓子痛了几天，然后就咳嗽了。那时候去看了家庭医生，开了点药吃了大概一周就好了。

Doctor：Has your cough symptoms completely disappeared after improvement?

那你的咳嗽症状在好转后完全消失了吗?

Patient：Yes，I stopped coughing after taking the medicine.

是的，在吃完药之后就没有再咳嗽了。

2. Dialogue 2 对话 2

Doctor：Do you have any digestive discomfort，such as stomach pain，indigestion，or loss of appetite?

你有没有消化系统方面的不适，比如胃痛、消化不良或者食欲不振?

Patient：I occasionally feel uncomfortable in my stomach，and sometimes I feel bloated and indigestible when eating.

我偶尔会感到胃部不舒服，有时候吃东西容易胀气，有点儿不消化的感觉。

Doctor：What is the approximate frequency of this discomfort? Is there a specific diet or time that can exacerbate these symptoms?

这种不适感出现的频率大概是怎样的? 有没有特定的饮食或时

间会加重这些症状?

Patient：Approximately once or twice a week，sometimes feeling even more uncomfortable after eating spicy or greasy food.

大概一周会有一两次,有时吃辛辣或油腻的食物后会感到更加不舒服。

3. Dialogue 3 对话 3

Doctor：Have you ever had any allergic symptoms or allergies to certain foods，drugs，or environments?

你曾经有过任何过敏症状或者对某些食物、药物或环境过敏吗?

Patient：I am allergic to pollen. In spring，my nose always itches and my eyes become red and swollen.

我对花粉过敏,在春天的时候鼻子总是特别痒,眼睛也会红肿。

Doctor：Besides pollen allergy，are there any other possible allergic symptoms，such as allergies to food or drugs?

除花粉过敏之外,有没有其他任何可能的过敏表现,比如对食物或药物过敏?

Patient：No，except for pollen allergy in spring，there is no special allergy to anything else at any other time.

没有,除了春天的花粉过敏,其他时候没有特别对其他东西过敏的情况。

4. Dialogue 4 对话 4

Doctor：How is your sleep condition? Is it easy to fall asleep at night? Do you have any insomnia or poor sleep quality?

你的睡眠情况如何? 晚上入睡是否容易? 有没有失眠或睡眠质量差的情况?

Patient：Sometimes it's difficult for me to fall asleep，especially when I've been under a lot of work pressure lately. Occasionally，there may be insomnia，but not frequently.

我有时候入睡比较困难,尤其是最近工作压力大的时候。偶尔会有失眠的情况,但不是经常。

Doctor：Besides sleep problems，have you recently felt any emotional fluctuations， such as anxiety， irritability， depression， and other emotional changes?

除了睡眠问题，你最近有没有感觉到情绪上的波动，比如焦虑、易怒、忧郁和其他情绪方面的变化?

Patient：I have been feeling a bit anxious and stressed recently， and some things in my work and life have made me feel a bit uneasy.

最近确实感到有些焦虑和压力大，工作和生活上的一些事情让我感到有些不安。

Chapter 3　The Western Medical Clinics

第 3 章　西医问诊

Section 1　The Internal Medicine
第 1 节　普通内科

Ⅰ. Dialogues 情景对话

1. Cold 感冒

Doctor：What seems to be the problem?

　　　　你哪儿不舒服(有什么问题)吗？

Patient：I think I have a cold, doctor.

　　　　我想我可能感冒了，医生。

Doctor：How long have you been sick?

　　　　你病了有多久了？

Patient：For two days.

　　　　两天了。

Doctor：What symptoms do you have?

　　　　你有些什么症状？

Patient：I have a runny nose and I ache all over.

　　　　流鼻涕，浑身痛。

Doctor：Do you have a fever?

　　　　发烧吗？

Patient：I haven't taken my temperature yet, but I feel feverish.

　　　　我没量过，但是我觉得发热。

Doctor：Do you have a cough?

咳嗽吗?

Patient：No，I don't.

不咳嗽。

Doctor：Do you have a sore throat?

嗓子痛吗?

Patient：Yes，my throat really hurts. It' also swollen.

是的,很痛。而且,我觉得嗓子也肿了。

Doctor：I want to look at your throat. Open your mouth. Please say "Ah".

我检查一下你的嗓子。请张大嘴说"啊"。

Patient："Ah""Ah"…

"啊""啊"……

Doctor：It's only a common cold. Nothing to worry about. I'll give you some medicine and write you a certificate for three days' leave. Have a good rest，and you will be fine in a few days.

没什么大事儿(不要紧的),只不过是普通感冒而已。我给你开点治感冒的药,顺便开三天的假条。你好好休息休息,用不了几天就会好的。

2. Hypertension 高血压

Patient：Doctor，I get terrible headaches.

医生,我头痛得厉害。

Doctor：When did they begin?

什么时候开始疼的?

Patient：About a week ago.

大约一个星期前。

Doctor：Does it help if you take aspirin?

你服用阿司匹林感觉有效吗?

Patient：No. They just seem to go away by themselves.

无效。疼痛好像是自然缓解的。

Doctor：Have you ever had this kind of headache before?

你以前有过这样的头痛吗?

Patient：I have had headaches off and on for the last few years, but none as bad as this.

近几年来我断断续续地头痛,但从来没有这次厉害。

Doctor：Had you visited a doctor before? And did he say anything about it?

你以前看过医生吗? 医生给你说过什么没有?

Patient：Three years ago I went to the local hospital for a swimming certificate. They just told me that I had hypertension.

三年前我去当地医院做游泳健康检查(办游泳证)时,医生曾告诉我说我有高血压。

Doctor：Have you ever had swollen ankles?

你的脚腕肿过没有?

Patient：Not that I can remember.

我没太注意过。

Doctor：What kind of treatment did you have in the past?

你以前做过什么治疗?

Patient：I took reserpine occasionally.

我偶尔服用利血平。

Doctor：Let me take your blood pressure firstly.

让我先量一下你的血压吧。

Patient：OK, thanks.

好的,谢谢。

Doctor：It's 200/120 mmHg (26.7/16.0 kPa). That's moderately high. I would like you to do a urinalysis, blood urea nitrogen test, chest X-ray and electrocardiogram examination.

200/120 毫米汞柱(26.7/16.0 千帕),你的血压有点偏高,最好做个尿常规化验、血尿素氮化验、X线胸片和心电图检查。

Patient：Oh, really? Is it serious?

是吗? 要不要紧?

Doctor：While… You should have a good rest, avoid nervous tension or stress, and give up smoking and alcohol. Don't be burdened with any thoughts. In addition, I'll give you some medicine.

嗯……你要好好休息,避免精神紧张,更不要有什么思想负担,记着忌烟、酒。另外,我给你开点药。

Patient：OK，I will.

好的，我听你的。

Doctor：Come back again next week for the results and another check of your blood pressure.

一周后来看化验结果，到时再复查个血压。

Ⅱ. Sentences 替换句型

(1) I can't stop coughing，doctor. And it started a week ago，but it has been getting worse since yesterday.

医生，我从一个星期前就一直咳嗽，从昨天起又加重了。

(2) I'm easily moved to anger with the onset of palpitation for the past two months，doctor.

医生，我最近两个月来爱发火，而且心慌。

(3) Would you please get undressed now? And let me examine you. Now，swallow，please.

好，脱下衣服我给你检查一下。请做一个吞咽动作，好吗?

(4) Do you cough up any phlegm?

你咳嗽时有痰吗?

(5) Just a small amount of phlegm，usually whitish. Occasionally I noticed some blood. This worried me，so I came to consult you.

只有少量白痰。偶尔我发现痰里带血。我有点害怕，所以就过来看病了。

(6) Let me examine you. Lie down on the bed please. Take your shoes off and unbutton your shirt please.

我给你检查一下，请脱下鞋子躺在床上，解开衣服扣子。

(7) Your heart seems to be normal. Your breathing is low. And I can hear moist rales over the left lung base. I'll take a white blood count and give you a fluoroscopic examination immediately.

你的心脏看来没什么大问题。呼吸音低。左肺底部能听到湿性啰音。我马上给你查个白细胞，再做个胸部透视。

(8) Here are the slips for blood test and fluoroscopic examination. First，please go to the cashier to pay the fee，then go to the laboratory for blood test and X-ray room for the fluoroscopic

examination. I'll wait here for the reports.

这是化验血和作胸部透视的单子。你先到收费处交费,然后到化验室验血,再到放射科去做胸部透视。我在这儿等你的检验结果。

(9) I suspect that you might have hyperthyroidism. Take this paper to the office, the nurse will arrange a time for you to have some thyroid function tests made.

我怀疑你得了甲状腺功能亢进。拿着这张化验单到办公室去,护士会安排时间给你做一些甲状腺功能的检查。

(10) I am sure it's pneumonia. Don't be careless. You had better be admitted to hospital and treated with penicillin (streptomycin). For the time being you should stop smoking. After several days you'll feel much better.

你肯定是得了肺炎了,不要大意,最好住院治疗,用青霉素(链霉素)效果就挺好的。不过你暂时不能吸烟,几天后病情一定会好转的。

(11) Here's your prescription. In addition, the affected toes should be rested and protected from any contact. Have regular meals, keep to a diet of salads and fruit, and eat very little meat. Avoid all alcohol.

这是你的处方。另外,患趾尽量少活动,尽量不要压它。饮食要有规律,应多吃蔬菜、水果,少吃肉类。不要喝酒。

(12) I have had a cough for about two years and I paid no attention to it because I thought it was from smoking. But two weeks ago I caught a cold. Since then I have felt very weak and feverish. My temperature is always a little higher in the afternoon.

我咳嗽两年了,但我没有太注意,因为我觉得这跟吸烟有关。可两周前我得了一次感冒后,总感到全身疲倦无力、发热,而且体温在下午总是高一些。

(13) Blood in the sputum strongly indicates the disease of tuberculosis. So we must take you a chest X-ray.

你痰中带血表明你得的很可能是结核病,因此你需要拍一张胸部 X 光片。

(14) Don't worry, Mr Smith. Nowadays, even those advanced cases with proper treatment can be cured within six months. But drug treatments should be continued (lasted) for almost two years.

不用担心，史密斯先生。目前即使是重症肺结核，只要治疗方法得当，半年内也可以完全康复。但单纯药物的治疗可能要持续两年之久。

（15）Please send a fresh specimen of your sputum for another testing. I'll prescribe isoniazid 0. 1 gm three times a day and injections of penicillin 1 gm once a day. By the way, you also need a good rest and good food.

请你送一个新鲜的痰标本再做个检查。我给你开药。异烟肼0.1克一天三次，青霉素注射1克一天一次。另外，你需要卧床休息、补充营养。

（16）Now I have it almost every day. It often awakens me two to three hours after I go to sleep.

我几乎每天都疼，常常是夜晚刚睡两三个小时就疼醒了。

（17）Your problem probably comes from a duodenal ulcer. You are suffering from shock due to bleeding. The medicine we have been using has not been effective, so we feel that it is necessary to perform an operation.

你可能是十二指肠溃疡。休克是因失血过多引起的。服药效果似乎不好，所以我们建议你手术治疗。

（18）Doctor, I suddenly developed a sharp pain in my upper abdomen.

医生，我上腹部突然剧痛。

（19）What kind of pain is it? Intermittent or persistent?

是怎样的疼？间歇性的还是持续性的呢？

（20）Does the pain go in a particular direction?

疼痛往某个方向窜吗？

（21）Can you describe the pain?

你能描述一下是怎么个疼法吗？

（22）The pain feels like a red-hot knife stabbing my toe.

疼得好像烧红的刀子在我脚趾上戳一样。

（23）It's a kind of sharp pain. It was off and on, but now it's pain all the time. And sometimes it goes towards my back.

是剧痛。本来是一阵一阵疼的，可现在是一直疼，有时疼痛还窜到我的背部。

（24）Since last midnight, it hurt so much that I couldn't sleep at all.

This morning I saw that the skin was red, hot and swollen.

从昨晚半夜开始,疼得我睡不着觉。今天早晨患处表皮又红又热又肿。

(25) According to your history, physical examination and laboratory tests, you have an acute panereatitis. It would be better if you could stay in hospital until you are well.

根据你的病史、体检和化验结果,你得的是急性胰腺炎。建议你最好住院接受治疗。

(26) I have felt weak recently. And these last few days I've felt much worse. I don't know what is the matter with me, doctor.

医生,我最近觉得乏力。这几天尤其严重。我不知道得了什么病。

(27) You look very pale. I'll give you a thorough check-up.

你脸色苍白。我给你详细检查一下吧。

(28) Come back the day after tomorrow for the results, please.

请后天来看结果吧。

(29) Have you noticed any lumps on your ears?

你是否注意过你耳朵上有小肿块?

(30) Has anyone in your family had the same trouble?

你家里有人得过这种病吗?

(31) My appetite's all right and I just feel tired. My legs are so weak sometimes, I can't even climb the stairs. Occasionally, I feel short of breath and giddy.

我食欲还好,只是感到疲劳。有时我的两腿无力,甚至不能爬楼梯;有时候我又觉得气短和头晕。

(32) According to the blood test, you are suffering from an iron deficiency anaemia, probably due to your heavy periods.

根据血液检查结果,你得的是缺铁性贫血,可能和你的月经过多有关。

(33) The results of the thyroid scanning and protein-bound-iodine show that you have hyperthyroidism.

根据甲状腺扫描和蛋白结合碘检查结果,你得的是甲状腺功能亢进。

(34) I think a subtotal thyroidectomy is necessary. And the operation will make a small scar on your neck.

我认为需要做个甲状腺次全切除术。而且手术会在你颈部留下一个小瘢痕。

(35) Is there any way to avoid surgery, doctor? If possible, I would rather not have surgery.

医生,有什么方法能避免手术吗? 如果可能的话,我不想做手术。

(36) Of course, antithyroid drugs, such as propylthiouracil and thiamazole, are used to control the symptoms. Their advantages are the avoidance of a surgical procedure with its attendant rare complications of recurrent laryngeal nerve paralysis or hypoparathyroidism, and reduced cost. But the major disadvantages of the medical treatment are the time required to gain control of the disease and the disease is rather prone to recur after treatment. Moreover, the drug therapy also has some side effects such as skin rash, fever, peripheral neuritis, and polyarteritis.

当然,抗甲状腺药物如丙硫氧嘧啶和甲巯咪唑可以控制症状。它们的优点是免得动手术,并防止由之引起的罕见并发症,如喉返神经麻痹或甲状旁腺功能减退等,而且费用低廉。但是药物治疗的主要缺点是控制疾病需要较长时间,治疗之后,很容易复发。而且药物疗法还有副作用,比如皮疹、发烧、末梢神经炎和多动脉炎。

(37) I am going to prescribe some iron tablets for you, which should be taken after meals or they will spoil your appetite. Then I would like you to see a gynecologist. We'll make an appointment for next Tuesday at 8:00 a.m.

我给你开一些补铁片剂,饭后服用,不然的话会影响你的食欲的。另外我想你还应该去妇科检查一下。你看给你约在下周二早晨8点钟,好吧。

(38) Recently I've been feeling very thirsty and passing a lot of urine. Is there any wrong with me, doctor?

医生,我最近总觉得口渴,尿量也多。是有什么病了吗?

(39) How is your appetite? And how do you feel otherwise?

你的胃口怎样? 健康状况好吗?

(40) In spite of increased intake of food, I lost 10 pounds in weight over a period of two months.

尽管我饭量增加,可两个月来我体重还是掉了10磅。

(41) I've lost weight despite my good appetite and I feel weak all the time.

尽管我食欲很好,可我的体重还是减轻了,整天还觉得很疲劳。

(42) Do you sleep well?

你睡得好吗?

(43) I have been suffering from insomnia lately.

我近来一直失眠。

(44) Doctor, I've a terrible pain in my foot.

医生,我的脚疼得厉害。

(45) I suddenly began to feel a severe pain in the joint of this toe.

我突然感到这个脚趾的关节很疼。

(46) Sorry to tell you that we cannot find any organic origin for this pain.

抱歉,对于这种疼痛,我们目前找不到任何器质性原因。

(47) Tell you the truth, Sir. On examination I could not find any striking abnormality.

实话告诉你先生,检查时我未能发现任何明显的异常。

(48) Have you been sweating as much as you usually do?

你最近出汗和往常一样多吗?

(49) My sweating has increased notably and I just can't stand warm weather at all.

我现在出汗的确比以前多很多,而且一到热天我就受不了了。

(50) Diabetes is a chronic disease due to poor functioning of the pancreas. It upsets the metabolism of sugar, fat and protein. Right now, it can't be cured, but it can be controlled so that you can enjoy life and feel well. You should stick to a special diet and avoid sugar and sweets, however.

糖尿病是一种由胰腺功能不良引起的慢性病,它主要是使糖、脂肪和蛋白质的代谢发生异常。目前此病虽然没有办法治愈,但是可以被控制,这样能使你的正常生活不受影响。糖尿病人需要坚持控制饮食,不吃糖和甜食。

(51) Smoking is harmful to anyone's health. Better give it up.

吸烟有害健康,我劝你戒烟。

(52) As a diabetic, how can I keep to a good diet?

我有糖尿病，该怎样制定一个良好的饮食方案呢？

（53） You can drink in moderation. As you know alcohol contains calories, what you have drunk must be counted in your diet（meal plan）.

你可适当喝一点酒。不过，酒精本身含有的热卡必须计算在你的食谱内。

(54) You should learn as much as you can about diabetes, have your urine tested regularly, stick to your diet, take your medicine on time and have some regular exercise. Then you can live a full, useful and meaningful life.

你应当尽量学习一些有关糖尿病的知识，定期检查小便，坚持按食谱膳食，按时服药，还要定量地运动，只要坚持你就能美满幸福地生活。

(55) Doctor, let me discuss it with my husband, then we'll decide what to choose. Is that all right?

医生，我可不可以跟我丈夫商量后，我们再决定采取什么办法呢？

Ⅲ. Words and Expressions 单词和短语

ankle joint 踝关节

ankle /'æŋkl/ *n.* 踝部

aorta /eɪ'ɔːtə/ *n.* 主动脉

appendix /ə'pendɪks/ *n.* 阑尾

arteria dorsalis pedis; dorsal artery of foot 足背动脉

artery /'ɑːtəri/ *n.* 动脉

back（dorsum）of hand 手背

beard /bɪəd/ *n.* 胡须

biceps /'baɪseps/ *n.*; bicipital muscle; musculus biceps 二头肌

blood capillary 毛细血管

blood vessel 血管

bone /bəʊn/ *n.* 骨

brain /breɪn/; encephalon /en'sefəlɒn/ *n.* 脑

bronchus /'brɒŋkəs/ *n.*（pl., bronchi /'brɒŋkaɪ/）支气管

brow /braʊ/; eyebrow /'aɪbraʊ/ *n.* 眉

carpal bone 腕骨

cecum /'siːkəm/ *n.* 盲肠

cerebral artery 脑动脉

cerebral ventricle 脑室

cerebrum /'serəbrəm/ *n.* 大脑

cheekbone /'tʃiːkbəʊn/ *n.* 颧骨

chest /tʃest/; breast /brest/ *n.* 胸

chin /tʃɪn/ *n.* 颏

collarbone /ˈkɒləbəʊn/；clavicula
　/kləˈvɪkjʊlə/；clavicle /ˈklævɪkl/ n. 锁骨
coronary artery 冠状动脉
deltoid /ˈdeltɔɪd/；deltoideus
　/delˈtɔɪdɪəs/ n. 三角肌
earlap /ˈɪəˌlæp/；earlobe /ˈɪələʊb/ n.
　耳垂
elbow /ˈelbəʊ/ n. 肘
elbow joint 肘关节
femoral vein 股静脉
fibula /ˈfɪbjələ/ n. 腓骨
finger /ˈfɪŋɡə/ n. 指
fingerling /ˈfɪŋɡəlɪŋ/ n. 指头
fingertip /ˈfɪŋɡətɪp/ n. 指尖
fist /fɪst/ n. 拳
forearm /ˈfɔːrɑːm/ n. 前臂
forefinger /ˈfɔːfɪŋɡə/ n. 食指
forehead /ˈfɔːhed/ n. 前额
fossa axillaris；axillary fossa 腋窝
gastrocnemius muscle；musculus
　gastrocnemius 腓肠肌
gluteus maximus muscle 大臀肌
greater trochanter；trochanter major
　大转子
groin /ɡrɔɪn/ n.；inguinal region 鼠蹊部
heel /hiːl/ n. 足心
hip /hɪp/；buttock /ˈbʌtək/ n. 臀部
humerus /ˈhjuːmərəs/ n. 肱骨
hypophysis /haɪˈpɒfɪsɪs/ n. glandula
　pituitaria；pituitary gland 垂体
iliac-crest 髂骨脊
iliac fossa；fossa iliaca 髂窝
iliac-spine 髂骨棘
inferior vena cava；vena cava inferior

下腔静脉
instep /ˈɪnstep/ n. 足背
intercostal muscle 肋间肌
internal and external oblique of
　abdomen muscle 腹内外斜肌
ischium /ˈɪskɪəm/ n. 坐骨
jaw /dʒɔː/ n. 下颌
jaw-joint 下颌关节
joint /dʒɔɪnt/；articulation
　/aːˌtɪkjʊˈleɪʃn/ n. 关节
jugular vein 颈静脉
knee /niː/ n. 膝
large intestine 大肠
lash /læʃ/；eyelash /ˈaɪlæʃ/ n. 眼睫毛
little finger；hypo-finger 小指
lymphatic vessel 淋巴管
median vein 正中静脉
meninges /məˈnɪndʒiːz/ n. 脑脊膜
mesentery /ˈmesəntəri/ n. 肠系膜
middle finger 中指
muscle /ˈmʌsl/ n. 肌肉
nail /neɪl/ n. 指甲
occiput /ˈɒksɪˌpʌt/ n. 枕部
palm /pɑːm/ n. 手掌
pectoralis major 胸大肌
pectoralis minor 胸小肌
pelvis /ˈpelvɪs/ n. 骨盆
portal vein 门静脉
pulmonary artery 肺动脉
pulmonary vein（vena）肺静脉
quadriceps femoris muscle 股四头肌肉
radial artery 桡动脉
radius /ˈreɪdɪəs/ n. 桡骨
ring finger 无名指

scapula /ˈskæpjʊlə/ *n.* 肩胛骨

shank /ʃæŋk/ *n.* 小腿

shoulders joint 肩关节

skull /skʌl/ *n.* 颅

small intestine 小肠

sole /səʊl/ *n.* 足里

spina iliaca posterior inferior 髂后下棘

spina iliaca posterior superior 髂后上棘

sternum /ˈstɜːnəm/ *n.* 胸骨

straight muscle of abdomen；
　musculus rectus abdominis 腹直肌

superior vena cava；vena cava
　superior 上腔静脉

tarsal bone 跗骨

temple /ˈtempl/ *n.* 颞

the upper arm；brachium /ˈbreɪkiəm/
　n. 上臂

thigh /θaɪ/ *n.* 大腿

thumb /θʌm/ *n.* 大拇指

thymus /ˈθaɪməs/ *n.* 胸腺

thyroid gland 甲状腺

tibia /ˈtɪbiə/ *n.* 胫骨

toe /təʊ/ *n.* 趾

triceps brachii muscle 三头肌

trunk /trʌŋk/ *n.* 躯干

ulna /ˈʌlnə/ *n.* 尺骨

urology /jʊəˈrɒlədʒi/ *n.* 泌尿学

vein /veɪn/ *n.* 静脉

vertex /ˈvɜːteks/ *n.* 顶

virology /vaɪˈrɒlədʒi/ *n.* 病毒学

waist /weɪst/；loin /lɔɪn/ *n.* 腰

windpipe /ˈwɪndpaɪp/；trachea
　/trəˈkiːə/ *n.* 气管

wrist joint 腕关节

wrist /rɪst/ *n.* 腕

Section 2　Surgery
第 2 节　普通外科

Ⅰ. Dialogues 情景对话

1. Open Injury 开放性损伤

Doctor：How were you injured?
　　　　你是怎样受伤的？
Patient：I tripped and fell, banging my forehead quite hard. My wife
　　　　wrapped a bandage around it to stop the bleeding.
　　　　我滑倒了，前额部碰得很重，我妻子用绷带给我缠上才止住了血。

Doctor：Did you lose a lot of blood?

　　　出血很多吗？

Patient：Not too much.

　　　不太多。

Doctor：Were you unconscious?

　　　受伤时你昏过去了吗？

Patient：No.

　　　没有。

Doctor：Did your nose or ears bleed after the accident?

　　　受伤时你的耳、鼻有没有出血呢？

Patient：No.

　　　没有。

Doctor：The wound is rather large, Sir. So I'll stitch it up.

　　　伤口很大，必须马上缝上。

Patient：Will it hurt, doctor?

　　　会疼吗？

Doctor：Oh, no. We'll give you a local anaesthetic. It won't be painful. You're a brave fellow, I think. Well, we're all finished. That wasn't so bad, was it?

　　　哦，我们会给你局部麻醉，不会疼的。我认为你很勇敢。好了，完工了，怎么样，不太疼吧？

Patient：No, not very.

　　　是的，不怎么痛。

Doctor：Have you had an anti-tetanus injection lately?

　　　你最近打过破伤风抗毒素针吗？

Patient：I think the only one I have had was about five years ago.

　　　我五年前打过一次。

Doctor：Well, I think you'd better have another one.

　　　哦，我想你需要重打一次了。

Patient：Whatever you say, doctor.

　　　好的，医生。就按你说的做吧。

Doctor：Come again after three days and we'll examine the wound.

　　　三天后再来复诊。

2. Gallstone 胆结石

Patient：Doctor，I suddenly felt a pain in the right upper side of my stomach.

医生，我突然觉得右上腹疼痛。

Doctor：When did it first start?

什么时候开始的?

Patient：About three days ago.

大约在三天前。

Doctor：Does the pain move anywhere else?

疼还向别的地方窜吗?

Patient：Yes，it goes towards my right shoulder.

是的，向右肩部窜。

Doctor：What kind of pain is it?

什么性质的疼痛?

Patient：It's colic at first，but soon it became constant.

先是绞疼，很快就变为持续性的疼了。

Doctor：Have you had any chill or temperature?

你发冷还是发烧?

Patient：I feel as though I have a temperature.

我觉得发烧。

Doctor：Which came first，the temperature or the pain?

发热在先还是疼痛在先?

Patient：The pain.

疼痛在先。

Doctor：How is your appetite?

你胃口好吗?

Patient：When I look at food，I feel sick.

我一看见食物就想吐。

Doctor：Have you vomited in the past three days?

三天来你吐过吗?

Patient：Yes，about 10 to 15 times. I always felt pain.

是的，一共吐了 10 到 15 次。我总感到疼。

Doctor：Have you vomited blood?

吐过血吗?

Patient：No. Just a kind of whitish, thick stuff.

没有。只是一些白的、黏稠的东西。

Doctor：Did you feel full after eating heavy or greasy food?

吃得过多或吃得油腻你肚子胀吗?

Patient：Yes，I went to two parties in succession three days ago. I felt bloated. Heavy eating seems to bring on the pain. Could this be the reason for it?

是的,三天前我连续参加了两次宴会。以后我就感到腹胀,暴食后就疼痛。这是发病的原因吗?

Doctor： Yes, overeating or drinking too much can cause these symptoms. And by the way, have your skin and eyeballs turned yellow?

是的,暴饮暴食可以引起这些症状。你的皮肤和眼球发黄过吗?

Patient：No.

没有。

Doctor：Have your stools been light in color?

你大便的颜色变浅过吗?

Patient：Yes, I found my stool was a sandy color yesterday.

是的,昨天我发现我的大便是沙土色的。

Doctor：Has your urine been dark?

你的尿色深吗?

Patient：Yes, just like tea.

是的,像茶一样。

Doctor：Let me examine you. Please lie down and relax. Take a deep breath. That's fine. You may have gallstones. We'll do an X-ray to see if that's the case.

我给你检查一下,躺下、放松、深呼吸,好的。你得的像是胆结石,不过还要拍个 X 光片确诊一下。

Patient：Would an operation be necessary?

需要手术吗?

Doctor：I can't say until I've seen the X-rays. You'd better come into hospital for a few days of observation.

在 X 光片结果出来之前，我还不能下结论。你最好住院观察几天吧。

3．Hemorrhoids（Piles）痔疮

Patient：I bleed quite a bit when I have a bowel movement. So I'm really worried about it，doctor.

我大便时出了不少血，我很担心，医生。

Doctor：What color is the blood?

血是什么颜色的？

Patient：It's bright red.

鲜红色的。

Doctor：Is it mixed with the stool?

血是和大便混在一起的吗？

Patient：No，it isn't.

不混在一起。

Doctor：Do you have constipation often?

你经常便秘吗？

Patient：Yes，all the time.

是的，经常便秘。

Doctor：Have there been any change in the pattern of your feces?

粪便形态有变化吗？

Patient：No.

没啥变化。

Doctor：Now，let's have a look at you. I'm going to examine you with an anoscope. Please undress and lie in the knee-elbow position. You've got hemorrhoids and a prolapse of the rectal mucosa.

我先用肛门镜给你做个肛门检查吧。请脱下裤子，跪着趴下。你有痔核，还有直肠黏膜脱垂呢。

Patient：Is there any way to cure it? If possible，I'd rather not have an operation.

用什么方法治疗呢？如果可能的话，我不想动手术。

Doctor：Don't worry. Here's a prescription. Use the suppositories and laxative. The bleeding should stop in two or three days.

别着急,这是你的处方。用一点坐药和泻药,过个两三天血就会止住的。

Patient：Anything else I should do?

我还要注意些什么吗？

Doctor：Eat more fruit or vegetables. Sit in warm water when you feel pain and if possible, avoid alcohol and spicy food.

多吃一些蔬菜或水果。肛门疼时可坐在热水盆里。尽量不要饮酒和吃辛辣食物。

Patient：Thank you. I'll follow your advice.

谢谢你的建议,我会照着做的。

Ⅱ. Sentences 替换句型

(1) I have a pain and swelling in my knee.

医生,我的膝关节又肿又疼。

(2) When did you first notice it?

什么时候开始觉得疼的？

(3) Have you ever had any swelling or pain in your other small joints such as your wrist, fingers, or toes?

其他小关节如腕、指、趾关节也疼,也肿吗？

(4) What kind of pain is it?

怎么个疼法？

(5) It seems a dull ache.

是那种隐隐约约的疼。

(6) Is it worse when the weather changes?

天气变化时疼得厉害吗？

(7) About two years ago, doctor. At first, the pain occurred only in the mornings right after I woke up, then it was off. But now the pain has become worse and more constant. Sometimes it disturbs my sleep.

医生,大约是在两年前。起先只有起床时疼,然后慢慢就缓解了,但是现在疼得越来越重,疼的时间也越来越长,有时还影响睡眠。

(8) Is the pain worse when you start to move after resting for a long time?

休息一段时间后,开始活动时疼痛加重吗?

(9) It's much worse in cloudy or wet weather, doctor.

医生,阴天或潮湿的时候会疼得厉害些。

(10) Did you run any temperature?

你发过烧吗?

(11) Have you lost weight lately?

最近你体重减轻了吗?

(12) If I massage it or put it in hot water, the pain seems to be lessened slightly.

如果我做按摩或把关节泡在热水里,疼得就轻些。

(13) Is it serious, doctor?

医生,我的病严重吗?

(14) The mass needs to be removed.

这个肿块需要摘除。

(15) The patient responded to the new treatment satisfactorily.

病人对这种新疗法非常满意。

(16) I am sorry I had to hurt you.

对不起,让你感觉很疼。

(17) I can't say. We need to make further examinations.

现在还很难说,得做进一步的检查。

(18) What can you do, doctor?

医生,那你准备怎么治疗呢?

(19) Walk across the room, please.

请从房间的这边走到那边。

(20) Honestly speaking, doctor. He is now used to walking with his artificial legs.

医生,说实话,他现在已经习惯用他的假肢走路了。

(21) Young children often react alarmingly to quite a mild head injury by having a convulsion.

年幼的孩子发生轻度头损伤时常伴有严重的痉挛反应。

(22) The sedimentation rate is normal, the rheumatoid factor is negative, and there is no anemia. The X-ray of your knees shows that the joint space is diminished. Beneath the cartilage there is sclerosis and cysts and the lipping of the margin of the joint. I

think you have osteoarthritis.

你的血沉正常,类风湿因子阴性,没有贫血,X 光片显示关节间隙变窄,关节软骨下有硬化和囊性变,膝关节边缘有唇样变,我想你得了骨关节炎。

(23) While, my friend suggested I have an operation.

我的朋友建议我做手术。

(24) I'll give you some Chinese traditional medicine pills. Apply a hot water pad over the knees. You can also have short-wave diathermy.

我给你开一点中药丸。你可以在膝关节上做热敷,还可以同时用超短波透热疗法。

(25) If you do, you would lose the movement of the knee. Total knee replacement has been used recently. If the pain is mild, then the treatment should be conservative. If it gets severe, then we will consider surgery.

如果动手术,你膝关节就活动不成了。近年来已使用全膝关节置换术了。如果中等程度的疼痛,还是以保守疗法为宜。要是疼痛厉害了,咱们再考虑动手术吧。

Ⅲ. Words and Expressions 单词和短语

abdomen /ˈæbdəmən/ n. 腹部
abscess of the lung 肺脓肿
actinomycosis of the bones 骨放射性菌病
actinomycosis of the thorax 胸廓放线菌病
acute lymphodenitis colli 急性颈淋巴结炎
adenalgia of the pituitary gland 垂体腺病
aneurysm /ˈænjərɪzəm/ n. 动脉瘤
appendicitis /əˌpendəˈsaɪtɪs/ n. 阑尾炎
arcus vertebrae 椎弓
arteriosclerotic gangrene 坏疽
arthritis gonorrheica 淋病性关节炎
arthritis rheumatism 风湿性关节炎
arthritis syphilitica 梅毒性关节炎

arthritis traumatica 外伤性关节炎
bandage /ˈbændɪdʒ/ n. 包扎;纱布
brain /breɪn/ n. 脑
brain osteoma 脑骨瘤
bronchial fistula 支气管瘘
burn /bɜːn/ n. 烫伤;灼伤
bursitis /ˌbɜːˈsaɪtɪs/ n. 滑囊炎
causalgia /kɔːˈzældʒə/ n. 灼痛
cerebral abscess 脑脓肿
cerebral embolism 脑栓塞
cerebritis /ˌserɪˈbraɪtɪs/ n. 大脑炎
cervical cyst 颈部囊肿
cervical fistula 颈部瘘
cervical vertebra 颈椎

change the bandage 换纱布

chondroma /kɒnˈdrəʊmə/ n. 软骨瘤

chronical bursitis 慢性滑囊炎

chronic empyema 陈旧性肺脓肿

chronic simple sialoadenitis 慢性单纯
　　性唾液腺炎

cicatricial stenosis；cicatricial
　　stricture 瘢痕性狭窄

clean the wound and refresh the
　　bandage 清创换药

coecum mobile 盲肠移动症

concussion cerebri 脑震荡

congenital malformation 先天畸形

congenital scoliosis 先天性脊柱侧凸

congenital torticollis 先天性斜颈

contracture /kəˈtræktʃə/ n. 挛缩

contusion cerebri 脑挫伤

contusion of the joint 关节挫伤

corn /kɔːn/；clavus /ˈkleɪvəs/ n. 鸡眼

corpus vertebrae 脊椎体

diabetic gangrene 糖尿病性坏疽

diaphragmatocele /daɪəfrəgˈmætəsiːl/
　　n. 膈疝

diverticulitis /ˌdaɪvəˌtɪkjʊˈlaɪtɪs/ n. 憩室炎

edema on the foot back 足背浮肿

edema on the hand back 手背水肿

elephantiasis /ˌelɪfənˈtaɪəsɪs/ n. 象皮病

embolism /ˈembəlɪzəm/ n. 栓子

empyema of thorax 脓胸

encephalitis /enˌsefəˈlaɪtɪs/ n. 脑炎；
　　大脑炎

encephalocele /enˈsefələʊˌsiːl/ n. 脑突
　　出；脑膨出

encysted peritonitis 包裹性腹膜炎

epiphysistis calcanea 跟骨髓炎

erythromelalgia /ʊˌriθrəʊməˈlældʒiə/
　　n. 皮红痛症；红斑性肢痛症

esophageal diverticulum 食管憩室

exophthalmic goiter 突眼性甲亢

fistula of the intestine 肠瘘

fistula of the vitello-intestinal duct 卵
　　黄肠管瘘

functional obstruction ileus 功能性肠梗阻

ganglion /ˈgæŋgliən/ n. 神经结节

general peritonitis 弥漫性腹膜炎

glioma /glaɪˈəʊmə/ n. 胶质病

goiter /ˈgɔɪtə/ n. 甲状腺肿

gunshot wound of the skull 颅创伤

hernia femoralis 股疝

hernia /ˈhɜːniə/ n. 疝

hernia inquinalis medialis（internia）
　　腹股沟内疝

hernia supravesicalis 膀胱上疝

hernia umbilicalis 脐疝

hernia ventralis 腹壁疝

hidradenitis axillaris purulenta 化脓
　　性毛囊炎（腋窝）

hydrarthrosis chronicus 慢性关节水肿

hydroma /haɪˈdrəʊmə/ n. 水囊瘤

idiopathic dilatation of the commom
　　bile duct 特发的胆总管扩张症

ileus intestinal obstruction 肠梗阻

ilues terminalis 小肠终部肠症

incarcerated hernia 嵌顿疝

inguinalis hernia 腹股沟疝

intracranial hemorrhage 颅内出血

jerking on snapping finger 弹拨指

juvenile gangrene 青年性坏疽

knee-jerk reflex 膝跳反射

leukemic lymphoma 白血病性淋巴瘤

local anesthesia 局部麻醉

local peritoneal abscess 局限性腹膜脓肿

lymphadenitis colli syphilitica 梅毒性颈淋巴炎

lymphadenitis /lɪmˌfædɪˈnaɪtɪs/ *n.* 淋巴结炎

lymphadenitis tuberculous colli 结核性颈淋巴结炎

lymphatitis *n.* 淋巴管炎

lymphogranuloma /ˌlɪmfəʊˌgrænjʊˈləʊmə/ *n.* 淋巴肉芽肿

lyphadenitis colli chronic 慢性颈淋巴结炎

mandible /ˈmændɪbl/ *n.* 小腭

mechanical obstruction ileus 机械性肠梗阻

mediastinal tumor *n.* 纵隔肿瘤

meningitis /ˌmenɪnˈdʒaɪtɪs/ *n.* 脑膜炎

Merckel's diverticulitis 麦克尔憩室炎

mixed tumor of the parotid gland 腮腺混合瘤

mucin cyst 黏液囊肿

muscular rheumatism 肌风湿

myositis ossificans 骨化性肌炎

navel /ˈneɪvl/；umbilicus /ʌmˈbɪlɪkəs/ *n.* 脐

omphalitis /ˌɔmfəˈlaɪtɪs/ *n.* 脐带炎

osteodystrophia ribros 肋骨骨营养障碍

osteomyelitis /ˌɒstɪəʊˌmaɪəˈlaɪtɪs/ *n.* 骨髓炎

pancreatic cyst 胰腺囊肿

pancreatic tumor 胰腺肿瘤

pancreatitis /ˌpæŋkrɪəˈtaɪtɪs/ *n.* 胰腺炎

paralytic ileus 麻痹性肠梗阻

paretic ileus 不完全麻痹性梗阻

periarthritis humeroscapularis 肩周炎

peri-pleural abscess 胸膜周围脓肿

peritonitis chronical fibrosa incapsulata 包裹性纤维性腹膜炎

peritonitis /ˌperɪtəˈnaɪtɪs/ *n.* 腹膜炎

presenile gangrene 中年期自发性坏疽

processus spinalis 脊(脊椎)突

processus transverses 横突

prolapse of brain 脑脱出

protruded intervertebral disk 椎间盘脱出病

psoitis /(p)səʊˈaɪtɪs/ *n.* 腰大肌炎

pulmonary fistula 肺瘘

purulenta osteomyelitis 化脓性骨髓炎

pylorospasm /paɪˈlɔːrəspæzəm/ *n.* 幽门痉挛

pyorrhea alveolaris 齿槽脓漏

rachischsis /rəˈkɪskɪˌsɪs/ *n.*；spina bifida 脊柱裂

ranula /ˈrænjʊlə/ *n.* 蛤蟆肿

rheumatoid arthritis 类风湿性关节炎

rupture of the achilles tendon 跟腱撕裂

salivary fistule 唾液瘘

salivary gland 唾液腺

scar torticollis 瘢痕性斜颈

scrotal hernia 阴囊疝

senile gangrene 老年性坏疽

sialolithiasis /saɪˌæləlɪˈθaɪəsɪs/ *n.* 唾石症

silent peritonitis 潜伏性腹膜炎

sinus thrombosis 窦血栓

skull /skʌl/ *n.* 颅骨；脑壳

spastic ileus 痉挛性肠梗阻

spinal irritation 脊椎过敏

spine & spinal column disease 脊椎（脊柱）疾病

spondylitis deformans 畸形性脊椎炎

spondylitis infectious acuta 急性传染性椎管炎

spondylitis syphilica 梅毒性脊椎炎

spondylitis tuberculosa 结核性脊椎炎

spondylitis typhosa 伤寒性脊椎炎

spondylolysis /ˈspɒndɪˈlɒlɪsɪs/ 脊椎分离

spontaneous gangrene 自发性坏疽

spontaneous hypoglycemia 自发性低血糖

sterilization /ˌsterɪəlaɪˈzeɪʃn/ n. 消毒；杀菌；绝育

stitch /stɪtʃ/ v. & n. 缝针

stomach sarcoma 胃肉瘤

struma /ˈstruːmə/ n. 甲状腺肿（炎）

subdural hemorrhage 硬脑膜下出血

symmetric gangrene 对称性坏疽

syphilis of the bone 骨梅毒

syphilis of the skull 颅骨梅毒

syphilis of the stomach 胃梅毒

take out the stitches 拆线

tendon sheath；vagina tendonitis 腱鞘（炎）

tendo-vaginitis gonorrhoeica 淋病性腱鞘炎

tendo-vaginitis purulenta 化脓性腱鞘炎

teratoma vertebral 脊椎畸胎瘤

thrombosis /θrɒmˈbəʊsɪs/ n. 血栓症

thrombus /ˈθrɒmbəs/ n. 血栓

thyroiditis /ˌθaɪrɔɪˈdaɪtɪs/ n. 甲状腺炎

tuberculosis of the bone 骨结核

tuberculosis of the peri-thorax 胸壁结核

tuberculosis of the rib 肋骨结核

tuberculous arthritis 结核性关节炎

tumor of brain 脑肿瘤

tumour of the pelvis 骨盆肿瘤

tumour of the spinal cord 脊椎肿瘤

typhoid osteochondritis of the rib 伤寒性肋骨软骨炎

ulcer bleeding 溃疡出血

ulcer on the leg 小腿溃疡

ulcus pepticus jejuni 空肠消化性出血

varicose veins 静脉曲张

vertebral tumor 脊椎肿瘤

Section 3　Orthopedics
第3节　整形外科

Ⅰ. Dialogues 情景对话

1. Tumor of the Breast 乳腺肿瘤

Doctor：Is there anything worrying you?

你有什么发愁的事吗?

Patient：Yes, doctor，I have a lump (mass) in my left breast.

是的,医生。我的左乳房上有一个肿块。

Doctor：How long have you felt it?

发现肿块有多久了?

Patient：About three weeks.

大约三个星期了。

Doctor：Have you had any pain in this area，especially during menstruation?

这块地方疼吗,特别是来月经的时候?

Patient：No.

不疼。

Doctor：Have you had any accident to this area?

这地方受过伤吗?

Patient：No.

没有。

Doctor：Have you had any discharge from it or any itching of the nipple?

乳头有什么分泌物吗? 痒吗?

Patient：No.

没有。

Doctor：Have you noticed any swelling under your left armpit?

你左侧腋窝下面肿不肿胀呢?

Patient：No.

　　不肿。

Doctor：Has anyone in your family ever had a lump or tumor of the breast?

　　你家里还有别的人乳房上长过肿块或瘤子吗？

Patient：No, not that I can remember.

　　没有，我记得没有。

Doctor：Do you mind if I examine you briefly?

　　我简单给你检查一下，好吗？

Patient：No, not at all.

　　好的。

Doctor：Would you please take off your blouse? That's fine. Sit up straight. Now rest your arm on mine. Let me examine your armpit. Put your right arm over your head. Now let's do the same with the left. Good. How old are you?

　　脱去衬衣。好。坐直，现在把你的胳膊搭在我的胳膊上。让我查查你的腋窝。把你的右胳膊放在脑后。左胳膊也同样做。好。你多大年纪了？

Patient：Fifty. Is it serious?

　　五十岁。我的病严重吗？

Doctor：Nothing serious. Just a cystic disease of the breast (adenofibroma). It's a benign hormone-dependent disease.

　　不严重，只是乳房囊腺病（腺纤维瘤），这是一种与内分泌有关的病。

Doctor：Do you have any relatives here?

　　在这儿你有亲戚吗？

Patient：Yes. My husband is just outside, shall I ask him to come in?

　　有。我丈夫就在外边，我可以叫他进来吗？

Doctor：Yes. Will you please go to the laboratory to check up a white blood cell count?

　　To patient's husband：As you know, your wife has a lump in her left breast. I think it could be a carcinoma of the breast. The only way to be certain is to do a biopsy. If she has cancer, she ought to have her breast removed. That's called a radical mastectomy.

可以,你现在到化验室去查一下白细胞。

对患者的丈夫说:你知道,你妻子的左乳房上有一个肿块。我们认为可能是乳腺癌。确诊的唯一手段是做活检。假如是癌的话,那她就可能摘除乳房。这叫乳瘤根除手术。

Husband: Please do everything you can to help her, doctor.

医生,请你尽一切可能治好她。

2. Fracture of the Lower Humerus 肱骨下段骨折

Patient: I have hurt my right elbow, doctor. Now I can't move it because of the pain.

医生,我的右肘受伤了,疼得动不了。

Doctor: How did it happen?

怎么引起的?

Patient: When I was getting into the bus in the morning, I fell on my elbow.

今天早晨上公共汽车时,我把肘部摔伤了。

Doctor: Is it still painful?

现在还疼吗?

Patient: Yes. Since the accident it has been stiff and looks black and blue. At times it feels numb.

疼,受伤后伤处僵硬,青一块紫一块。有时还觉得麻木。

Doctor: Can you feel this, when I put it in your hand?

我现在放你手上,你有感觉吗?

Patient: Yes.

有。

Doctor: I'm afraid you may have broken your elbow. I'll send you to the X-ray department to check. Oh, look, the X-ray reveals a fracture of the lower humerus. We'll give you a "U" type plaster cast on your elbow and shoulder.

你的肘关节可能骨折了,现在我送你去放射科检查一下吧。X光片显示肱骨下段骨折。现在在你肘部和肩膀上要打个"U"型石膏托。

Patient：How long will I have to have it?

这石膏托要戴多久？

Doctor：About six weeks.

大约六个星期吧。

Patient：Is there anything else I should do?

我还需要注意点什么吗？

Doctor：You'd better rest in bed and keep your elbow higher than your heart. Move your finger joints from time to time, and keep an eye on the color of the fingers. If you have pain and numbness or if the color of the fingers turns pale or dark，come right away.

你最好卧床休息,将患肘尽量放在高于心脏的部位,还要经常活动指关节,注意手指颜色的变化。如果手指疼、发麻,或者颜色发白、发暗,马上再来诊治。

Ⅱ. Sentences 替换句型

(1) I can't lift my right arm，doctor.

医生,我抬不起我的右臂了。

(2) Bend your left leg，please.

请弯一下你的左腿。

(3) Roll over on to your tummy.

翻身,趴在那儿。

(4) Take a deep breath and hold it.

深呼吸,然后屏住气。

(5) Turn over on to your left side，madame.

请转向你的左侧,夫人。

(6) Take all your clothes off and lie on the couch under the blanket.

脱掉你的衣服,躺在铺毛毯的检查床上。

(7) The lungs are subject to several diseases which are treatable by surgery.

肺病是外科能够治疗的几种疾病之一。

(8) We're going to pass this tube into your back passage.

我们要把这管子送入你的肛门。

(9) I'm going to give you an injection for the pain in a minute.

我一会儿给你打止痛针。

(10) Have you had your skin test yet?

你还没做皮肤试验吗？

(11) The doctor will now stitch the wound.

医生现在就要缝合伤口。

(12) This wound needs to be dressed.

这个伤口需要包扎。

(13) The nurse removed the stitches.

护士拆去了缝线。

(14) The anaesthetist was intubating the patient while the houseman was setting up an intravenous infusion.

麻醉师正在给病人插管的同时,住院医生给病人静脉输液。

(15) I sponged the boy's cut knee, and bandaged his leg.

我用海绵擦了擦男孩割伤的膝盖,并给他的腿打了绷带。

(16) He had his leg dislocated by his footing. And the doctor pulled the joint back into position.

他跌了一跤,腿关节脱了臼,医生已经把关节推回到原来的位置了。

(17) Would you mind my colleague having a look at your leg?

我的同事看一下你的腿部,你不介意吧?

(18) I'm afraid you'll need another two operations. It's a long job, I'm afraid, but it should put you on your feet again.

我想你还需要两次手术,这恐怕是个长期的工作,但是那将使你重新站起来。

(19) Has she come round yet?

她还没有恢复知觉吗?

(20) Be careful that the woman was thin, dehydrated and shocked with marked tenderness over the lower abdomen.

大家请注意,这个妇女消瘦、脱水,而且下腹部明显有压痛现象。

(21) Doctor, I can't bear it any more and I want something to ease this pain.

医生,我实在受不了了,我想要一些止痛药。

(22) She was unable to eat any solid food for weeks.

她几周内不能吃任何硬食。

(23) Some speech defects can be improved by correct positioning of the

teeth and tongue.

某些言语缺陷可以通过矫正牙齿和舌头的位置进行改善。

（24）I can hear better now. I've got my hearing-aid.

现在我的听力好点了，我已戴上助听器。

（25）After operation，when did you first notice you had difficulty in swallowing?

手术后，你什么时候发现有吞咽困难的？

（26）The ideal time for having children is when a woman is young enough physically and old enough emotionally.

要孩子理想的时间是一个妇女从体格上说还年轻，从情感方面讲已经成熟。

（27）The 24-year-old woman had her uterus removed.

这个 24 岁的妇女摘除了她的子宫。

（28）He is going to have his plaster taken off next week.

他下周就要拆掉石膏了。

（29）He is going to have an artificial limb fitted.

他要安装一个义肢。

（30）If it bleeds a lot during the night，ring 120 and an ambulance will bring you here.

如果夜间出血很多，打电话给 120，救护车会把你送到这儿的。

Ⅲ. Words and Expressions 单词和短语

anemic /ə'ni:mɪk/ *adj*. 贫血的

anisocoria /ænˌaɪsəʊ'kəʊriə/ *n*. 左右不对称（瞳孔）

ankylosis /ˌæŋkɪ'ləʊsɪs/ *n*. 僵直

anxious /'æŋkʃəs/ *adj*.惊恐的

apathetic /ˌæpə'θetɪk/ *adj*. 淡漠的

asymmetric /ˌeɪsɪ'metrɪk/ *adj*. 非对称的

aural discharge；otorrhea /əʊtə'ri:ə/ *n*. 耳漏

auricle /'ɔ:rɪkl/ *n*. 耳廓

bone of the foot 足骨

circular /'sɜ:kjələ/ *adj*. 环形的

cleft of the face 面裂

cleft palate 腭裂

club foot 畸形足

colour of face 面色

cornea /'kɔ:niə/ *n*. 角膜

corneal reflex 角膜反射

coxae valga 髋外翻

coxae vara 髋内翻

cyanotic /ˌsaɪə'nɒtɪk/ *adj*. 紫（青）绀样

deaf /def/ *adj*. 聋

derangement of the knee joint 膝关节位移

eardrum /ˈɪədrʌm/; drumhead
/ˈdrʌmˌhed/ n. 鼓膜

edema /ɪˈdiːmə/; dropsy /ˈdrɒpsi/ n. 浮肿

expression /ɪkˈspreʃən/ n. 面貌;表情

eyelid /ˈaɪlɪd/ n. 眼睑

facies abdominalis 腹膜炎面貌

facies adenoid 腺样体面貌

facies pertussica (pertussis) 百日咳面貌

fibroadenoma mamma 乳腺纤维瘤

flat foot 扁平足

flushed cheek 颊面红润

frost-bite 冻伤

genus valgum 膝外翻

genus varum 膝内翻

gynecomastia /ˌgaɪnɪkəʊˈmæstɪə/ n.
(男子的)女性化乳房

hallux valgus 外翻趾

hard of hearing 重听

hare lip 兔唇

hyperemic /ˌhaɪpəˈriːmɪk/ adj. 充血的

idiotic /ˌɪdiˈɒtɪk/ adj. 白痴的

irregular /ɪˈregjələ/ adj. 不规则的

mammary gland 乳腺

mamma tumor 乳腺肿瘤

mask-like 假面状

mastitis /mæsˈtaɪtɪs/ n. 乳腺炎

mastoid /ˈmæstɔɪd/ n. 乳突

mastoptosis /mɑːsˈtɒptəʊsɪs/ n. 乳房
下垂

miotic /maɪˈɒtɪk/ adj. 瞳孔缩小的

mouth pallor 口周苍白

mydriatic /ˌmɪdrɪˈætɪk/ adj. 扩瞳的

nasal discharge 鼻涕

nasal obstruction 鼻闭

oedematous /ɪˈdiːmətəs/ adj. 水肿的

painful /ˈpeɪnful/ adj. 疼痛的

pale /peɪl/ adj. 苍白的

palpebral conjunctiva 眼睑结膜

papillary reaction to light 对光反射
(瞳孔)

parotid gland 腮腺

pes equinovarus 马蹄足

plastic operation 整形手术

ptosis /ˈtəʊsɪs/ n. 下垂

pupil /ˈpjuːpl/ n. 瞳孔

retroauricular /retrəʊjuːˈrɪkjʊlə/ adj.
耳后的

rhinolalia /ˌraɪnəʊˈleɪlɪə/ n. 鼻音

saddle nose 鞍鼻

sardonic laugh 痛笑

tinnitus /ˈtɪnɪtəs/ n. 耳鸣

torticollis /ˌtɔːtɪˈkɒlɪs/ n. 斜颈

turgid edematous 浮肿状

xerotic /zɪˈrɒtɪk/ adj. 干燥症的

Section 4　Obstetrics and Gynecology

第4节　妇产科

Ⅰ. Dialogues 情景对话

1. Early Pregnancy 早孕

Doctor：What can I do for you, madame?

　　　　夫人,哪儿不舒服吗(需要我帮什么忙吗)?

Patient：My period is 18 days late.

　　　　我的月经都晚了18天了。

Doctor：How about your menstrual cycles?

　　　　那你的月经周期是多少天呢?

Patient：Usually 30 days apart, but sometimes three to five days late.

　　　　正常情况下是30天,不过有时会推迟个3—5天。

Doctor：When was your last period?

　　　　你最后一次月经是什么时候?

Patient：September 16th, which was on time. I don't know for sure (for certain) whether I'm pregnant or not, so I would like you to check it for me.

　　　　9月16日,是正常时间。所以我也不知道现在是不是怀孕了,想请你给我查一查。

Doctor：Have you had any discomfort?

　　　　你还有哪儿不舒服吗?

Patient：Yes. I have swelling pain of my breasts.

　　　　乳房胀疼。

Doctor：And how about your appetite?

　　　　胃口怎样?

Patient：Not quite well (It has been poor). I feel nauseous in the morning, but there is no vomiting.

胃口不好。早晨还感到有些恶心,不过没有吐。

Doctor：Let me make a pelvic examination for you.

来,我给你做个盆腔检查吧。

Patient：OK. Thank you very much.

好的,谢谢。

Doctor：Oh, your uterus is enlarged and feels soft, indicating (showing) a pregnancy of about six weeks. Can you give us some urine for a further test?

啊哟,你的子宫柔软,而且增大不少,像是怀孕六周的样子。为了确诊,你去留点尿做个早孕检查好吗?

Patient：Yes.

好的。

Doctor：The urine pregnancy test turned out to be positive. You are pregnant. So take care of yourself.

妊娠检验结果显示是阳性。你怀孕了,请多保重。

Patient：Oh, my God. Thanks a lot.

噢,天哪,太好了,多谢。

2. Antenatal Care 产前检查

Patient：Doctor, I'm pregnant, would you please give me an examination?

医生,我怀孕了,你能给我做个检查吗?

Doctor：Take off your shoes so that we can weigh and measure you, then take the blood pressure.

好的,脱了鞋子,我们先给你测个身高、体重,再给你量一下血压。

Patient：OK, I'll.

好的。

Doctor：When was your last menstruation?

你末次月经是什么时候?

Patient：It was June 14th, 2006.

2006 年 6 月 14 日。

Doctor：Are your menstrual cycles regular?

你的月经周期规律吗?

Patient：Yes，they are.

规律。

Doctor：Then your due date will be March 21st，2007.

那你的预产期大概在 2007 年 3 月 21 日。

Patient：I have a poor appetite，and have been vomiting after meals for two months. But it's much better now.

我的食欲不好，已经有两个月了，吃完就吐，不过现在好多了。

Doctor：Did you have any illness before pregancy?

怀孕前你得过什么病吗?

Patient：No，I'm quite healthy.

没有，我身体很好。

Doctor：What problems（troubles）have you ever had during this pregnancy? Have you had bleeding，watery discharge，pain in your lower abdomen and legs，etc. ?

这次怀孕你出现过什么问题吗? 有没有过阴道出血、水性分泌物、下腹部疼痛及腿疼的现象呢?

Patient：I don't have any problems. But I felt a little pain in my legs when I was tired.

没什么情况，就是累的时候腿疼过。

Doctor：And is there any multiple pregnancy，hypertension，tuberculosis，diabetes or hereditary diseases in your family?

你家族里有没有人生过多胞胎，患过高血压、结核病或其他遗传病的?

Patient：I was one of a pair of twins，and my mother and younger sister died during the delivery because of profuse bleeding.

我本人就是双胞胎其中的一个。我母亲和妹妹是在分娩的时候因出血过多死亡的。

Doctor：Let me give you a thorough examination. You have been pregnant for three months. The findings of the physical examination are all normal. The pelvis is big enough. I'll give you these sheets for routine blood and urine examination，liver function tests and blood grouping. Keep these sheets for floroscopy of the chest four months from now on. Come back in two weeks for a check-up and then once every month during the first six months of pregnancy and every two weeks for the next three months, and once a week in the last month. You should take more nourishment such as eggs, vegetables, fruit, milk, meat, vitamins, etc. You should avoid sexual relations in the early three months and the last month of pregnancy.

我给你彻底检查一下。你怀孕三个月了。体格检查正常。骨盆大小正常。我给你开些单子做一下常规的血、尿检查,以及肝功能和血型的检查。这些胸部透视单要保存四个月。两周后请来复查。以后的检查分别是:在妊娠最初六个月内每月复查一次,以后的三个月内每两周复查一次,最后的一个月内每周复查一次。你应当多吃些营养品,如蛋类、蔬菜、水果、牛奶、肉类、维生素等。妊娠最初三个月内和妊娠最后一个月还要避免性生活。

Patient: All right. I'll do as you advise (have said).

好的,谢谢你的建议。

3. In Labor 临产

Patient: Doctor, I noticed some bloody discharge this morning. But this is more than 10 days (fortnight) before my due date.

医生,我今天早上见红了。离预产期还有 10 天(两个星期)呢。

Doctor: Have you had any pain in your abdomen?

你肚子感到疼吗?

Patient: Yes, but it's mild and not regular.

疼,但不是很疼,疼得也没规律。

Doctor: When did you feel the pain (the pain start)?

从什么时候开始疼的?

Patient: It's been off and on during the past three or four days.

有时疼有时不疼,已经三四天了。

Doctor: Have you had any watery discharge?

下部流过水吗?

Patient: No, I didn't find (notice) it.

没发现。

Doctor: Is this your first pregnancy?

你这是第一次怀孕吗?

Patient：No，I had one (boy, daughter) two years ago.

不是,两年前我生过一个孩子(男孩、女孩)。

Doctor：Were there some difficulties in the first delivery?

那你第一次生孩子觉得困难(难产)吗?

Patient：En… The course of labor was quick, but I bled a lot soon after the baby was born.

嗯……产程很快,但小孩出生后不久,我就出了很多血。

Doctor：Did you receive a blood transfusion at that time?

当时输血了吗?

Patient：Yes，they gave me 400cc of fresh blood.

是的,输了400毫升的血。

Doctor：And do you know what was the cause (reason) of the bleeding?

你知道出血原因吗?

Patient：I was told that the placenta remained in the uterus for more than 30 minutes.

我听说是因为胎盘滞留在子宫中时间太长,超过30分钟吧。

Doctor：I'll give you an examination. The fetus is in a good position and the head is deeply engaged. The fetal heart is strong and the beat is regular. There is slight bleeding from the vagina. You are now in the preliminary stage of labor. Don't worry about the bleeding. You should stay in the hospital for observation. And labor will start later on…

我给你检查一下。胎儿位置很好,头位已经固定,胎心搏动规律、有力。阴道有少量出血,你已经临产了,不用担心。你该住院观察了,很快就会生的……

Doctor：Do you feel the contractions regularly?

你觉得宫缩有规律了吗?

Patient：Yes，they have been regular since 9 o'clock this morning.

从今天早上9点钟就开始规律了。

Doctor：How long is the interval between two contractions, and how many minutes does it last?

那两次宫缩间隔几分钟? 每次持续多长时间呢?

Patient：I don't know.

我不太清楚。

Doctor：I'll do you a rectal examination. It will make you a little uncomfortable. Oh, the cervix is open about five centimeters. Your baby will be delivered today.

我给你做个肛查，可能会有点不舒服。噢，宫口已经开了五厘米了。你今天可能就要生了。

Patient：Really? I hope so.

真的吗？但愿能早点生。

4. Dysmenorrhea 痛经

Patient：Doctor, my next period is due to start in a few days, but I have cramps already. I have been suffering from cramps every mouth for the last eight years. I always feel awful just before my period.

医生，我的月经还有几天才来，但是肚子现在就开始痛起来了。已经八年了，每月都这样，每次来月经前我都很害怕。

Doctor：Are you a student?

你是个学生吗？

Patient：Yes, I'm a medical student. I have severe premenstrual pain, so that I can hardly concentrate on my studies.

是的，我是医学院的学生，我的经前疼痛很严重，这种疼痛很影响我学习。

Doctor：How many days does the pain last?

疼痛持续几天？

Patient：It lasts for three to five days and disappears on the 2nd day of periods.

一般要疼个三到五天，来月经的第二天就不疼了。

Doctor：Do you have severe headaches?

伴随有头痛的症状吗？

Patient：Yes, I have headaches, but not too bad.

有，但是疼得不厉害。

Doctor：Do you have pains in your back or stomach?

腰部、胃部疼吗？

Patient：I have backaches and my legs feel heavy. My whole body feels swollen.

是的,腰疼,腿发沉。另外我还觉得全身发胀。

Doctor：Then probably your legs are also a bit swollen.

那你的腿也一定有点肿吧。

Patient：Yes, is it serious, doctor?

是的,严重吗?

Doctor：Well, in your case you suffer from so-called dysmenorrhea accompanied by premenstrual stress.

嗯,你患的是痛经,还有经前紧张综合征。

Patient：Is there any medicine for it?

可以治吗?

Doctor：Let's try some hormone extracts or some medicine for muscle relaxation, diuresis and analgesics.

我们试着用激素类药物,也可以用些松弛肌肉的药、利尿剂和止疼药。

Patient：Is there any herbal medicine for it?

吃中药管用吗?

Doctor：Oh，there are several kinds of Chinese traditional medicines, and acupuncture works also.

噢,有几种中药管用,针灸治疗也行。

Patient：I prefer getting acupuncture, doctor.

医生,我愿意针灸治疗。

Doctor：That's all right. I will give you acupuncture treatments.

那好吧。我来给你针灸。

Patient：I feel much better after acupuncture. Thank you.

针灸后感觉很舒服了,谢谢你。

5. Postpartum Hypogalactia 产后缺乳

Patient：Doctor, it's been a week since the baby was born, and I don't have sufficient milk.

医生,生完孩子一周了,奶水少。

Doctor：Cesarean delivery or natural delivery? Did you bleed a lot? How about the amount of lochia? Have you experienced postpartum depression? Are your breasts swelling and painful? How about the color of the milk? Does it look thick and sticky or just thin and clear? How about your body constitution? Have you ever suffered from anemia? Do you mind that if I give you a breast palpation?

请问是剖宫产还是顺产？生产时出血多吗？现在恶露多不多？有没有产后情绪不好？乳房有没有胀痛？乳汁什么颜色？稠厚的还是清稀的？平时体质怎么样？以前有过贫血吗？是否能接受给你做个乳房触诊？

Patient：I gave birth by natural delivery. There wasn't much bleeding. There is little lochia now. But I can't sleep very well, and I feel a little depressed. My breasts usually feel swelling and painful; sometimes my temperature will be abnormal, with 38. 3℃ being the peak. The color of the milk is white. My constitution is all right, and I haven't suffered from anemia. You can give me a breast palpation.

是顺产,生孩子时出血不多。现在恶露也不多。有时候睡眠不好,确实情绪上有点低落。乳房胀痛,有时候体温不正常,最高38.3℃。乳汁是白色的,平时体质还好,以前没有贫血。你可以给我做个乳房检查。

Doctor：Both breasts are swollen and hard. How is your diet situation? How is your appetite? Let me see your tongue, and feel your pulse.

双侧乳房胀硬。你饮食怎么样？有食欲吗？我看看你的舌苔,把把脉。

Patient：I have no appetite.

不想吃饭,没有食欲。

Doctor：OK. Your tongue fur is all right, thin and yellowish fur, thready and slippery pulse. You are suffering from postpartum hypogalactia, which can be dialectically diagnosed as liver depression and qi stagnation. It can be treated with Chinese medicine and external application.

好的。舌质正常,苔薄黄,脉弦滑。你患的是产后缺乳,辨证为肝郁气滞证,服用中药加外敷综合治疗。

Patient：OK，please write out the prescription，and I will fetch the medicine.

好的，你给我开方吧，我去拿药。

6. Postmenopausal Syndromes 绝经前后诸症

Doctor：Do you have other symptoms? Is your back sour? Do you have bitter taste and dry throat? How about your defecation and urination? Have your ever done any physical examination?

别的还有什么不舒服吗？腰背酸困吗？口干口苦有没有？大便小便怎么样？做过什么检查吗？

Patient：I can feel my back sour，my eyes dry，my taste bitter and my throat dry. I am fearful of cold as well as heat. Sometimes my skin feels dry and itchy. I have constipation and my urine looks yellowish. I have done the color Doppler ultrasound examination，and it reveals that the size of my womb is normal，but the endometrium seems to be thin. I also had six endocrine index examinations，which shows the estrogen level is low，the other indexes being normal.

腰背酸困，眼睛干涩，口干口苦，怕冷又怕热。皮肤有时候干痒。大便干，小便有点黄。做过彩超，结果说是"子宫大小正常，内膜薄"。查内分泌六项，雌激素水平低，检查其他的都正常。

Doctor：OK. Your tongue is red with less white coating, and your pulse is weak. You are suffering from postmenopausal syndromes plus previous menopausal syndromes. You can take hormone by means of western medicine therapy to relieve your discomfort.

好的。看你舌红少苔，脉细数，你患的是绝经前后诸症，加上先前的更年期综合征，可以服用西药激素缓解不适。

Patient：I don't want to take the hormone. Can I use the Chinese medicine treatment?

我不想服用激素，能否服用中药治疗一下呢？

Doctor：Yes. In Chinese medicine your symptoms can be diagnosed as deficiency of yin bringing about the interior heat syndrome. You can take the medicine which can nourish yin and clear heat.

可以的,中医是阴虚内热证,可以服用滋阴清热的中药。

Patient:OK, thank you.

好的,谢谢你。

Ⅱ. Sentences 替换句型

(1) What troubles(problems), such as dizziness, nausea, vomiting, headache or blurring of your vision, did you have during this pregnancy?

你这次怀孕出现过像头晕、恶心、呕吐、头痛或视力模糊等现象吗?

(2) I'm suffering from nausea and vomiting. I can't take any food or even water, especially in the morning.

我恶心想吐,特别是早晨,吃不成东西,连水也喝不了。

(3) Nausea started about three weeks ago, but wasn't so severe. I have been suffering from terrible nausea and vomiting this week, and I feel very weak.

我恶心大概有三个星期了,但不是太厉害。可从这个星期起,我又恶心又吐,感到身体很虚。

(4) Are you trying to eat? If you want to be relieved, try to eat something that can be easily digested, in small amounts, and intermittently. It's better for you to keep something in your stomach. Besides, you are now at the end of your third month of pregancy, so this malaise will soon be over.

你试着吃点东西吗? 你要是不想吐,你必须得试着不停地、少量地吃点易消化的食物。胃里有东西了,自然就不恶心了。另外,你现在怀孕都快三个月了,妊娠反应很快就过去了。

(5) I try to eat, but I immediately throw up, especially, I feel like vomiting even when I smell the food.

我试着吃点,但很快就吐了,尤其是一闻到食品的味道就想吐。

(6) In that case, the cold but not greasy food is much better for you. That's true, it's always worse in the morning, therefore, you'd better have some snacks ready so you can take a bit if you wake up at night.

要是这样的话,你吃点清淡的冷食会好些。是的,孕吐往往是早晨厉害些,因此你最好备些零食,晚上醒时可以吃点。

（7）In that case, I'll give you a glucose infusion at once, but you should try to take some food yourself. Anyway, we can give injection of vitamins, glucose, or some antiementic drugs, if necessary. Morning sickness is one of the discomforts you must face when becoming a mother. It's calculated that about 80% pregnant women have different degrees of morning sickness. On the other hand, if you can't bear (endure, stand) it, I can give you a shot or admit you to the hospital (to stay in the hospital).

如果是这样的话,我就给你静脉点滴葡萄糖了,但你自己也还是要想办法吃的。我们可以给你注射些维生素、葡萄糖,必要时让你吃些止吐药。孕吐是成为母亲时必须面对的不适之一。据统计80%的孕妇都有不同程度的孕吐现象。你要是真的受不了,也可以打针或住院。

（8）I've had a headache since yesterday. And, doctor, my feet have been swollen for a week. In the past two days, it has become (turned) worse, besides, my fingers have become swollen, too.

医生,我的头从昨天起就开始疼了。而且,我的脚已经肿胀一个星期了,尤其这两天,肿得更厉害了,手也有些肿了。

（9）I'll take your blood pressure firstly. It's 160/90 mmHg (21.3/1.2 kPa). In addition to this bleeding, your eyelids are swollen seriously, too. You must(had better) stay in the hospital and receive proper treatments.

我先给你量个血压吧。160/90毫米汞柱(21.3/1.2千帕)。除了阴道出血,我看你的眼皮也肿得厉害。你必须(最好)住院进行治疗。

（10）Please give some urine for a routine examination. Your urine albumin is positive with two plus. And you have high pressure, edema and albumin checked in your urine, too. It is called toxemia of pregnancy, a complication produced(made) by(along with) pregnancy itself. You should omit salt from your diet. Appropriate treatment is needed, so I advise you to be (should be) admitted to the hospital immediately. Otherwise you are at risk (in danger, it may become worse).

留点尿做个常规检查。尿蛋白两个加号。高血压、水肿、蛋白尿,你得了妊娠毒血症,也就是由怀孕本身引起的并发症。你应该忌盐,而且马上住院接受治疗,否则的话,会危及生命。

(11) Doctor, I missed two periods already, but I have some bleeding today, and together with some pain in the lower abdomen.

医生,我已经两个月没来月经了,今天阴道突然有点出血,而且下腹部疼痛。

(12) How many pregnancies have you had?

你怀过几次孕?

(13) I had only one abortion three years ago, but no child.

三年前只流过一次产,现在还没孩子。

(14) When did you start menstruation? And what is the amount of your bleeding? Is it profuse or not? And when was your last period?

你的初潮是什么时候? 你经血量怎样,多吗? 你末次月经是什么时候?

(15) The bleeding is quite heavy (so much), so I change my pads almost every hour, but there isn't any pain.

经血量很多,几乎每小时得换一次卫生巾,但是肚子不疼。

(16) My menstruation is regular (normal) now, but it used to be somewhat (a little, slight) late before I was (got) married.

我结婚前月经经常错后,不过现在正常了。

(17) The pregnancy test is positive, now tell me please where the pain is and what it's like?

你的妊娠检验是阳性的,现在跟我说说你什么地方疼,怎么个疼法呢?

(18) The pain occurs in the central part of my lower abdomen, and it comes in attacks. Each attack lasts for only several minutes and is accompanied with (together with, along with) vaginal bleeding while the pain lasts.

下腹部中间一阵一阵地疼,每次疼痛都持续几分钟,阴道还出血。

(19) The bleeding is more severe than usual and the attacks of pain recur every five to eight minutes.

出血量增多,阵发性腹痛五到八分钟一次。

(20) The cervix is already open about six centimeters. And part of the fetus can be seen in the cervix. The fetus will come out soon. I'll prepare the blood for you in case a blood transfusion is needed. I

say, you should be admitted to the hospital immediately.

宫口已开六厘米,而且可见胎头了。马上住院准备生产,还要备够足够的血液以备失血时输用。

（21） It seems that you are pregnant with threatened miscarriage (abortion), and sexual intercourse is forbidden in order for you to remain pregnant. And you should also stay in bed except for taking some medicine, eating or going to the toilet. Remember to go to the emergency clinic immediately whenever the bleeding is (turns, becomes) much more severe than usual.

你有先兆流产的迹象。要想保胎,除服药、吃饭、上厕所外,要绝对卧床休息,避免性生活。如果出血量增多,请立即来看急诊。

（22） I have had lower abdominal pains off and on in recent three months ever since the abortion. And the vaginal discharge has been a little more profuse than before with an unpleasant odor.

从上次流产过后,我的下腹部已经时不时疼痛三个月了,阴道分泌物比以前多,而且还有味儿。

（23） What's the colour and the character of your discharge? Is there any unpleasant odor?

你的分泌物是什么样、什么颜色的? 有什么特殊的气味吗?

（24） I had gushes of vaginal discharge this morning. It's yellow, thick and creamy, but has no special odor. Since I don't feel quite well, I think perhaps something is wrong.

今早我发现阴道有一股分泌物流出,黄色、稠奶酪样的,虽没什么怪味儿,但我感觉不舒服,我想肯定有什么事了。

（25） Is your vagina itching and burning, or do you have any pain in your vagina?

你的阴道疼、痒,有灼烧感吗?

（26） Has recently there been any change in your menstruation?

你的月经最近有什么变化吗?

（27） Usually my periods last about a week and they seem heavy. Sometimes there are clots. During my period, I feel a lot of pain.

我的月经一般持续一周左右,量很多。有时有血块。在整个经期我都感到疼痛。

（28） Is your menstruation normal? And have you ever had any female diseases, such as pelvic inflammation, cervicitis or polyp of the cervix, etc.?

月经正常吗？你以前得过妇科病吗，比如盆腔炎、宫颈炎、宫颈息肉等？

(29) Empty your bladder and I'll give you a pelvic examination. Please take off your shoes and panties, lie down on the examining table. Oh, you have a typical vaginal moniliosis. Wait, I'll take some of your discharge for examination under the microscope… Oh, typical monilia are found. But don't worry, since it can be cured with proper suppositories. Every evening, put one suppository into your vagina after washing and continue to do the same just for two weeks. Then come back for a check-up three days after you have finished the medicine.

请排空膀胱，脱了鞋和内裤，躺到床上去，我给你做个内查。哦，像是典型的阴道念珠菌感染。等会儿，我取点分泌物再做个显微镜检查……哦，果然是的，镜下可见念珠菌。不过不要紧的，使用合适的栓剂的话，这病可以治愈。回去后每晚清洗后阴道内放一粒栓剂，持续两周给药。停药三天后再来复诊一次。

(30) Doctor, my periods have always been irregular. And it's so terrible that I have had vaginal bleeding for eight days beginning (starting from) five days after the last period ended. Although the problem is somewhat improved after I have received many treatments, both Chinese traditional and western medicine, yet, the trouble recurred frequently.

医生，我的月经周期紊乱。从上次月经过后的第五天开始我又出血了，到今天已经八天了。虽然我中西医都看过，病情有所好转，可老是反复发作。

(31) I'm having a lot of trouble with my periods. And I have dizzy spells when I get up.

我来月经时很不舒服。而且起床时感觉一阵一阵地头晕。

(32) Doctor, my periods became irregular too within the last three months. Bleeding was heavy and always lasted up to one or two weeks, and sometimes it was delayed for 20 to 30 days.

医生，我的月经周期最近三个月也总不规律，出血量多，而且持续时间长,有时长达一两个星期,甚至有时还后推二三十天才来。

(33) Doctor,I have borne no child since my marriage eight years ago. And my periods are not regular,they are always half a month or one month late,the bleeding is scanty too. In the past three months,the amount of blood lost has diminished to about one-third of previous (former) periods. And besides,for no reason,I have gained weight for the last six months.

医生,我结婚八年来没生过小孩。我的月经周期非常不准,常常晚来半个月或一个月,经血量也少。而且最近三个月少得只有过去的三分之一。莫名其妙的是,我近半年来体重增加不少。

(34) Mostly,the sterility(infertility) is due to the husband,whose sperm is perhaps normal in number and activity,but with more abnormality rate. Then,how about the health of your husband? And has your husband had his semen examined?

大多数的不孕症原因在丈夫身上,比如他的精子数量、活性正常,可是畸形率很高。那么你丈夫健康状况如何? 是否查过精液呢?

(35) Firstly,I'll give you an injection once a day for three days,after that come back and I'll give you a thorough examination,including a pelvic examination,vaginal smear for estrogen,cervical mucus and BBT at the same time. Now,in my opinion,it's probably what is called the functional uterine bleeding and hormone imbalance may be the cause of the bleeding. Then we'll find out for sure (certain) what the problem (your trouble) is. In that case, it's surely cured(treated) with hormone,so take it easy.

你先打三天的针,每天一针。三天后来做个全面的检查,有盆腔检查,阴道涂片雌激素水平检查,再查个宫颈,测个基础体温。现在我怀疑是内分泌失调型功能性子宫出血,等彻底查完了,可用激素治愈,这一点你放心。

(36) Before the birth of my child,my periods always came with a regular 30-day-interval. But I don't know why my periods have changed (become) so irregular after the delivery,sometimes three days earlier,and sometimes five or six days later,and even one month late.

生小孩儿前我月经还挺正常的,30 天来一次。生完孩子后,也不知道什么原因月经非常没有规律了,有时提前三天,有时错后五六天,有时甚至还晚来一个月呢。

(37) Doctor, I have been feeling (have had; have touched) a mass (masses) on the left side (right side, both sides) of the lower part of my abdomen for almost three months, and it (they) has (have) grown (turned, become) bigger (larger) than before, I think.

医生,已经有三个月了,我的左(右、两侧)腹部能摸到肿块,最近感觉又长得特别快。

(38) When it started it was the size of an egg (apple, orange) and became as big as the head of a newborn baby in the last four weeks. It's soft and quite movable from side to side.

开始时还像鸡蛋(橘子、苹果)那么大,可短短四个星期就长得像小孩儿头这么大了,摸上去软软的,还会动来动去的。

(39) You have an ovarian cyst (an ovarian tumor). Look, there is a mass beside the uterus in the right quadrant, about eight centimeters in diameter. It's quite movable, when I touched it just now you said there was no pain.

是卵巢囊肿(肿瘤)。看,在子宫右侧区域有个直径大约八厘米的肿块,刚才我摸时,活动性很好,而且你说也不疼。

(40) It's an abortion after a pregancy of two months. Since the fetus didn't come out completely, the doctor had to operate on me. Afterwards, I had a low grade fever about 37.5 to 37.9℃ for almost half a month. They gave me some injections and the temperature returned (withdrew) to normal.

我怀孕两个月时,不完全流产,医生只得给我做清宫手术。术后在37.5—37.9℃之间低烧持续近半个月,后来打了一些针烧才退。

(41) The menstruation is controlled by sex hormones. During breast feeding, the human prolactin inhabits (prohibits, adjust) the production of estrogen and progesterone which regulate your menstruation. I think you had better stop the breat feeding now, and then your periods will soon be regular. Otherwise, you may come back for a check-up.

我想你现在最好能给孩子断奶,这样你的月经周期会很快恢复,因为妇女的月经是由性激素来控制调节的,可是在哺乳期间,身体中的催乳素会抑制雌激素和孕酮的产生,而二者可以调控月经。孩子断奶后,如果效果不理想,你再来复查。

(42) That is impossible for me to be pregnant, since my husband hasn't been with me for more than three months. So I think stopping breast feeding perhaps is a good way for me, and now I don't worry about missing my periods anymore.

我丈夫不在家已经三个多月了,所以怀孕是不可能的。医生,我现在不担心月经不来的问题了,我想也该给孩子断奶了。

(43) What methods of contraception have you used before, contraceptive pills or an intrauterine device?

你以前用过什么避孕方法,口服避孕药还是放节育环呢?

(44) Commonly speaking, contraceptive pills don't have any side effects, except for those who suffer from diabetes or liver troubles. And tell me how far apart your menstrual cycles are, then I'll provide you with some pills and explain how to take them.

一般来说,口服避孕药没什么毒副作用,但是肝病、糖尿病人应慎用。请告诉我你两次月经之间一般相隔多少天,然后我给你开药,跟你说怎么服用。

(45) I'll give you enough pills for twenty-two days. The day that your menstruation starts is counted (regarded) as the first day of the cycle, remember to take one pill each day from the fifth day and for twenty-two days thereafter. And once you stop taking it, the ovulation will be normal, and of course, your natural menstruation cycle resumes.

我给你开了 22 天的药量。记住来月经的第一天是一个服药周期的第一天,你从第五天开始每天服一片,连续服用 22 天。当然,一旦停药,排卵、月经周期就都会恢复正常。

(46) To get more effections, you'd better take it in the evening before sleep. Anyhow you will (must) take it regularly, or it will be ineffective. And it's normal your period will start one or two days after you have stopped taking it. Then the day is again counted as the first day of the cycle and on the fifth day after that you will resume taking the pills.

记住每天晚上睡觉前按时口服,不能漏服,这样避孕效果才会更好。停药一两天月经就会来,这可又是新一个服药周期的第一天,还是像从前一样,从第五天开始服药。

(47) A woman cannot rely on the safe period of birth control if her periods are irregular.

如果妇女的月经不规则,那么就不能依靠安全期控制生育。

(48) She used to have a lot of pain with her periods, but she doesn't now. She's on the pill.

她过去患有严重的痛经,但是现在不痛了,她正在服避孕药。

(49) Eight patients had been using oral contraception.

这八个病人一直采用口服避孕法。

(50) We cannot do this treatment if you are menstruating.

如果你正在月经期间,我们就不能做这种治疗了。

(51) The woman had been complaining of regular contractions for some hours. Twelve hours after admission a baby was born. Dr. Sayers lifted the baby onto the scales.

这名女性抱怨说她有规律宫缩已经几个小时了。住院 12 小时以后,孩子出生了。塞耶斯医生把婴儿抱到体重器上称重。

(52) Did you have any complications when your other babies were born?

你生其他孩子时有并发症吗?

(53) She has three months to go yet before her baby is due.

她的预产期还有三个月。

(54) She must have her baby in hospital as she has had four miscarriages.

她必须在医院生孩子,因为她已经流产四次了。

(55) Pregnant women are often sick in the early morning in the first trimester.

妊娠最初三个月孕妇通常会在清晨恶心。

(56) Both children and adults, especially pregnant women, frequently have infections of the urinary tract.

儿童和成人,特别是孕妇经常患有尿道感染。

(57) The majority of pregnant women are probably still given iron tablets whether they are needed or not.

不管需要与否,大多数孕妇仍在服用补铁剂。

（58）Women with a history of menstrual dysfunction may be predisposed to amenorrhoea when contraceptive medication is discontinued.

有月经不调病史的女性停吃避孕药之后易出现闭经。

（59）I'll make an appointment for you and do a special test to see whether your tubes are blocked or not.

我给你约个时间，做个输卵管检查，看是不是堵塞。

（60）Women whose growth has been stunted and whose health has been impaired by malnutrition during childhood may be irreparably damaged by the time they reach motherhood.

童年因营养不良而生长受阻、健康受损的女性做母亲时可能难免会受到损害。

Ⅲ. Words and Expressions 单词和短语

abortion /əˈbɔːʃən/；miscarriage /ˈmɪskærɪdʒ/ n. 流产

amnion /ˈæmniən/ n. 羊膜

amniotic fluid 羊水

annexitis /æˈneksaɪtɪs/ n. 附件炎

bartholin gland 前庭大腺

birth /bɜːθ/ n. 生产；分娩；出生

birth canal 产道

breast /brest/ n. 乳房

breech presentation 骨盆端位（臀位）

cancer /ˈkænsə/ n.；carcinoma /ˌkɑːsɪˈnəumə/ n.；malignant newgrowth 癌

catheterization /ˌkæθɪtəraɪˈzeɪʃən/ n. 尿管插入

cervical catarrh 颈管炎

cervical dilatation 宫颈扩张

cervix tear 宫颈撕裂

cervix uteri 子宫颈

cesarean section 剖宫产

chorioepithelioma /ˌkɔːriːəuˌepɪˌθiːliˈəumə/ n. 绒毛膜上皮癌

climacteric bleeding 更年期出血

corpus luteum；yellow body of ovary 黄体

corpus uteri 宫体

decidua /dɪˈsɪdjuə/ n. 脱膜

deformity /dɪˈfɔːməti/ n. 畸形

descensus uteri 子宫下垂

dry nurse 保姆

eclampsia of pregnancy 子痫

edema of pregnancy 妊娠浮肿

endometritis /ˌendəumɪˈtraɪtɪs/ n. 子宫内膜炎

endometrium /ˌendəuˈmiːtriəm/ n. 子宫内膜

ergot /ˈɜːgət/ n. 麦角

erosion of cervix; cervical erosion 宫颈口糜烂

external urethral ostium 宫外口

extrauterine pregnancy 宫外孕

fallopian tube 输卵管

fetal heart sound 胎心音

follicular hormone 卵泡激素

fomentation /ˌfəumenˈteɪʃən/ n. 热敷

foot position 足位

forceps delivery 产钳分娩

forceps /ˈfɔːseps/ n. 产钳

functional uterus bleeding 子宫功能出血

genitals /ˈdʒenɪtlz/ n. 外生殖器

gravid uterus; pregnant uterus 妊娠子宫

gynecology /ˈɡaɪnəˈkɒlədʒi/ n. 妇科学

hematosalpinx /heməˈtəuzælpɪŋks/ n. 输卵管血肿

housewife /ˈhauswaɪf/ n. 家庭主妇

hydramnion /haɪˈdræmnɪɒn/ n. 羊水过多

hyperemesis /ˌhaɪpərˈemɪsɪs/ n.; vomiting of pregnancy 妊娠呕吐

hypogastric region 下腹部

incomplete abortion 不全流产

infant /ˈɪnfənt/ n. 新生儿

interruption of the pregnancy 中断妊娠

intoxication of the pregnancy 妊娠中毒

labium /ˈleɪbiəm/ n. 阴唇

labor pains; delivery pains 阵缩

lactation /lækˈteɪʃn/ n.; breast-feeding 哺乳

laminary tent 断头屏障

laparoscope /ˈlæpərəˌskəup/ n. 腹腔镜

laparoscopy /ˌlæpəˈrɒskəpi/ n. 腹腔镜检查

laparotomy /ˌlæpəˈrɒtəmi/ n. 剖腹手术

lochia /ˈlɒkiə/ n. 恶露

mammary gland 乳腺

mammilla /mæˈmɪlə/ n. 乳头

mastitis /mæsˈtaɪtɪs/ n. 乳腺炎

meconium /mɪˈkəuniəm/ n. 胎粪

menses /ˈmensiːz/; menstruation /ˌmenstruˈeɪʃn/ n. 月经期

micturition /ˌmɪktjuˈrɪʃn/ n. 排尿

midwife /ˈmɪdwaɪf/ n. 助产士

mother milk 母乳

multipara /mʌlˈtɪpərə/; pluripara /pluˈrɪpərə/ n. 经产妇

myoma of uteri 子宫肌瘤

navel cord 脐带

neonatal cephalohematoma 新生儿血肿

neonatal icterus 新生儿黄疸

nullipara /nʌˈlɪpərə/ n. 未产妇

obstetrics /əbˈstetrɪks/ n. 产科学

occipital position 枕位

ovarian cyst 卵巢囊肿

ovarian hypofunction 输卵管功能减退

ovariotomy /əuˌveərɪˈɒtəmi/ n. 卵巢摘除术

ovary /ˈəuvəri/ n. 卵巢

parametritis /ˌpærəmɪˈtraɪtɪs/ n. 宫周炎

pelvis /ˈpelvɪs/ n. 骨盆

pelvis-peritonitis 盆腔腹膜炎

perineal tear 会阴裂伤

perineum /ˌperɪˈniːəm/ n. 会阴

perineum support 保护会阴

placental forceps 胎盘钳

placenta /pləˈsentə/ n. 胎盘

position of head 头位

pregnancy /ˈpregnənsi/；gestation /dʒeˈsteɪʃn/； conception /kənˈsepʃn/ *n.* 受孕

pregnancy kidney 妊娠肾

premature birth 早产

pubic hair 阴毛

puerperal fever 产褥热

retroflexion uteri 子宫后倾

rotation /rəʊˈteɪʃən/ *n.* 转胎术

rupture of the womb 子宫破裂

salpingitis /ˌsælpɪnˈdʒaɪtɪs/ *n.* 输卵管炎

salpingography /ˌsælpɪŋˈgɒgrəfi/ *n.* 输卵管造影术

salpingo-oophorectomy 输卵管卵巢摘除术

sign of pregnancy 妊娠表现

sterility /stəˈrɪləti/ *n.* 不孕症

still birth 死产

supravaginal amputation of uterus 颈上宫摘术

tape measure 带尺

threatened abortion 危险流产

throes /θrəʊz/ *n.*； labour pains； travail /ˈtræveɪl/ *n.* 阵痛

total extirpation of uterus 子宫全摘

toxemia of pregnancy/hypertensive state of pregnancy 妊娠中毒症/妊娠高血压

transverse presentation 横位

tubal pregnancy 输卵管妊娠

tubal sterillization；tubal ligation 输卵管结扎术

twin /twɪn/ *n.* 双生儿

uterine artery 子宫动脉

uterine glands 子宫腺

uterine speculum 宫镜

uterus /ˈjuːtərəs/ *n.* 子宫

vagina /vəˈdʒaɪnə/ *n.* 阴道

washing /ˈwɒʃɪŋ/ *n.* 洗涤

wet nurse 乳母

Section 5　Urology
第 5 节　泌尿科

I. Dialogue 情景对话

1. Acute Pyelonephritis 急性肾盂肾炎

Patient：Doctor, I feel much pain when urinating.
　　　　医生，我排尿时感觉很痛。

Doctor：How long have you had it?

有多久了?

Patient：About two or three days.

大概有两三天了。

Doctor：What kind of pain is it?

是什么样的疼痛?

Patient：It's a kind of burning pain. It seems to be getting worse.

是一种烧灼痛。而且好像越来越严重。

Doctor：Any other symptoms?

还有其他什么症状吗?

Patient：I have a terrible headache and a backache. I feel feverish and shivery. I also want to pass water more often than usual.

我的头和腰疼得也厉害。我有时发烧有时发冷。另外,我还有尿频现象。

Doctor：How many times do you have to pass urine each day?

你每天排尿次数多少呢?

Patient：I can't say. Almost hourly.

我说不清。几乎每小时一次吧。

Doctor：Have you any blood in your urine?

你尿里带血吗?

Patient：I don't know.

我也不知道。

Doctor：You may have an acute pyelonephritis, a kind of urinary tract infection. And I want a routine urine and a mid-stream clear catch urinalysis. I'll also send a urine specimen for culture and sensitivity.

你可能得的是急性肾盂肾炎,是一种尿路感染。你要先去取个中段尿液,做个尿常规检查。再送个尿标本做培养和敏感试验。

Patient：What shall I do?

我该怎么办呢?

Doctor：Don't worry. You should rest in bed and drink plenty of water. You need injections and also some tablets.

别着急。你应卧床休息,多喝水,接受一些注射和口服药物。

Patient：When should I come back?

我什么时候再来复诊呢?

Doctor：I would like to see you in three days. If the symptoms get worse, come to the emergency clinic immediately.

三天后再来吧。如果病情加重,你就马上来看急诊。

Patient：OK, thank you, doctor.

好的,谢谢你,医生。

2. Chronic Prostatitis 慢性前列腺炎

Patient：I have not been feeling well for some time, doctor, and I seem to be losing my usual pep and vigor.

医生,我最近一段时间感到精神和体力好像都不行了。

Doctor：I beg your pardon. I didn't quite get you. Please speak more slowly, I know only a little English.

请你再说一遍好吗,我没有完全听懂你的话,请你讲得慢一点,我的英文不太好。

Patient：Oh, I am sorry, doctor. I mean, I seem to get tired very easily and feel discomfort in the lower abdomen, the back and the penis, and I have noticed a gradual loss of sexual desire over the past few months.

对不起,医生。我是说我这段时间,总是感到很疲劳,下腹部、腰部和小便的地方不舒服。同时我还发现近几个月性欲逐渐减退。

Doctor：Have you ever noticed a creamy discharge at the end of your penis before you begin to urinate in the morning?

你早晨小便时是否注意到小便口上有白色分泌物?

Patient：Yes, I have. What do you think is the matter, doctor?

有,医生这是怎么回事呢?

Doctor：I suspect that you might have chronic prostatitis. In order to make sure, I think you should have a three-glass urine test made as well as an examination of the prostatic secretion.

我想你可能得了慢性前列腺炎。为了进一步明确给你诊断,你要去做一下尿三杯试验,还要做前列腺液检查。

Patient：How can I do these?

怎样做呢?

Doctor：Now，I'll do a rectal examination for you to take the prostatic secretion for microscopic examination. Well，I'll tell you how to do it. Take three bottles to the bathroom when you pass urine，put a little at the beginning in one bottle，then a little at the middle in the second bottle，and then a little at the end in the third bottle. Send the specimens to the laboratory，then come back.

现在我先给你做一个肛门检查，取点前列腺分泌液做一个显微镜下检查。然后我告诉你下一步怎么做：你拿三个尿瓶子到厕所去，排尿时，取开始的一点尿放在第一个瓶子里，中段的尿放在第二个瓶子里，末段的尿接到第三个瓶子里。将这些标本送到化验室后再回来。

Patient：What did you find on the examination，doctor?

医生，检查发现什么了吗？

Doctor：We found a lot of white cells and clumping of leukocytes of your prostatic secretion. The urine also contains a lot of white blood cells in the first portion of the urine.

是的，检查发现你的前列腺液中有相当多的白细胞，甚至有白细胞丛生现象。在你的第一段尿检盘中同样也发现了白细胞。

Patient：What do you think is the matter?

这些又说明了什么问题呢？

Doctor：These findings support my primary diagnosis.

这些检查结果都证实了我的初步诊断。

Patient：Is it serious?

严重吗？

Doctor：No，if we can manage it properly.

不太严重，不过如果能正确处理那就更不用担心了。

Patient：Please tell me what should be done.

那就请告诉我该怎样治疗吧。

Doctor：I'll give you antibacterial treatment，but prostatic massage and hip baths are probably even more important. Chinese medicine will do you good too.

我给你用抗生素治疗，但是前列腺按摩和热水坐浴也很重要。中药对你这病的治疗很有好处。

Patient：Any other things I should do?

我还有什么其他需要注意的吗？

Doctor：If possible, alcoholic beverages and spicy food should be avoided. Normal frequency of sexual intercourse is not considered harmful since it promotes emptying of the prostate.

如有可能,尽量避免饮酒和吃刺激性的食物。正常的性交没有任何坏处,它反而可以促进前列腺排空。

3. Urinary Tract Infection 泌尿道感染

Parent：Doctor, my baby ran a high temperature suddenly last night and cried all night.

医生,我孩子昨天晚上突然发高烧并且整夜都哭闹。

Doctor：Is there anything else unusual?

还有什么和平时不一样的呢？

Parent：She cries each time she passes water.

她每次小便时都要哭。

Doctor：Does she urinate more often than usual?

她比平时小便次数多吗？

Parent：Yes, very often.

是的,小便次数挺多的。

Doctor：What color is her urine?

尿液是什么颜色的呢？

Parent：It's cloudy.

是混浊的。

Doctor：Please give us a specimen of her urine for a further examination right away.

请你现在就给她留个尿标本去化验一下吧。

Parent：Here is the result, doctor. And is there anything abnormal?

医生,这是化验结果,你看正常吗？

Doctor：Yes, there is, madame. And has she been ill like this before?

有点小问题,夫人。她以前得过这样的病吗？

Parent：No, this is the first time.

没有,这是第一次。

Doctor：I think she is suffering from a urinary tract infection.

她这是泌尿道感染。

Parent：Well，doctor. Will she be all right?

那她能治好吗，医生?

Doctor：Yes，madame. There is nothing to worry about. Give her the medicine regularly and see that she drinks plenty of fluids. Bring her back here in one week.

能治好，夫人，别着急。但是她必须按时服药，大量饮水。一周后带她再来复查吧。

Ⅱ. Sentences 替换句型

(1) I've been having trouble with passing water，doctor. I mean that the stream is weak and doesn't start immediately.

我小便不利，医生。我的意思是尿不通畅，马上还尿不出来。

(2) I have been suffering from it for about half an year. And it seems worse after drinking wine.

大约有半年了，而且每次喝酒后感觉症状加重了些。

(3) Do you have any pain during urination?

你小便时疼吗?

(4) How long have you noticed this discharge?

你发现这种分泌物已经多久了?

(5) Do you pass water more often than you used to?

你排尿比过去更频繁吗?

(6) Have you ever passed any blood in your urine?

你尿里有血吗?

(7) I have passed red-colored urine.

我的尿是红颜色的。

(8) Is this urine red-colored throughout the stream?

排出的尿全都是红色的吗?

(9) How many times a night do you have to pass water?

你一晚上得尿几次?

(10) About five or six times a night. While as for daytime, I think there are at least 15 to 20 times，but each time only a little bit.

晚上一般得尿五六次。可是白天呢,至少要有 15 到 20 次,而每次也就是尿那么一点点。

（11） It's a severe burning sensation all the time I'm passing water, doctor.

医生,我整个排尿过程都有烧灼疼痛感。

（12） Have you noticed any discharge at the tip of your penis before you begin to urinate in the morning?

早晨你起床后排尿时,有没有发现尿道口上有分泌物呢?

（13） We would like to have a urine specimen to examine it, take this paper to the office. The nurse will tell you what to do. Wait for the result please, then come back.

我们想让给你做个尿标本检查,你拿着这张化验单到化验室去。那儿的护士会告诉你怎样做的。等化验结果出来后你再到我这儿来。

（14） I think you have a prostatic hypertrophy（prostatitis, a urinary stone）.

有可能你得了前列腺肥大（前列腺炎、泌尿系结石）了。

（15） I'll do a rectal examination for you. Don't be afraid. Please undress and lie in a knee-chest position.

我给你做一下直肠检查。不要紧张,脱去裤子,跪着趴下。

（16） Have you ever had syphilis before?

你以前得过梅毒吗?

（17） Have vou ever had a pimple on your penis?

你阴茎上长过疙瘩吗?

（18） Have you had gonorrhea? You must tell me the truth, so that I can treat you properly.

你得过淋病吗? 请你如实告诉我你的病况,这样我才能给你对症治疗。

（19） I've had gonorrhea several years before, but that was cured.

我好几年前得过淋病,而且早已治好了。

（20） Diagnosis is based on the history, physical signs, physical examination and laboratory confirmation of the clinical diagnosis.

诊断建立在病史、体征、身体检查和化验证实临床诊断的基础之上。

（21） In a month's time you will have finished your course of drugs.

再有一个月,你就完成你的药物疗程了。

(22) If you breathe this gas, it will help relieve the pain.

如果你吸入这种气体,它将帮助缓解疼痛。

(23) This drug is used for treating bacterial infections.

这种药物用于治疗细菌性感染。

(24) This new drug does not produce side effects.

这种新药不产生副作用。

(25) They've still not sent us the results of the investigations.

他们还没有把那个观察结果送给我们。

Ⅲ. Words and Expressions 单词和短语

abscess of the kidney; renal abscess 肾脓肿

acute nephritis 急性肾炎

after the act 排尿后

aggravation by movement 运动而加剧

anuria /əˈnjʊəriə/ n. 无尿

attack of acute pain (to groin) 急性痛发作(放射至鼠蹊部)

bladder /ˈblædə/ n. 膀胱

bougie /ˈbuːʒi/ n. 探子

B ultrasonic examination B 超检查

calyx /ˈkeɪlɪks/ n. 肾盂

chronic nephritis 慢性肾炎

cloudy urine 尿混浊

colic /ˈkɒlɪk/ n. 绞痛

contracted kidney 肾萎缩

CT scan CT 扫描

cystic kidney 囊性肾

cystitis /sɪˈstaɪtɪs/ n. 膀胱炎

cystoscope /ˈsɪstəˌskəʊp/ n. 膀胱镜

cystoscopy /sɪsˈtɒskəpi/ n. 膀胱镜检查

diseases of urinary organs 泌尿器疾病

during the act 排尿时

dysuria /dɪsˈjʊəriə/ n. 排尿困难

engorged kidney 肾肿大

enuresis 遗尿症

epididymitis /ˌepɪˌdɪdiˈmaɪtɪs/ n. 附睾炎

eunuchism /ˈjuːnəˌkɪzəm/; anorchidism /æˈnɔːrkɪdɪzəm/ n. 无睾症

filariasis /ˌfɪləˈraɪəsɪs/ n. 丝虫病

floating (wandering) kidney 游走肾

frequency of urination 尿次

glomerulonephritis /ˌglɒmerʊləʊnɪˈfraɪtɪs/ n. 肾小球肾炎

hematuria /ˌhiːməˈtjʊəriə/ n. 血尿

hydrocele testis 阴囊积水

hydronephrosis /ˌhaɪdrəʊnɪˈfrəʊsɪs/ n. 肾积水

hyperplasia of the prostate 前列腺肥大症

incontinence /ɪnˈkɒntɪnəns/ n. 失禁

incontinent /ɪnˈkɒntɪnənt/ adj. 失禁的

inflammation of renal pelvis; pyelitis /ˌpaɪəˈlaɪtɪs/ n. 肾盂炎

kidney /ˈkɪdni/ *n.* 肾

lumbago /lʌmˈbeɪɡəʊ/ *n.* ; pain in the lumbar region 腰痛

masturbation /ˌmæstəˈbeɪʃn/ *n.* 手淫

MRI（magnetic resonance imaging） 核磁成像术

nephritis /nɪˈfraɪtɪs/ *n.* 肾炎

nephrolithiasis /ˌnefrəʊlɪˈθaɪəsɪs/ *n.* 肾结石

nephrolith /ˈnefrəlɪθ/ *n.* 肾石

nephro phthisis; tuberculosis of the kidney 肾结核

nephroptosis /ˌnefrɒpˈtəʊsɪs/ *n.* 肾下垂

nephrosclerosis /nefrəˌskləˈrəʊsɪs/ *n.* 肾硬化症

nephrosis /nɪˈfrəʊsɪs/ *n.* 肾病

oliguria /ˌɒlɪˈɡjʊəriə/ *n.* 尿少

orchitis /ɔːˈkaɪtɪs/ *n.* 睾丸炎

pain in micturition/urination 排尿痛

penis /ˈpiːnɪs/ *n.* 阴茎

phimosis /faɪˈməʊsɪs/ *n.* 包茎

pollakiuria /ˌpɒləkɪˈjʊəriə/ *n.* 尿频

polycystic kidney 多囊肾

polyuria /ˌpɒlɪˈjʊəriə/ *n.* 多尿

prostate /ˈprɒsteɪt/ *n.* 前列腺

pyelography /ˌpaɪəˈlɒɡrəfi/ *n.* 肾盂造影

pyuria /paɪˈjʊəriə/ *n.* 脓尿

renal colic 肾绞痛

renal pelvis 肾盂

retention of urine; uroschesis /jʊərɒˈskiːsɪs/ *n.* 尿潴留

scrotum /ˈskrəʊtəm/ *n.* 阴囊

semen /ˈsiːmen/ *n.* 精液

sperm /spɜːm/ *n.* 精子

tenderness and pain 过敏和痛

tenesmus of the bladder 膀胱里急后重感

testicle pain 睾丸痛

testis /ˈtestɪs/ ; testicle /ˈtestɪkl/ *n.* 睾丸

tuberculosis of bladder; cystophthisis /sɪstəʊˈθaɪsɪs/ *n.* 膀胱结核

tumor of kidney 肾肿瘤

tumor of the bladder 膀胱肿瘤

TV-cystoscope 电视膀胱镜

ulceration of the genitalia 生殖器溃疡

ultrasonic examination 超声波检查

uremia /jʊəˈriːmiə/ *n.* 尿毒症

ureteral colic 尿道绞痛

ureter /jʊˈriːtə/ *n.* 输尿管

urethra /jʊˈriːθrə/ *n.* 尿道

urethral catheterization 导尿法

urethral discharge 尿道病理排泄物

urethritis /ˌjʊərəˈθraɪtɪs/ *n.* 尿道炎

urinary tract 尿路

urine /ˈjʊərɪn/ *n.* 尿

urogenital organ 泌尿生殖器官

urology /jʊəˈrɒlədʒi/ *n.* 泌尿科

venereal warts 性病性疣

vesical hernia 膀胱疝

Section 6　Pediatrics
第6节　小儿科

Ⅰ. Dialogues 情景对话

1. Crying 啼哭

Parent：Doctor，my child cried the whole night. He wouldn't sleep at all，and I don't know what's the matter with him.

医生,我的孩子整夜都哭,一直都不睡觉,我不知道他怎么了。

Doctor：Did he cry in spells? Was there any vomiting? And what about his bowel movement?

他是断断续续地哭吗? 呕吐吗? 另外,他的大便怎样?

Parent：Yes，he cried in spells. He perspired a lot when he cried. He vomited twice. And he had two stools today. They contained undigested food.

是的,他哭一阵,停一阵。哭的时候还出很多汗。吐了两次。今天大便了两次,里面还有一些没消化的食物。

Doctor：I think he cried because of abdominal discomfort. Don't worry，Madame，let me examine him and see what it is.

那他哭的原因可能是因为肚子不舒服。我先给他查查,看看是怎么回事吧。

Parent：All right.

好吧。

Doctor：It's nothing serious. The pain is probably due to indigestion. I'll give him a sedative to quiet him down. Don't give him too much to eat. If he continues to cry，bring him back.

看来没什么大问题,是消化不良引起的啼哭。我给他开一点镇静剂使他安静下来,但是别再给他吃太多东西了。要是他还继续哭,再带他来看看。

Parent：OK，I will. Thank you, doctor.

明白了。医生，谢谢你。

2. Upper Respiratory Tract Infection 上呼吸道感染

Parent：My child is coughing, sneezing and has a running nose, doctor.

医生，我孩子咳嗽，打喷嚏. 流鼻涕。

Doctor：How long has he been ill?

有几天了？

Parent：For two days.

两天了。

Doctor：Does he have a temperature?

发烧吗？

Parent：Yes, it's 38℃.

发烧，38℃。

Doctor：How much has he been coughing? And has he any sputum?

咳得厉害吗？有痰吗？

Parent：No. He has a bad, dry cough, especially at night. He hasn't been sleeping well. Sometimes, he has vomited after coughing.

没有痰。他咳得厉害，是干咳，尤其在晚上。他一直没睡好。有时咳后就吐。

Doctor：Has he a sore throat?

嗓子疼吗？

Parent：Yes. He has difficulty in eating solid foods. He can only drink water.

是的，嗓子疼，吃东西困难，只能喝水。

Doctor：Is anyone else also ill in your family?

家里还有其他人得同样的病吗？

Parent：His sister had it a few days ago.

前几天她妹妹也得了同样的病。

Doctor：Most likely it's a virus infection. I'll give you a prescription. The white tablet is for his fever. Give him one tablet when his temperature is above 38℃，but not more than once every four hours. The other medicine is for his cough. Give him one teaspoonful three times a day. If he is worse, bring him back anytime.

可能是病毒引起的感染。我给你开个处方。白色药片是退热的。若体温超过 38℃,就给他吃一片,但必须间隔四小时以上才能再吃一次。另一种是止咳糖浆,每次一茶匙,一天三次。如果服药后不见好,随时带他来看。

3. Bronchial Asthma, Asthmatic Bronchitis 支气管哮喘、哮喘性支气管炎

Parent：Doctor, my child has been coughing and wheezing for three days. He hasn't been sleeping well at night.

医生,我孩子又咳又喘已经三天了,他晚上也总睡不好觉。

Doctor：Is the cough very bad? Much sputum? Any temperature?

咳嗽得厉害吗? 痰多吗? 发烧吗?

Parent：He has a bad dry cough. At the end of the coughing spell, he has some sputum. He has no temperature.

是干咳,但是咳得非常厉害。咳到最后咳出一些痰。他不发烧。

Doctor：Can he lie flat? And do his lips appear blue?

他能平躺吗? 嘴唇发紫吗?

Parent：When the attack is severe, he can't lie flat. Both his lips and nails appear blue.

他发作厉害时,不能平躺,嘴唇和指甲都发紫。

Doctor：Has he ever had attacks like these before?

他以前有类似的发作吗?

Parent：He has had them for two years.

经常发作已经两年了。

Doctor：Can you tell me what you think his attacks may be related to? Cold? Specific foods? Does he have more in a particular season?

你能告诉我你以为他的发作和什么有关吗? 寒冷? 还是吃过什么特殊食物? 或者他在某个特定季节发作得较频繁呢?

Parent：I really don't know what causes them, doctor.

医生,我真的不知道是什么原因引起的。

Doctor：Did he ever have asthmatic attacks in your country?

他在你们国内时喘过吗?

Parent：Yes，he had some attacks，but now he is getting worse. All the medicines give only a temporary relief. Can you suggest something better for him，doctor?

在我们国家时的确发作过几次，但是现在比以前更严重了。所有的药都只是暂时有效，医生，你有什么更好的办法吗?

Doctor：I think he is allergic to something，and so should be examined in the allergy clinic firstly.

我想他可能是对什么东西过敏，最好先带他去变态反应科检查一下。

4. Pneumonia 肺炎

Parent：Doctor，my child has a temperature and cough for three days. Yesteraday he became much worse.

医生，我孩子发烧咳嗽已经三天了。昨天起好像情况加重了。

Doctor：Has he any difficulty in breathing? And does he complain of chest pains? Does he play as usual?

他呼吸困难吗? 胸痛吗? 还是和平常一样地玩吗?

Parent：He's weak，and can't breathe easily. He looks very pale.

他虚弱无力，呼吸困难，脸色苍白。

Doctor：I'll examine his lungs. Most likely it's pneumonia. Let him have a fluoroscopy check. Yes，he has pneumonia.

我检查一下他的肺部，像是肺炎。给他再做个 X 线检查吧。不错，他得了肺炎。

Parent：Is it serious? Is there any danger，doctor?

病情严重吗? 有危险吗，医生?

Doctor：I think he should be admitted to hospital for further treatment.

我建议他住院治疗。

Parent：I have other children at home. I have to take care of them too. Is it possible to have him treated in the out patient clinic?

我家里还有别的孩子需要我照硕。这孩子如果在门诊部治疗行吗?

Doctor：Yes，I would like to give him penicillin injections twice a day for two days. Is he allergic to penicillin?

没问题,可以的。我要给他注射青霉素,一天两次,共两天。他对青霉素过敏吗?

Parent：No, he isn't. But how should I take care of him at home?

不,他不过敏。可是,在家我应当怎样照顾他呢?

Doctor：It's important for the air to be a little humid, madame. It makes it easier for him to cough up the sputum. If he has difficulty in breathing, raise his head a little bit with a pillow or half-sit him up in bed. Better turn him from side to side once every two to three hours. Give him easily digested food and lots of water to drink. Give him medicine regularly and come back to the clinic for his injections twice a day. If his condition gets worse, bring him back anytime. Otherwise come back to see me the day after tomorrow.

夫人,很重要的一点是要让房间里的空气潮湿一些,这样他的痰比较容易咳出。遇到他呼吸困难时,可以用枕头将他头部抬高一点或是让他采用半坐的卧位。最好每两三个小时给他翻一次身。还要给他吃一些易消化的食物,让他多喝水。记着按时服药,每天到门诊来注射两次药。如果病情不见好转,要随时再带他来看。如果情况还好的话,那就后天再来看一次吧。

5. Infectious Mononucleosis 传染性单核细胞增多症

Doctor：What's wrong with the child?

这孩子怎么了?

Parent：He started to run a temperature four days ago. Yesterday he developed a skin rash. His neck is also swollen.

他四天前就开始发烧了。昨天身上起了疹子,脖子也肿了。

Doctor：Does he have a temperature every day? Is it very high? Does he shiver before the fever? Did you give him any medicine?

他是每天都发烧吗? 烧得高吗? 发烧以前感觉发冷吗? 你还给他吃过什么药吗?

Parent：He has had a temperature every day. It's lower in the morning. Aspirin helped to bring it down, but then it went up again. I didn't give him any medicine except aspirin. And he wasn't shivering any more.

最近几天他每天都发烧，早晨起来低一些，吃完阿司匹林后烧就退了，但是很快就又烧起来了，除阿司匹林以外，我没给他吃过别的什么药。他也不觉得发冷。

Doctor：Is there pain in the neck? Can he move his neck freely? Any other symptoms? Is he very lively? Does he play as usual?

他感觉脖子疼吗？脖子能自如转动吗？另外，他还有什么别的症状吗？他活泼吗？还像平时一样玩吗？

Parent：His neck is a bit swollen, but not painful. He is quite active as usual, but his appetite is not so good.

他脖子有点肿，但是不疼。他还是像平时一样爱玩、好动，只是胃口不怎么好。

Doctor：Are there any other children in the same school or kindergarten with a similar trouble?

在他学校或幼儿园里的孩子中有发现类似的情况吗？

Parent：A few other children are running a temperature, but they do not have skin rashes or swollen necks.

有几个孩子也发烧，但是他们身上都没起疹子，脖子也不肿。

Doctor：Let me examine him. His neck and axillary lymph glands are swollen. His tonsils are enlarged and red with little white spots. His liver and spleen are also slightly enlarged.

我来给他检查一下吧。脖子和腋下淋巴结都肿了；扁桃体又大又红，还有些脓点。还有，他的肝、脾也都有点增大。

Parent：What's wrong with him, doctor?

医生，他得了什么病啊？

Doctor：There are several possibilities, for example, acute purulent tonsilitis, infectious mononucleosis, hepatitis and other diseases. It is necessary to make a few tests. Today we'll do a blood test, and this is the slip. Please take it to the laboratory for a blood test. After that, wait in the sitting room for the result.

有几种可能性，比如急性化脓性扁桃体炎、传染性单核细胞增多症、肝炎或其他的疾病。要确诊的话，还要做几个化验。今天先查个血吧。这是化验单，请带他到化验室去查血，在候诊室等着拿结果。

Parent：Here is the result，doctor．What does it say?

医生,这是化验结果。怎样啊?

Doctor：According to the lab report, he is most probably suffering from infectious mononucleosis．We have to do another blood test to confirm it．Please bring him back tomorrow morning without his breakfast．After the test，he can eat.

根据化验报告,他得的可能是传染性单核细胞增多症。为了明确诊断,还得再做个血化验。请明天早晨空腹再来查血,一定要在取血后再让他吃饭。

Parent：OK，I know.

好的,我知道了。

Doctor：How is your child today? Is he a little better?

今天孩子怎样? 感觉好一些了吗?

Parent：He still has a temperature，doctor，his face looks pale，he is very weak，and his eyes are also red and swollen．The medicine didn't seem to help him．He's been sick for almost one week now．What is the result of the blood test?

医生,他还发烧,面色苍白,也很虚弱,两眼又红又肿的。你开的药看起来对他不怎么有效。他已经病了一个星期了。血化验的结果怎样啊?

Doctor：It shows he's most likely suffering from infectious mononucleosis.

他得的就是传染性单核细胞增多症。

Parent：Is that serious? When will he recover? What should I do?

那严重吗? 什么时候才能好呢? 我该怎么办呢?

Doctor：It's a virus infection．It usually lasts two to four weeks, sometimes even longer．The fever may last one to three weeks. There is no medicine specially effective against virus infection.

这是一种病毒感染。一般需要两到四个星期才能好,有时甚至更长些。发烧可能会持续一到三个星期。对于病毒感染,没有什么特效药物。

Parent：Does he need any medicine more?

那他还需要再吃些药吗?

Doctor：I'll give you some to help lower his fever, increase his appetite and prevent secondary infection.

我给他开点药,帮助降降体温,促进食欲,预防继发感染。

Parent：Should he stay in bed, doctor?

医生,他需要卧床休息吗?

Doctor：Yes, until his temperature is normal, and give him easily digested food to eat and plenty of fluids to drink.

是的,他需要卧床,直到烧退以后才能起床,给他吃些易消化的食物,还要多喝水。

Parent：Is it infectious?

这病传染吗?

Doctor：Yes, but not highly infectious. If possible, try to keep him away from other children.

传染,但不厉害。如果有条件,还是和其他孩子分开好。

Ⅱ. Sentences 替换句型

(1) In that case, you should feed your baby with your own milk and cow's milk together.

要是这样的话,你的孩子应该母乳、牛奶混合喂养。

(2) Have you ever had any serious illness before you gave birth to the baby, such as allergies, liver or kidney troubles (diseases), hypertension, etc. ?

你生这个孩子前,有没有得过严重的,像过敏、肝炎、肾病、高血压这些疾病呢?

(3) It's difficult to examine his abdomen satisfactorily when he cries. I'll give him a little sedative and examine him when he quiets down.

因为孩子哭的时候很难把腹部检查清楚,我给他一点镇静药,等他安静下来再检查。

(4) He may be suffering from some illness, but it's difficult to say at the moment. We would like to admit him a few hours for observation.

目前很难确定他有什么病。我们希望他留在这里观察几个小时。

(5) My child has been vomiting frequently, doctor. And usually after

taking food.

医生,我孩子他总是吐,而且通常是在进食以后吐。

(6) When did it start? How frequently? And does he vomit a large or small amount each time?

是从什么时候开始的? 一天大概几次? 那么每次吐的量多还是少呢?

(7) It started about ten days ago. He vomits about five times a day.

有十天了。一天大概吐五次左右。

(8) Does she have a cough? And is she afraid of light?

她咳嗽吗? 还有,她怕光吗?

(9) Has she been vaccinated against measles? When was she vaccinated?

她接种过麻疹疫苗吗? 什么时候接种的?

(10) Rheumatic fever is a bacterial infection whose victims are usually children.

风湿热是一种细菌性感染,其患者通常是儿童。

(11) My baby has been running a low temperature for two days, doctor. This morning I noticed there was a rash all over her body.

医生,我孩子发低烧有两天了。今天早晨我发现她全身都起了疹子。

(12) My son had his tooth filled.

我儿子的牙齿已经补过了。

(13) By watching the child at play, the psychiatrist found the boy was seriously disturbed emotionally.

精神病医生通过观察这个男孩玩耍,发现他在感情上受过严重创伤。

(14) Do children need to be vaccinated?

孩子们需要打预防针吗?

(15) The child had bouts of shaking of the limbs.

这个儿童患阵发性四肢抽搐。

(16) The child needn't go to hospital, he can go everyday as an outpatient.

这个孩子不必住院,他可以作为门诊病人每天来看病就行了。

(17) Children often have an exaggerated febrile response to infection.

儿童经常有一种对感染逾常的发热反应。

(18) The eight-year-old still wets his bed.

这个八岁的孩子还尿床。

(19) Malnutrition is still the most important health problem among the world's children.

营养不良仍然是世界很多国家儿童中最重要的健康问题。

(20) The child eats too much and is overweight，he must lose weight.

这个孩子吃得太多，太重了，他必须减肥。

(21) The nurse sponged the child's body to reduce the temperature.

护士用海绵给这个孩子擦身体来达到降温的效果。

(22) Is the stool watery（very loose，large in amount）? Is there pus，blood or mucus in it?

大便呈水样（很稀，量很多）吗？里面有没有脓、血或黏液？

(23) The glands behind her ears and head are swollen. With that and her rash I think she's got German measles.

她耳后的淋巴结和枕部的淋巴结都肿了。还有她身上出的疹子，我认为她得了风疹。

(24) His stools are quite loose with milk curd and undigested food in them.

他的大便很稀，还有奶瓣和不消化的食物。

(25) Is his stool normal? Has he got diarrhea? Or is he losing weight?

大便正常吗？他腹泻吗？或者说他的体重减轻了吗？

(26) His appetite is good and everything else seems to be all right.

他的胃口很好，别的似乎也都很正常。

(27) Don't worry，madame. In two or three days the symptoms will disappear. Your daughter doesn't need any medicine.

不必担心，夫人。过两三天症状就会消失的。你女儿不需服什么药的。

(28) Most likely his vomiting is due to your improper feeding. Usually after feeding, the baby should be held erect over your shoulder and patted gently on the back，so that any swallowed air can come out. After burping him，put him in his crip on his right side with his head slightly raised. If he should vomit，you should turn him on to his side with his face down，so he can't inhale his vomits.

他的呕吐看来是喂养不当引起的。每次给孩子喂完奶后，应该把孩子竖起来，靠在你的肩膀上，然后轻轻拍他的后背。这样孩子吃奶时吞咽的空气才可以排出来。等他打完嗝以后,让孩子向右侧躺,头稍微抬高一点。如果他吐的话,赶快让他的脸朝下,这样他就不会呛着了。

(29) He's probably got indigestion. Please stop all food except milk. Try to give him a little less milk than usual. Now, I'll prescribe some medicine for him.

他可能是消化不良了。先把所有的辅食停了,只给孩子吃奶,而且还要减少一点奶量。我给他开点药。

(30) New symptoms may appear, such as headaches, vomiting, bleeding spots on the skin and jaundice. If his general condition is satisfactory and he is not getting worse, don't bother him to come everyday. But do come back after he has finished the medicine. Anything new develops you can bring him here anytime.

在生病的过程中,有时会有新的症状出现,比如头痛、呕吐、皮肤上出现出血点、黄疸等。如果他的情况有好转就不必每天来门诊了。将药吃完以后再来复查。如果出现任何新的症状可以随时再来。

Ⅲ. Words and Expressions 单词和短语

1. Disease of Respiratory System 呼吸器官疾病

acidosis /ˌæsɪˈdəʊsɪs/ n. 酸中毒

acute bronchitis 急性支气管炎

acute pneumonia 急性肺炎

alkalosis /ˌælkəˈləʊsɪs/ n. 碱中毒

atelectasis of the lung; atelectasis /ˌætəˈlektəsɪs/ n.; pulmonary atelectasis 肺不张

avitaminosis /æˌvɪtəmɪˈnəʊsɪs/ n. 维生素缺乏(症)

beriberi /ˌberiˈberi/ n. 脚气病

bronchial asthma 支气管哮喘

bronchiectasis /ˌbrɒŋkɪˈektəsɪs/ n. 支气管扩张

bronchostenosis /ˌbrɒntʃəʊsəˈnəʊsɪs/ n. 支气管狭窄

buonchopneumonia /ˌbrɒŋkəʊnjuːˈməʊniə/ n. 支气管肺炎

catarrhal pneumonia 卡他性肺炎

central pneumonia 中央性肺炎

cheesy pneumonia 干酪性肺炎

chronic bronchitis 慢性支气管炎

corpulence /ˈkɔːpjələns/; obesity /əʊˈbiːsəti/ n. 肥胖症

croupous bronchitis 格鲁布性支气管炎

croupous pneumonia 格鲁布性肺炎

diabetes insipidus 尿崩症

diabetes mellitus 糖尿病

disease of bronchus 支气管疾病

diseases of lung 肺病

diseases of metabolism 新陈代谢病

diseases of pleura 胸膜病

dry pleuritis 干性胸膜炎

empyema /ˌempaɪˈiːmə/ n. 脓胸

fibrous bronchitis 纤维性支气管炎

fibrous pneumonia 纤维性肺炎

gout /ɡaʊt/ n. 痛风

hemoptysis /hɪˈmɒptɪsɪs/ n.; blood
　　spitting 咯血

hemorrhagic pleuritis 出血性胸膜炎

hypostatic pneumonia 坠积性肺炎

interstitial lobular pleuritis 叶间性胸膜炎

lobular pneumonia 小叶性肺炎

mediastinal pleuritis 纵隔性胸膜炎

mediastinal tumour 纵隔肿瘤

moist pleuritis; wet pleurisy;
　　pleurisy with effusion 湿性胸膜炎

oedematous pneumonia 水肿性肺炎

osteomalacia /ˌɒstɪəʊməˈleɪʃɪə/ n. 骨
　　软化(症)

pleuritis /plʊəˈraɪtɪs/ n. 胸膜炎

pneumothorax /ˌnjuːməʊˈθɔːræks/ n.
　　肺气肿

pulmonary carcinoma; cancer of lung 肺癌

pulmonary distome; lung fluke 肺吸虫

pulmonary edema 肺水肿

pulmonary emphysema 肺气肿

pulmonary gangrene of the lung 肺坏疽

pulmonary lung abscess 肺脓肿

pulmonary phthisis; lung phthisis 肺痨

pulmonary tuberculosis (TB) 肺结核

purulent bronchitis 脓性支气管炎

rickets /ˈrɪkɪts/; rachitis /rəˈkaɪtɪs/ n.
　　佝偻病

sappurative pleuritis 脓化胸膜炎

scurvy /ˈskɜːvi/ n. 坏血症

septic bronchitis 腐败性支气管炎

2. Diseases of Endocrine System
　　内分泌病

acromegaly /ˌækrəʊˈmegəli/ n. 肢端
　　肥大症

Addison's disease 艾迪生病

audible /ˈɔːdəbl/ adj. 可听到的

auscultation /ˌɔːskəlˈteɪʃən/ n. 听诊法

basedow disease 突眼性甲状腺肿

breathing sound 呼吸音

bronchial breathing; vesicular
　　breathing 支气管音(肺泡音)

bronchophony /bˈrɒntʃəfəni/ n. 支气管音

capacity of lungs 肺活量

clear /klɪə/ adj. 清

coarse /kɔːs/ adj. 大

cracked-pot sound 破壶音

crepitation /ˌkrepɪˈteɪʃn/ n. 捻发音

dry rales 干性啰音

dull /dʌl/ adj. 浊

expiration prolonged 呼出音延长

inaudible /ɪnˈɔːdəbl/ adj. 听不到的

lung /lʌŋ/ n. 肺

medium /ˈmiːdiəm/ adj. 中

moist rales 湿性啰音

myxedema /ˌmɪksɪˈdiːmə/ n. 黏液肿

nonresonant /ˌnɒnˈrezənənt/; toneless
　　/ˈtəʊnləs/ adj. 无响性的

notes of percussion 叩诊所见

rale /rɑːl/ *n*. 啰音

resonant /ˈrezənənt/ *adj.*；consonant /ˈkɒnsənənt/ *adj.*；with resonance 有响性的

rough /rʌf/；coarse /kɔːs/ *adj*. 粗糙的

sharp /ʃɑːp/ *adj*. 尖锐

sibilant /ˈsɪbɪlənt/ *adj*. 咝咝作声的

splashing sound 震荡音

tetany /ˈtetəni/ *n*. 抽搐

tympany /ˈtɪmpəni/ *n*. 鼓胀

upper-liver border/lung-liver border 肝上界/肺肝界

vocal fremitus 嗓音震荡

vocal resonance 嗓音共鸣

Section 7　Otolaryngology
第7节　耳鼻喉科

Part 1　Ear Clinic
第1部分　耳科

Ⅰ. Dialogues 情景对话

1. Chronic Suppurative Otitis Media 慢性化脓性中耳炎

Patient：Doctor，my ear drum was perforated when I swam at the sea shore.

医生,我在海边游泳的时候,我的耳鼓膜穿孔了。

Doctor：Please tell me what kind of secretion was discharged from your ears. Was it pussy, mucous, bloody or with a bad smell?

请告诉我从你耳朵里流出来的是什么样的分泌物。是脓的,黏的,带血的,还是带臭味的?

Patient：My right ear started to run with foul smelling pus after an attack of measles when I was young.

我记得小时候出过麻疹之后,我的右耳就开始往外流带臭味的脓了。

Doctor：Upon examination I find that you are suffering from a chronic suppurative infection of your middle ear.

刚才检查，我发现你的中耳有慢性化脓性感染。

Patient：I can hardly hear what people say, and I have had occasional earaches ever since pus flowed out of my ears.

自从我的耳朵流脓之后，别人说的话我听不清，有时还耳朵疼。

Doctor：Does the earache occur deep inside or just at the orifice of your ear?

你觉得哪里耳疼，是在耳朵深处呢还是在耳朵口上呢？

Patient：It seems to be a pulsating ache located deep in my ear.

好像是在我耳朵深处，而且还是跳动着的那种疼。

Doctor：There is a lot of pus and pieces of white debris in your middle ear cavity. I am afraid that a bony destruction is taking place in the mastoid. A mastoid operation is necessary to eliminate the possibility of intracranial complications.

你的中耳腔里有很多脓和白色的坏死碎屑。我担心在乳突部有骨质破坏。为了消除引起颅内并发症的可能性，我建议你最好做乳突手术。

2. Diseases of the External Ear 外耳病

Patient：Doctor, I have a throbbing pain in my left ear. It hurts terribly when I touch it. My affected ear can't touch the pillow when I lie in bed.

医生，我的左耳一跳一跳地疼，尤其是我碰着它的时候疼得要命。我躺在床上的时候，这只耳朵连枕头也不能沾。

Doctor：Did any dirty water get into your ears when you took a shower bath or went swimming in the pool?

你在淋浴或者游泳的时候有没有脏水进到耳朵里呢？

Patient：My ears became terribly painful after some dirty water got into them when I went swimming the day before yesterday.

我前天去游泳，耳朵里的确进了些脏水，之后，两只耳朵就剧烈地疼起来了。

Doctor：Your ear canal is almost completely impacted with a big mass of ear wax. I will clean it for you with a curette and a pair of forceps. Please keep your head in a fixed position and don't move.

你的耳道几乎让一大块耳屎给堵满了，我先用挖耳勺和镊子给你取出来。请把头靠在一个固定的位置上，不要乱动。

Patient：I picked out my ear wax with a match stick by myself last night. I felt a pain and there was moisture inside my ear the next morning.

昨天晚上我自己用火柴棍掏耳屎。第二天早晨我就觉得很疼，而且还觉得耳朵里潮乎乎的。

Doctor：There are several small boils around the opening of your left ear canal. It may give you very sharp pain. I'll make an incision and drain the pus for you.

那是因为在你左耳道口的周围长有几个小疖子，也许就是这个让你疼得厉害。我待会儿给这几个疖子切开，把脓导出来。

3. Hard of Hearing 重听

Patient：Doctor, I haven't been able to hear well for some time and it seems to get worse as I get older.

医生，我听力不好已经有些时候了，而且似乎年岁愈大，听力也愈差了。

Doctor：Can you tell me which kind of sounds you find more difficult to hear? Spoken or musical sounds?

你能不能告诉我什么样的声音你听起来更困难？是说话的声音，还是音乐的声音？

Patient：Spoken, and my ears are buzzing constantly. I cannot sleep properly at night.

说话的声音。而且，我的耳朵还不断地嗡嗡作响。晚上我的睡眠也不好。

Doctor：I would like to test your hearing ability with a tuning fork (an electro-audiometer). The electro-audiogram shows that yours is a type of nerve deafness (conduction deafness, mixed type deafness).

我想用音仪(电测听仪)测试一下你的听力。你的电测听图表明你患的是神经性耳聋(传导性耳聋，混合性耳聋)。

Part 2　Nose Clinic
第 2 部分　鼻科

1. Allergic Rhinitis 过敏性鼻炎

Patient：Doctor，every morning I suffer from a running nose with a profuse watery discharge. And sometimes，my nose itches badly inside，sometimes this is accompanied by itching in my eyes，ears and throat.

医生，每天早晨我总要流大量清鼻涕。而且有时，我的鼻子里痒得厉害，有时连眼睛、耳朵和嗓子一齐痒。

Doctor：When and where does your nose bother you most?

那什么时候、在什么地方你的鼻子会觉得最难受？

Patient：It's strange that all the trouble with my nose disappears after a rain shower，but it gets worse when the wind blows hard.

很奇怪，只要是下了一场雨之后，我鼻子不舒服的症状就会消失，但是在大风天的时候它就变得更重。

Doctor：Do you get these attacks seasonally or all year round?

你的这种发作是季节性的还是常年都是如此呢？

Patient：For the past few years，I have had repeated violent sneezing attacks starting in late July and lasting till the end of October.

近些年来，从七月底开始到十月底为止，我总是反复剧烈地打喷嚏。

Doctor：Do any one of your family members suffer from a similar allergic condition?

那在你的家庭成员中，还有别人有过类似的过敏情况吗？

Patient：As I remember，my mother and my little sister，they both had severe asthmatic attacks in their childhood.

据我所知，我的妈妈和小妹在童年时期都得过严重的哮喘病。

Doctor：Were you sensitive to other things previously，for example，drugs and foods?

你以前还对什么别的东西过敏吗，比如药物、食品类的？

Patient：Oh，yes，I am sensitive to penicillin and I usually have abdominal pain after eating crabs. What is the trouble with my nose, doctor?

噢,是的,我对青霉素过敏,而且一吃螃蟹就肚子疼。那医生,我的鼻子是怎么回事儿呢?

Doctor：The mucous membrane of your nose appears markedly pale and edematous. And according to your case history, as you have presented it to me, I believe that you are suffering from allergic rhinits.

你鼻黏膜显得特别苍白并且还有些水肿。根据你所提供的病史,我想你得的是过敏性鼻炎。

Patient：What treatment do you suggest?

你打算怎么给我治疗呢?

Doctor：With your approval, I shall give you a series of specific skin tests at first. This will help us to identify the substances to which you are allergic.

如果你同意的话,我想先给你进行一组特异性的皮肤试验,看看你对什么东西过敏。

Patient：OK, no problem. Does it hurt?

好的,没问题。会疼吗?

Doctor：It won't hurt you very much, and it will feel no worse than a mosquito bite. The result of the skin tests will show up in fifteen minutes.

这种试验对你不会造成多大的痛苦,就跟被蚊子叮咬差不多。十五分钟后就可以看皮肤试验的结果了。

Patient：OK, I'll wait here.

好的,我就在这儿等了。

Doctor：The special tests we have done show a strong positive reaction to house dust, pollens, moulds and house mite. I would like to give you a course of desensitization therapy. It should be regularly injected subcutaneously twice a week. By the way, the course of desensitization takes a relatively long time. I hope you will be patient and cooperate with us.

我们做的特殊试验表明你对室内尘土、花粉、霉菌和家螨都有强阳性反应。我准备给你做一个疗程的脱敏治疗,每周按时皮下注射两次。顺便说一下,脱敏治疗需要比较长的时间,我希望你能耐心地和我们配合。

2. Suppurative Sinusitis 化脓性鼻窦炎

Patient：Doctor，my nose is running with a discharge of a yellow substance and I suffer from a dull headache every morning and evening. I wonder if something is wrong with my sinuses.

医生,我的鼻子总是流着一种黄色的分泌物,每天早晚都感到头部隐隐地疼,我想可能是我的鼻窦出毛病了吧。

Doctor：Does your nose run only on one side or on both?

那你的鼻子,是一侧流鼻涕呢,还是两侧都流呢?

Patient：It seems to run on both sides，but I don't remember clearly since a pussy discharge flows from my nose all the time. And a postnasal drip with a foul smell bothers me very much.

好像是两侧都流,但我也记不清楚了,因为脓鼻涕老是从鼻子里流着。而且,这种带臭味的鼻涕从鼻子后面流到嗓子里,会更让我感到苦恼。

Doctor：Does it hurt when I tap your forehead?

我拍打你前脑门儿的时候你觉得疼吗?

Patient：No.

不疼。

Doctor：Is it painful when I apply pressure on your cheeks? Tell me which side hurts more.

当我这样按压你的脸颊时疼不疼呢? 告诉我哪边疼得厉害些。

Patient：It seems the left side hurts more. In addition，I can't sleep well because I must always keep my mouth open to breathe when I lie down. As I can't breathe through my nose freely，I can't sleep and smell either.

好像左边疼得厉害。还有就是我睡眠也不好,因为我一躺下就得张着嘴呼吸。因为我不能通畅地用鼻子呼吸,所以我睡不好觉,嗅觉也不灵。

Doctor：You are suffering from a suppurative maxillary (frontal，ethmoidal) sinusitis，but it's of a mild nature. I think you will recover pretty soon after some conservative treatment.

你患的是化脓性上颌窦(额窦,筛窦)炎,但症状还是比较轻的。我想经过一些保守治疗会很快恢复的。

Patient：What's your advice then, doctor?

那么,医生你有些什么建议呢?

Doctor：I will give you a sinus puncture and irrigation in order to clean up the pus inside the sinus cavity.

我准备给你做一次穿刺和冲洗,先把窦腔里的脓液清洗干净。

Patient：What will be the best time for my sinus operation?

我的鼻窦手术什么时候做最好?

Doctor：The sinus operation had better be postponed till after a period of supportive treatment. (I believe that your sinus infection will completely subside within a short period of time after you return home.)

鼻窦手术最好顺延到辅助治疗一个阶段之后。(我相信你的鼻窦感染会在你回家后短时间内完全消除的。)

3. Deviation of Nasal Septum 鼻中隔偏斜

Patient：Ever since childhood I have had great difficulty in breathing through my right nostril, doctor.

医生,自从童年以来,我右侧的鼻孔通气总是很困难。

Doctor：Let me examine it for you. Yes, your nasal septum is markedly deviated to the right side. And there is a bony ridge at the bottom of your nasal septum.

来让我给你做个检查吧。啊哟,你的鼻中隔明显地向右偏斜。而且,你鼻中隔底部还有一个骨脊。

Patient：What?

怎么回事儿呢?

Doctor：Emm… There is a bulging spur situated in the portion of your septum, sir.

嗯,你鼻子的中央有一个隆起的骨刺,先生。

Patient：My nose bleeds frequently, especially in winter time. Do you think it's also the result of nasal septum deviation?

我的鼻子经常出血,尤其是在冬天。你认为这也是鼻中隔偏斜引起的吗?

Doctor: I think so. A bony spine has penetrated right into your nasal concha. It may cause repeated nose-bleeding. There is an active bleeding point right on the surface of your nasal septum. I will try to stop it with a cotton sponge (electric cautery, chemical burn).

是的。有根骨刺正好长在你的鼻甲上。它可能会引起鼻子的反复出血。检查看到,在你鼻中隔表面的确有一个活动性的出血点。我来用棉球(电烙,化学烧灼)把它止住吧。

Patient: My head often feels heavy. I can't concentrate when my work requires a mental effort. Two years ago when I fell from a ladder, my nose was traumatized and became obstructed.

我的头经常感到昏沉沉的。工作需要用脑子的时候,精神老是集中不起来。两年前,我从梯子上摔下来时鼻子受了伤,而且变得更堵了。

Doctor: The deviation of your nasal septum is just a mild one. There is no need for any operation at this time. (I would suggest a submucous resection of your nasal septum in order to correct the deviation. For the sake of safety, a blood and urine examination should be made before the operation.)

你的鼻中隔偏斜还很轻微,目前无需手术。(为了矫正偏斜,我建议你做一次鼻中隔黏膜下切除手术。为安全起见,手术前应先做血和尿的检查。)

Part 3　Throat Clinic
第3部分　喉科

1. Tonsillitis and Enlarged Adenoids 扁桃体炎和腺样增殖体肥大

Patient: I felt listless and had an acute sore throat this morning, then ran a fever of 40℃ after lunch.

今天早晨我感到不舒服而且嗓子疼得厉害,午饭以后发烧到40℃。

Doctor：Your tonsils are very much congested and enlarged with several white spots spreading over their surface. My diagnosis is acute lacunar tonsillitis.

你的扁桃体充血而且非常肥大，在它表面上还散布着几个小白点。我的诊断是急性陷窝性扁桃体炎。

Patient：By the way, doctor, my son always keeps his mouth open and his nose is running all the time. Moreover he snores loudly when he falls asleep. When I wash his face, I can feel a small round mass just beneath his chin. I don't know what it is.

还有，医生，我儿子老是张着嘴，经常流鼻涕，而且睡着时鼾声很大。我给他洗脸的时候，发现他的下巴底下有一个小圆鼓包儿。我不知道是什么。

Doctor：Let me have a look, too.

那让我也给他检查一下吧。

Patient：Anything wrong with him, doctor?

有事吗，医生？

Doctor：Your child has enlarged adenoid and tonsils. As they frequently become infected, an operation is advisable. Children with a tonsil infection always have enlarged lymph nodes in the region of the neck.

孩子的腺样增殖体和扁桃体都增大。如果它们时常感染，可以考虑手术。有扁桃体炎的孩子脖子上经常有增大的淋巴结。

Patient：OK, doctor, but what can I do then?

好吧，那我该做点什么呢，医生？

Doctor：Except for limited amounts of water, any intake of food for him should be restricted within six hours prior to the operation.

手术前六个小时，除喝点水之外，让他禁进任何饮食。

2. Pharyngitis 咽炎

Patient：Doctor, my throat has been dry and irritated all winter. I have a dry cough and a slight pain in my throat. It gets worse after smoking or prolonged talking.

医生，我的嗓子整个冬季都发干而且感觉不舒服，我有时还干咳嗽,嗓子还有点疼,抽烟和说话时间长了病情就加重。

Doctor：Let me check for you. There is nothing seriously wrong with your throat except chronic pharyngitis.

让我看看,你的嗓子没有什么大病,只是有点慢性咽炎。

Patient：I noticed a number of enlarged nodules over my neck region. Sometimes I run a low grade fever.

我的颈部还有不少增大的结节,有时还发低烧。

Doctor：Your throat is bright red and is markedly swollen. The lymphogranules of your posterior pharyngeal wall show a slight increase in number and size.

你的嗓子红肿明显,在咽后壁上的淋巴颗粒稍有增大和增多。

Patient：I have felt a foreign body in my throat during the past three months. And I am afraid there is a tumor growth inside.

近三个月来,我嗓子里总有异物感,我担心里面长肿瘤了。

Doctor：All the trouble in your throat may be due to a pharyngeal neurasthenia. It's wise to treat your throat ailment through establishing regular daily habits rather than relying on medicines.

你的嗓子不舒服可能都是由于咽喉部神经官能症引起的。治疗这种嗓子疼最好的办法就是养成规律生活的好习惯,这比单纯依赖药品治疗效果要好得多。

Ⅱ. Sentences 替换句型

(1) I suggest that your ear operation be postponed until there is complete control of the suppuration for at least three months to half a year.

我建议你的耳郭手术推延至少三个月到半年,等化脓完全控制之后再做。

(2) It is difficult to predict whether normal hearing will be restored or not after the tympanoplastic operation.

很难预测经过鼓室成形手术后,正常听力还能不能恢复。

(3) Be sure not to blow your nose too violently, otherwise the discharge in your nose may be pushed into your ears to reinfect the middle

ear.

切忌使劲擤鼻子,否则你鼻子里的分泌物可能被挤到耳朵里去,这样反而会使中耳重新感染。

(4) For three days already, doctor, my ears are almost entirely plugged up and are ringing all the time. I can only hear sound as if I were confined in a closed cabin.

医生,我的耳朵几乎完全被堵塞住了,而且还不停地耳鸣,都已经三天了。声音听来,感觉好像是我自己被关在一个密闭的小舱里似的。

(5) Doctor, I notice murmuring sound just like water flowing in my ear whenever I get up from bed or move my head abruptly. I can't hear sounds from the outside clearly, but there is a loud noise when I speak myself.

医生,当我从床上坐起或者突然移动头部的时候,我总能听到一种好像有水在我耳朵里流动似的潺潺声。我对外界的声音也听不清楚,但是我自己说话的时候,却感觉有很响的嘈杂声。

(6) I can see a fluid shadow through your ear drum that indicates there are some secretions behind the drum.

透过你的鼓膜我可以看到一个液体的阴影,这说明在鼓膜的后面还有些分泌物。

(7) My examination shows that you are suffering from secretory otitis media. It's a kind of nonseptic inflammation of the middle ear which produces mucous secretion instead of pus.

我的检查表明你患有分泌性中耳炎。这是一种中耳的非化脓性感染,也就是说,它只产生黏液但不化脓。

(8) Excuse me, doctor, I am not quite clear as to the meaning of "secretory otitis media".

对不起,医生,我对分泌性中耳炎的意思还不太清楚。

(9) The fluid inside your tympanum should be withdrawn right away. An ear drum puncture should be performed in order to aspirate as much of the fluid as possible.

鼓室腔里面的液体应立即抽出来。为了尽量把液体抽净,应该做鼓膜穿刺。

(10) If the secretion within the tympanum dries up spontaneously it will interfere with the vibration of your drum and influence your

hearing permanently.

如果让鼓室腔里的分泌物自行干涸，可能就会干扰你鼓膜的震动，这样反而会长期地影响你的听力。

(11) I advise you to do some eustachian tube inflation by yourself in the following way. Please block your nose with your fingers, close your mouth and hold your breath, then blow through your nose vigorously until a small amount of air penetrates into your ears.

我建议你用下述方法自己做做欧氏管吹胀练习。请你用手捏住鼻子，闭起嘴，屏住气，然后用力从鼻子鼓气，直到感觉有少量的空气进入你的耳朵里。

(12) Doctor, I heard a ticking sound in my ear when the plane took off in Tokyo.

医生，当飞机从东京起飞的时候，我耳朵里立刻就听见嘀嘀嗒嗒的响声。

(13) I noticed a fullness in my ear associated with a sharp pain inside right after the plane landed at the Beijing Airport.

飞机在北京机场着陆之后，我就感到耳朵发闷，并且疼痛得厉害。

(14) Doctor, I felt a sharp pain in my ear when I left the cabin of the plane, so I came here with my interpreter for a consultation.

医生，当我从机舱里一出来，我的耳朵里就感到刺痛，所以我就带着翻译来这里看病了。

(15) According to your case history and the symptoms described to me, I believe that you are suffering from aero-otitis.

根据你的病史和你给我描述的症状，我认为你患的是航空性中耳炎。

(16) Would you please explain to me the cause of aero-otitis, doctor?

医生，你给我讲一讲航空性中耳炎发病的原因，行吗？

(17) Well, simply speaking, aero-otitis is simply caused by the sudden imbalance of the air pressure inside and outside the middle ear.

嗯，简单的说，航空性中耳炎就是由中耳内外的压力骤然失去平衡造成的。

(18) All of your complaints may subside after an ear drum massage and tube inflation. Now please take a mouthful of water and swallow it immediately when I ask you to swallow.

你的这些不适,通过鼓膜按摩和耳咽管吹气之后可能症状会消除了。现在你含口水在嘴里,听我的指令,我让你咽时你要马上咽下去。

(19) Do you feel better since I manipulated the drum for you a minute ago?

我刚给你的鼓膜做了简单的处理,你现在觉得好些了吗?

(20) It's dramatic, doctor, all the symptoms disappeared right after your manipulation.

太神奇了,你的操作一结束,一切症状就都消失了。

(21) In order to maintain the pressure balance of your ear, I suggest you use some nose drops and take a piece of chewing gum before the plane lands on your next journey.

我建议你在下次旅行的时候,用些滴鼻药,而在飞机着陆前嚼块儿口香糖,这样就能很好地保持耳内压力的平衡了。

(22) Physiotherapy will be beneficial to promote reduction of the inflammatory process and to get rid of the pain.

理疗对消炎和止疼都有促进作用。

(23) Since last night, doctor, I've been suffering from a sudden decrease of hearing accompanied by vertigo.

医生,从昨晚开始,我的听力突然下降,还伴有头晕。

(24) What's the pitch of your ear ringing? Is it in high or in low tones?

你耳鸣的音调是怎样的? 是高调还是低调?

(25) Does the impairment of your hearing occur constantly or intermittently?

你的听力减退是持续性的还是间歇性的?

(26) A tympanoplastic operation may elevate your hearing level to a certain extent. The hearing gain after surgery depends upon the degree of destruction of the conduction apparatus of your middle ear.

鼓室成形手术可能会使听力提高一些。至于手术后听力恢复多少,这完全要看你中耳传导器官破坏的程度了。

(27) Doctor, I always notice a constriction in the chest and shortness of breath following a fit of sneezing.

医生,每次在打过一阵喷嚏之后,我总觉得胸部发紧,呼吸短促。

(28) Strangely enough, doctor, my nose becomes worse whenever I drive to the countryside or go across a field grown with an abundance of wild plants.

很奇怪的,医生,我只要一乘车下乡或者只要穿过一片长满野草、野花的田野,我的鼻子就感觉不舒服了。

(29) I suffer a lot if I breathe in dust, tobacco smoke, coal fumes, insecticides or something with a particular odor.

我要是一吸进灰尘、香烟和煤烟的气味,以及杀虫药或其他带特别气味的东西,我就感觉很难受。

(30) Usually my eyes get teary and I have a badly running nose when I drive outside or go to a picnic in the suburbs.

平时我总泪汪汪的,尤其是,当我一开车出门或在郊外野餐时,我的鼻涕就淌得更厉害了。

(31) Your nose is completely stopped with multiple polyps.

你的鼻子被好多个息肉完全堵住了。

(32) Inside of your nose cavity there is a profuse accumulation of mucous secretions.

你的鼻腔里积满了大量的黏鼻涕。

(33) Your case is diagnosed as acute suppuration of the left frontal sinus. You will have to get some electric diathermy at first, followed by antibiotic therapy.

你的情况诊断为左侧急性化脓性前额窦炎。你必须先做电透热治疗,然后进行抗生素治疗。

(34) The X-ray film shows that there are fluid levels in both of your maxillary sinuses. Your sinus is badly infected. It would be best to perform an operation after admission to the hospital.

X线片显示你两侧的上颌窦里都有液平面。你的鼻窦发炎很厉害,最好住院做手术。

(35) Since the sinus cavity is filled with polyps, they should be surgically removed.

由于窦腔已被息肉充满,因此应该用手术把息肉摘除。

(36) The inflamed sinus has become a focus of infection in your body. Any focus of infection may affect one's joints, muscles, kidneys, even the heart, thus I suggest it be removed.

发炎的鼻窦已经在你身上成为一个病灶,任何病灶性感染都有可能危害人的关节、肌肉、肾脏,甚至心脏,所以我建议清除它。

（37） One week has elapsed since your sinus operation. The postoperative course seems very smooth. I think that you may be discharged from hospital the day after tomorrow if nothing particular happens.

你的鼻窦手术已经做过一个星期了,术后的过程看来很顺利。如果不发生什么特殊情况,我想后天你就可以出院了。

（38） When you speak, your voice has a nasal tone. There must be some obstruction in your nose. Let me see. Your nasal turbinate appears enlarged. Apparently this is obstructing your nasal passage.

你说话时鼻音很重,你鼻子里一定有些堵塞。让我给你看看。你的鼻甲肥大,这显然是把你的鼻道给堵住了。

（39） I have had a stuffy nose for three years and it has become worse in the past five months.

我的鼻子堵塞已经三年了,近五个月来更加严重了。

（40） A thick and sticky discharge always remains in my nose. It's difficult to blow it out. I get a dull headache whenever I catch cold.

我的鼻子里经常有一种粘稠的分泌物,不容易清理干净,只要一感冒,我的头就隐隐地疼。

（41） How about your ability to smell?

你的嗅觉怎样?

（42） I can smell properly if my nasal passage is open, but I lose my smelling ability when my nose is blocked.

当我鼻子通畅的时候闻得很好,但是如果鼻子堵了,嗅觉也就失灵了。

（43） Does your nose get worse in winter time?

你的鼻子到了冬季是不是就更严重了?

（44） Yes, the weather in Beijing is rather cold and dry in winter. And I do feel uncomfortable.

是的,北京的气候到了冬季很冷而且干燥,我的确感觉非常不舒服。

（45） I'm giving you one bottle of ephedrine. You may use it if the nose is blocked. Two to three drops will be enough for each side.

我现在给你一瓶麻黄素。当你感觉鼻子堵的时候可以用它,每侧滴上两到三滴就够了。

(46) The best way to prevent acute infection of your nose is to avoid catching cold.

预防你鼻子发炎最好的办法就是防止感冒了。

(47) I intend to perform an electric cauterization for your hypertrophic nasal mucosa.

我想给你肥厚的鼻黏膜做一次电烧灼手术。

(48) Your nose trouble is only in its early stage now. I think that you'll soon be cured if you follow these therapeutic instructions.

你的鼻病目前还不严重,如果能按这种治疗方案去做,我想很快就会痊愈的。

(49) Since your congested nasal mucosa does not respond properly to medicine, I advise you to have a partial resection operation performed for your hypertrophic lower turbinate.

鉴于你的鼻黏膜充血严重,而且已不能对药物产生正常的反应,我建议你做下鼻甲的肥厚部分切除手术。

(50) My nose feels dry all the time, could you please give me a check-up, doctor?

医生,我的鼻子老是发干,请你给我检查检查好吗?

(51) Upon examination I find an atrophic change has taken place in your nose. Did you notice any bad odor in your nose?

根据检查,我发现你的鼻子有萎缩性病变。你觉得鼻子里有臭味吗?

(52) Since my teens, I've had a foul smell in my nose. People have told me that when I breathe my nose emits a rather foul odor, but I myself can't notice it at all.

我从十几岁起,鼻子里就有臭味。别人告诉我说,我呼吸时,鼻子里会散发出很臭的味道,但是我自己一点也感觉不到。

(53) I suppose you are suffering from atrophic rhinitis. It is a chronic condition commonly seen in young females. It may take a long time for recovery. What kind of discharge appears in your nose?

我想你得的是萎缩性鼻炎。它是一种常见于青年女性的慢性病,恢复起来很费时间。你鼻子的分泌物是怎样的呢?

(54) Every morning I blow big gray yellow casts out of my nose. I can't breathe freely through my nose. From time to time this is accompanied by an insidious headache. What shall I do for this condition, doctor?

每天早晨,我鼻子里都能擤出大块灰黄色的结痂。而且我还不能通畅地用鼻子呼吸,还时常伴有慢慢加剧的头痛。这种情况我该怎么办呢,医生?

(55) It would be beneficial to irrigate your nose with warm salt water once a day. An atrophic condition of the nose may sometimes be improved with better nutrition. Avoiding contact with dust and irritating fumes may help you to get rid of the atrophic inflammation of your nose.

每天用温盐水冲洗一次鼻腔对改善你的病情是会有好处的。有时鼻子的萎缩状况可以通过改善营养而有所好转。要避免接触尘土和刺激性的气味,这样的话,也会有助于你消除鼻子的萎缩性炎症。

(56) My throat is so sore that my voice has undergone a change. I can't eat anything, especially solid and hot food.

我的嗓子痛得连发音都变了,我什么东西也吃不下去,尤其是硬而烫的食物。

(57) You had better stay in bed and take a soft or liquid diet for two or three days. Please give up smoking till the infection is over. And I'll give you penicillin injections, some lozenges to suck, and something to gargle with.

你最好卧床休息两三天,吃软的或流质食物。到感染消除之后再抽烟。你需要注射青霉素,含些糖锭剂,用些漱口药。

(58) Avoid catching cold, avoid smoking and don't eat irritating foods of any sort. It will help your throat to get better fast. I advise you to have your infected tonsils removed later.

不要抽烟,避免受凉和吃任何刺激性的食物。这样你的嗓子就能好得快了。我建议你以后把发炎的扁桃体切除掉。

(59) Generally speaking, the tonsillectomy can be finished within half an hour. Please keep on breathing normally and cooperate with me during the operation.

一般说来,扁桃体切除手术在半小时之内就可以完成,请你在手术时保持正常呼吸，并好好和我配合。

（60）Give up smoking and avoid excessive use of your voice. This will improve the condition of your throat. I'm going to prescribe a bottle of gargle solution and a packet of sucking lozenges.

希望你戒烟，避免过度使用嗓子。这对你嗓子的病情会有好处。今天我给你开一瓶漱口药和一包含化糖锭。

Ⅲ. Words and Expressions 单词和短语

acute mastoiditis 急性乳突炎

acute otitis media 急性中耳炎

acute rhinitis 急性鼻炎

acute sinusitis; sinus infection 急性鼻窦炎

acute tonsillitis 急性扁桃体炎

adenoid /'ædɪˌnɔɪd/ n. 腺样体

air douche 咽鼓管通气

allergic rhinitis 变态性反应性鼻炎

anterior-rhinoscopy 前鼻镜检查

aspiration /ˌæspə'reɪʃn/ n. 吸出疗法

atrophic rhinitis simple 单纯性萎缩性鼻炎

aural discharge 耳漏

blowing the nose 擤鼻

body of gland 腺体

brain abscess 脑脓肿

chronic otitis media 慢性中耳炎

cleaning of the nasal cavity 清拭鼻腔

cleaning /'kliːnɪŋ/ n. 清拭

cochlear implant 耳蜗埋植

cochlea /'kɒklɪə/ n. 耳蜗

cone-shaped light reflex 锥形光反射

cryotherapy /ˌkraɪəʊ'θerəpi/ n.; freezing therapy 冷冻疗法

deaf-muteness 聋哑症

deafness /'defnəs/ n. 聋

deviation of the nasal septum 鼻中隔偏曲

disturbance of olfaction 嗅觉障碍

earache /'ɪəreɪk/; otalgia /əʊ'tældʒiə/ n. 耳痛

eczema of auricle 耳廓湿疹

ethmoid air cells 筛窦（气房）

ethmoidal sinusitis 筛窦炎

ethmoidal sinus 筛窦

eustachian tube 咽鼓管；欧氏管

examination with conversation voice 谈话语言检查

examination with ear speculum 耳镜检查

examination with whispered voice 口耳语言检查

external auditory tract 外耳道

external ear 外耳

external nose 外鼻

facial paresis 面神经瘫痪

fenestration /ˌfenɪ'streɪʃən/ n. 开窗术

fetid atrophic rhinitis or ozaena 臭鼻症

foreign body 异物

frontal sinusitis 额窦炎

frontal sinus 额窦

functional endonasal sinus surgery (FESS) 功能性鼻内窥镜手术

furuncle of the nose 鼻疖

furunculosis of external canal 耳疖

handle of malleus 锤骨柄

headache /'hedeɪk/ *n*. 头痛

hypertrophic rhinitis 肥大性鼻炎

impacted cerumen 耵聍栓塞

instillation /ˌɪnstɪ'leɪʃən/ *n*. 滴药

insufflation /ˌɪnsə'fleɪʃən/ *n*. 吹粉

internal ear 内耳

irrigation /ˌɪrɪ'geɪʃən/ *n*. 洗鼻

labyrinthitis /ˌlæbərɪn'θaɪtɪs/ *n*. 内耳炎

laser treatment 激光疗法

malleus /'mælɪəs/ *n*. 锤骨

mastoid process 乳突

maxillary sinusitis 上颌窦炎

maxillary sinus 上颌窦

microwave therapy 微波疗法

middle ear 中耳

mucous(secretoy, exudative) otitis media 黏液性(分泌性、渗出性)中耳炎

lateral rhinotomy 鼻侧切开术

myringotomy /ˌmɪrɪŋ'ɡɒtəmi/ *n*. 鼓膜切开术

nasal cavity 鼻腔

nasal diphtheria 鼻白喉

nasal discharge 鼻漏

nasal fiberscope or fiber opticscope 纤维鼻内窥镜

nasal hemorrhage 鼻出血

nasal obstruction 鼻塞

nasal polypectomy 鼻息肉摘除术

otogenic complication; otogenic intracranial complication 耳源性并发症

otogenic facial paralysis 耳源性面瘫

otogenic sepsis 耳源性毒血症

otogenic sinus thrombosis 耳源性血栓

otology /əʊ'tɒlədʒi/ *n*. 耳科

otosclerosis /ˌəʊtəʊsklə'rəʊsɪs/ *n*. 耳硬化

pain upon swallowing 吞咽痛

painting /'peɪntɪŋ/ *n*. 涂药法

paracentesis /ˌpærəsen'tiːsɪs/ *n*. 鼓膜切开

paranasal sinus 鼻窦

pars tensa 紧张部

pharynx /'færɪŋks/; throat /θrəʊt/ *n*. 咽

puncture for examination 穿刺诊断

respiratory function 呼吸功能

rhinogenic intraorbital and intracranial complications 鼻源性眶内和颅内并发症

rhinoplasty /'raɪnəʊˌplæsti/ *n*. 鼻成形术

saddle nose 鞍鼻

shrapnell's membrane; pars flaccida 松弛部

semicircular canal 半规管

septoplasty /septəʊp'læsti/ *n*. 鼻中隔成形术

short process of malleus 锤骨短突起

simple acute catarrhal pharyngitis 单纯性急性咽炎

sphenoid sinusitis 蝶窦炎

sphenoidal sinus 蝶窦

spontaneous pain 自发性痛

stapes /'steɪpiːz/ *n*. 镫骨

incus /'ɪŋkəs/ *n*. 砧骨

tympanic membrane 鼓膜

tympanotomy /tɪmpəˈnɒtəmi/;
  myringotomy /ˌmɪrɪŋˈɡɒtəmi/
  n. 鼓膜切开术
ultrasound eletrophoresis 超声药导疗法

umbo /ˈʌmbəʊ/ *n*. 脐
vertigo /ˈvɜːtɪɡəʊ/ *n*. 眩晕
vestibule /ˈvestɪˌbjuːl/ *n*. 前庭
wet pack 湿布包裹

Section 8 Ophthalmology
第8节 眼科

Ⅰ. Dialogues 情景对话

1. Acute Infective Conjunctivitis 急性感染性结膜炎

Patient：Doctor，my right eye has been red for two days. And it's very uncomfortable.

医生，我的右眼红了两天了，难受极了。

Doctor：Is there any discharge?

有分泌物吗？

Patient：Yes, a lot, especially in the morning.

有，很多分泌物，特别是在早晨。

Doctor：Do you have good eyesight?

你视力好吗？

Patient：Yes.

好的，不错。

Doctor：Please look down，and let me have a look. You have acute infective conjunctivitis. I'll write a prescription for you. Get the eye drops and ointment from the pharmacy and apply them as directed. It'll clear up in three or four days.

请向下看，让我给你看看。这是急性感染性结膜炎。我给你开一个处方。请到药房去取眼药水和眼药膏，按医嘱应用。过三四天炎症就会消失的。

Patient：Shall I come again?

我需要再来吗？

Doctor：Please come back in three days. Besides，acute conjunctivitis is a contagious disease，so keep your towels and pillowcases separate from those of other people.

三天后来复诊一下。此外，急性结膜炎是一种传染病，要把你的毛巾和枕头套跟别人的分开使用。

Patient：Oh，I see，doctor. Thank you very much.

好的，谢谢你，医生，我知道了。

2. External Stye 外麦粒肿

Patient：Doctor，there's a red swelling on my left eye and it's been hurting me for two days.

医生，我的左眼红肿，已经疼了两天了。

Doctor：Yes. The upper lid is badly swollen. There is a pustule on the lid margin and some pus can be seen in the centre of it. It ought to be incised at once. Do you agree to that?

是的。你的上眼睑肿得很厉害，眼睑边缘能看到有一个脓疱，中央部分已经有些脓了，必须马上切开。你同意吗？

Patient：Of course，but will it hurt?

当然同意，但是疼吗？

Doctor：Hardly，don't worry about it. It's just like a mosquito bite. There，all the pus is out. There's a pad，and a prescription to buy some eye drops. Please come back tomorrow morning and let me see your eye.

别担心，几乎不疼，只不过像蚊子叮一口那样。好的，现在脓都排出来了。戴个眼罩。拿药方去买些眼药。请明天上午再来复诊一次。

Patient：All right，doctor，thanks.

好的，谢谢医生。

3. A Foreign Body in the Cornea 角膜异物

Patient：Doctor，I feel something in my right（left）eye，and it's been hurting me since yesterday.

医生,我觉得我的右(左)眼里好像有东西,从昨天开始就一直感觉磨着疼。

Doctor：Please look straight ahead (look down or look up). There is a foreign body on the cornea. I'm going to put a few drops of dicaine into your eye. Don't move, look straight ahead. Now I've removed the foreign body. Have a look at it.

请你向前(向上或向下)看。角膜上是有个东西。我给你滴上几滴地卡因。不要动,向前看。现在你瞧这个异物已经取出来了。

Patient：Oh, it is so small, yet it hurt me so much.

哦,这么小一点,不过可真把我给疼坏了。

Doctor：I'll check your cornea with a slit-lamp to see whether there is anything left on it. Please open your eyes and look straight ahead. There is an abrasion on the surface of your cornea. I'll put some antibiotic eye drops into your eye. Now I'll put on an eye-pad, so that the abrasion will heal quickly.

我现在用裂隙灯给你再检查一下角膜,看看还有什么留在上面没有。请睁开眼向前看,噢,角膜浅层有明显的擦伤。我给你往眼睛里滴一些抗生素眼药水。戴个眼罩,这样角膜擦伤就会很快愈合。

Patient：Thank you, doctor.

谢谢你,医生。

Doctor：Well, please come tomorrow morning. I'll check it again then.

请你明天早晨再来,我还要给你检查一次。

Patient：OK, no problem, doctor.

好的,医生。

(The next day)

(第二天)

Doctor：Is the pain less severe?

疼痛减轻了些吧?

Patient：Yes, doctor. I don't feel anything now.

是的,医生。我感觉一点也不疼了。

Doctor：Now I'll take off the eye-pad and apply a corneal stain with a drop of "fluorescein". I'll have a look at it now with the slit-lamp. The abrasion has healed. There's no need for the pad. But you still have to continue the eye drops for two more days.

我给你摘掉眼罩,做个角膜"荧光素"染色,在裂隙灯下再检查检查。现在角膜擦伤已完全愈合,不需要戴眼罩了。但是你还得继续滴两天眼药水。

4. Central Serous Chorioretinopathy 中心浆液性脉络膜视网膜病变

Patient：Doctor, I don't know what's wrong with my eyes. The focal point of what I see is dark. I can see better around the perimeter than in the middle. Things look small and blurred.

医生,我也不知道我的眼睛怎么了。我看到的所有东西的中心点都是黑黑的,看中心点的周围显得稍好点儿。所有东西看起来好像变小了点,而且还有点模糊不清。

Doctor：Have you noticed any change in your vision?

你注意到最近视力有什么变化吗?

Patient：My eyesight is worse. Perhaps I'm far-sighted.

有,视力减退很多。我感觉可能有点远视了吧。

Doctor：Is it only one eye or both?

是一只,还是两只呢?

Patient：Only one eye. The other day I happened to notice it, when the other eye was covered.

一只眼。有一天我遮着另一只眼睛看东西时,才碰巧察觉眼睛有问题的。

Doctor：You seem to be fit and healthy, but I wonder if you've been doing too much lately.

你看上去身体很健康,但我不知道你最近是不是有点过于劳累了。

Patient：Yes, I'm so overworked. I never get enough sleep. I'm healthy enough, but I always feel tired.

是的,我的工作太忙,总是加班,所以睡眠不足。我身体很健康,但我总是感到疲乏得很。

Doctor：Are you forcing yourself to do too much or can't you relax?

是工作过度紧张还是情绪有波动,不会自我放松呀?

Patient：Well，both. I suppose I'm under a lot of stress.

都有。我认为我的工作压力很大。

Doctor：I see. Let me examine you. You are suffering from central serous chorioretinopathy.

明白了,让我给你检查一下吧。你得了中心浆液性脉络膜视网膜病变。

Patient：Oh，what can you give me for it?

哦,怎么治疗呢?

Doctor：I'll give you an injection and some medicine to take.

你需要打针、口服些药物了。

Patient：How long does it take to clear up, doctor?

医生,那多长时间能治愈呢?

Doctor：Generally speaking，it should be all right within three months. Then your vision will return to normal. A relapse is common，however，if it does occur，black spots will remain in your eyes. You must pay attention to your health. Don't overdo things and learn to relax.

一般来说,三个月基本可以治愈,视力可恢复到正常。但这种病会经常复发,也就是说,黑点又会重新出现。你必须关注自己的健康。你需要注意休息,避免过度疲劳。

Patient：I see, I'll try to be careful. (All right, I'll take your advice.)

好,我一定注意。(好,就按你说的办。)

5. Checking the Eyes for Glasses 配眼镜

Patient：My eyesight is not good，doctor. I can't see distances clearly.

医生,我的视力不好。远距离的东西看不清。

Doctor：Then I'll examine your eyes. Please sit down here，cover one eye with this patch. Look at the mirror. Which way is the letter "E" facing，up or down，right or left? Please tell me. You seem to be short-sighted. You ought to wear glasses.

让我先检查一下你的视力吧。请坐在这里,用这个眼罩遮住一只眼。看着镜子,看看"E"开口向哪一边,上或下,右或左? 请告诉我。你的眼睛是近视了,应该戴眼镜了。

Patient：Can you test them right now?

现在能给我验光吗?

Doctor：It takes at least an hour or so, and before the test you must put some eyedrops into your eyes to dilate the pupils. I'll prescribe some eyedrops for you. Please put one drop into your eyes every five minutes six times tomorrow before you come. Please come at eight o'clock.

验光至少需要 1 个小时,而且验光前必须点散瞳药,我给你开些眼药水,明天上午来之前每 5 分钟点一次,共 6 次。请你 8 点钟来,可以吗?

Patient：All right.

好。

Doctor：Have you used the eyedrops six times already?

你点够 6 次眼药水了吗?

Patient：Yes. Everything's blurred.

点够了,什么东西都模模糊糊的,看不清。

Doctor：That's because your pupils are dilated. Sit down and I'll test your eyes now. Look at the line. Which one is better? This one or that one?

这是因为你的瞳孔散开了。请坐下来查视力。请看这一行。你感觉哪个镜片看得清楚些? 这个好还是那个好?

Patient：The second one is better.

第二个好些。

Doctor：And how is it with this piece of glass?

戴上这个镜片好些了吗?

Patient：It's better.

好一些。

Doctor：You are short-sighted. Your right eye is at 325 degrees, your left at 175 degrees. Please sit down here and read a few pages of *Beijing Review* with this pair of glasses. How do you feel? Do you want them?

你的眼睛是近视。右眼 325 度,左眼 175 度。现在请你戴上这副眼镜读几面《北京周报》试试看。你觉得怎样? 这副眼镜合适吗?

Patient：I'll take them.

我就要这副了。

Doctor：Please look straight ahead，let me check the distance between the pupils. It is 58 mm. Here is the prescription for your glasses.

请你往前看，我量一下你瞳孔的距离。58 毫米。这是你的配镜处方。

Ⅱ. Sentences 替换句型

（1）You must wear the patch all the time，it will make your other eye work and feel better.

你必须一直戴眼罩，它会使你用另一只眼睛看东西并感觉好点。

（2）Keep your head still and follow my finger with your eyes.

你的头保持不动，你的眼睛随我的手指转动。

（3）The woman complained of reduced vision and increasing pain in the affected eye.

这个妇女诉说病眼视力下降，疼痛加重。

（4）My eyes hurt and feel as if there is grit in them. It seems to be my eyelashes. I pull them out，but they still get in my eyes.

我眼睛疼，仿佛里面有沙子，我感觉也许是我的睫毛就给拔出来了，可它们还是往里长。

（5）Oh，it's trichiasis (ingrowing eyelashes). That is to say that your eyelashes are uneven and ingrowing. Your eyelid is curved inward，so the eyelashes touch the cornea and irritate it. You had better have a minor operation. That will solve the problem.

噢，这是倒睫。也就是因为你的睫毛长得不齐而且往里长。眼皮的边缘往里卷，睫毛触着并刺激了你的角膜。最好做个小手术。这样就解决问题了。

（6）Doctor，I would like my eyes tested for a driving license.

医生，为了领驾驶证，我需要检查一下眼睛。

（7）All right. We have to check your long distance vision. Let me also check you for color blindness. Since you have red and green color blindness，I'm afraid you can't pass the test.

好的，你需要检查一下远视力和色盲。你有红绿色盲，我怕你领不到驾驶证了。

(8) Please re-check them. In our country the doctor said I only have a color weakness, so that I could drive a car. I can see clearly for a long time.

请你再检查一次吧。在我们国家,医生说我只是色弱,可以开车。而我也一直看得很清楚呀。

(9) I would check up again. It's unlucky. Actually you have blindness, so you can't drive a car.

我再检查一次。抱歉,你的确是色盲,所以你不能开车。

(10) Doctor, a lump has been growing slowly here on my right lid for about two months, what is it?

医生,最近两个月来我的右眼皮上慢慢地起了个疙瘩,你看是怎么回事呢?

(11) It is a "tarsal cyst" or so-called "chalazion". Better have it removed. It's only a minor operation. An incision will be made on the inside of the lid, there will be no scar on the skin. It will heal in a couple of days. If you agree to have it removed, we can make the appointment now. Can you come on Thursday afternoon?

这是"睑板腺囊肿"或叫"霰粒肿"。最好将它切除掉。这只是个小手术。在眼皮里面作切口,在外皮上就不会留伤疤。两天就可长好。如果你同意手术,我们就可约好时间。本星期四下午你能来吗?

(12) All right. What time is convenient, doctor?

好吧,医生。你看几点钟来合适?

(13) Please come at two o'clock sharp. Here is a prescription for eye drops. Please put them into your right eye four times a day before the operation.

请两点钟准时来吧,这是眼药水的处方,手术前请你点右眼,一天四次。

Ⅲ. Words and Expressions 单词和短语

accommodation /əˌkɒməˈdeɪʃən/ n. 调节
anisometropia /ˌænaɪsəʊməˈtrəʊpiə/ n. (两眼)屈光参差
amblyopia /ˌæmblɪˈəʊpiə/ n. 弱视

artificial eye；glass eye 义眼

asthenopia /ˌæsθɪˈnəupiə/ n. 眼疲劳

astigmatism /əˈstɪgməˌtɪzəm/ n. 散光

binocular vision 双眼视

blepharitis ciliaris 睑缘炎

blepharoptosis /blefæˈrɒptəusɪs/ n. 睑下垂

blindness /ˈblaɪndnɪs/ n. 盲

cataract /ˈkætəˌrækt/ n. 白内障

catarrhal conjunctivitis 卡他性结膜炎

chalazion /kəˈleɪziən/ n. 霰粒肿

choroid /ˈkɔːrɔɪd/ n. 脉络膜

ciliary body 睫状体

colour-blindness 色盲

colour-sense 色觉(感)

conjunctiva /ˌkɒndʒʌŋkˈtaɪvə/ n. 结膜

convergence /kənˈvɜːdʒəns/ n. 辐辏

cornea /ˈkɔːniə/ n. 角膜

dacryocystitis /deɪkriːəˈsɪstaɪtɪs/ n. 泪囊炎

dark room 暗室

diabetic retinitis 糖尿病性视网膜炎

diffuse retina chorioiditis 弥漫性视网膜脉络膜炎

dim vision 视力模糊

diplopia /dɪˈpləupiə/ n. 复视

disturbance of vision 视力障碍

ectropion /ekˈtrəupɪˌɒn/ n. 睑外翻

emmetropia /ˌemɪˈtrəupiə/ n. 正视

entropion /enˈtrəupiən/ n. 睑内翻

exophthalmus /ˌeksɒfˈθælməs/ n. 眼球突出；突眼

eye ball 眼球

eye ground 眼底

eye shield tears 眼水

eye-discharge 眼粪

eyeglass /ˈaɪˌglɑːs/ n. 眼镜

eyelid /ˈaɪˌlɪd/；palpebra /ˈpælpəbrə/ n. 眼睑

follicular conjunctivitis 滤泡性结膜炎

glaucoma /glɔːˈkəumə/ n. 青光眼

gonorrheal ophthalmia 淋病性眼炎

hemianopsia /ˌhemiænˈəupiə/ n. 偏盲

vitreous hemorrhage n. 玻璃体出血

hordeolum /ˌhɔːdɪˈəuləm/；stye /staɪ/ n. 麦粒肿

hypermetropia /ˌhaɪpəməˈtrəupiə/ n.；far sight 远视

interstitial keratitis 实质性角膜炎

intraocular tension 眼压

iridocyclitis /ˌɪrɪdəusɪˈklaɪtɪs/ n. 虹膜睫状体炎

iris /ˈaɪəris/ n. 虹膜

iritis /aɪˈraɪtɪs/ n. 虹膜炎

lacrimation /ˌlækrɪˈmeɪʃən/ n. 溢泪

lens /lenz/ n. 镜片

muscae volitantes 飞蚊症

myopic /maɪˈɒpɪk/ adj.；short-sighted 近视

nephritic /neˈfrɪtɪk/ n. 肾炎的

night-blindness 夜盲

oblique illumination 斜照法

ophthalmology /ˌɒfθælˈmɒlədʒi/ n. 眼科学

optic nerve atrophy 视神经萎缩

optic neuritis 视神经炎

orbit /ˈɔːbɪt/ n. 轨道；眼眶

panophthalmia /ˌpænɒfˈθælmiə/ n. 全眼球炎

papilloedema /ˌpæpɪləʊəˈdiːmə/ n. 乳头水肿

paralysis of the ocular muscles; ophthalmoplegia /ɒfˌθælməˈpliːdʒiə/ 眼肌麻痹

photophobia /ˌfəʊtəʊˈfəʊbiə/ n. 怕光

pigmentary retinitis 变性色素视网膜

presbyopia /ˌprezbɪˈəʊpiə/ n. 老花眼

pterygium /təˈrɪdʒiəm/ n. 翼状胬肉

pupil lens 瞳孔

refraction /rɪˈfrækʃən/ n. 折射

retinal angiosclerosis 视网膜动脉硬化

retinal hemorrhage 视网膜出血

retina /ˈretɪnə/ n. 视网膜

scotoma /skɒˈtəʊmə/ n.; blind spot 盲点

sciascopy /saɪˈæskəpi/ n. 视网膜镜检查

sclera /ˈsklɪərə/ n. 巩膜

scleritis /sklɪəˈraɪtɪs/; sclerotitis /ˌsklɪərəʊˈtaɪtɪs/ n. 巩膜炎

sclerosing keratitis 硬性化角膜炎

serpiginous /sɜːˈpɪdʒɪnəs/ n. 匐行性角膜炎

eyesight /ˈaɪˌsaɪt/ n.; visual acuity 视力

strabismus /strəˈbɪzməs/ n. 斜视

stricture of the dacronasal duct 鼻泪管狭窄

superficial keratitis 表层性角膜炎

sympathetic ophthalmia 交感性眼炎

central chorioretinitis 中心性网膜脉络膜炎

thrombosis of the central retinal vein 中心视网膜静脉血栓

trachoma /trəˈkəʊmə/ n. 沙眼

transillumination /ˈtrænsɪˌljuːmɪˈneɪʃən/ n. 透照法

trichiasis /trɪˈkaɪəsɪs/ n. 倒睫

vernal or spring conjunctivitis 春季结膜炎

visual field; field of vision 视野

vitreous body 玻璃体

vitreous opacity 玻璃体混浊

xerosis of conjunctiva 结膜干燥症

Section 9　Stomatology
第9节　口腔科

I . Dialogues 情景对话

1. Inflammation of the Gums (Gingivitis) 牙龈炎

Patient：Doctor，my gums bleed and my mouth is emitting a bad smell.
　　　　医生，我的牙龈总出血，还发出一种臭味。

Doctor：How long have you had this condition?
　　　　这情况有多久了?

Patient：Since about a year ago.
　　　　差不多一年了。

Doctor：Does the bleeding occur by itself or is it induced by some irritation? That is to say，do your gums bleed when you brush your teeth，when you eat，or do they bleed for no apparent reason at all?
　　　　是无缘无故就出血，还是由什么刺激的呢? 也就是说，是刷牙、吃东西引起的出血，还是没有任何明显的原因就出血了呢?

Patient：I don't know. All I know is that it seems to happen very often.
　　　　我也不清楚。我只知道它经常出血。

Doctor：Have you noticed any bleeding spots on your skin?
　　　　你的皮肤上发现有出血点吗?

Patient：No.
　　　　没有。

Doctor：Let me do a check-up. H'm，there is a lot of dental calculus on the teeth and this may cause inflammation and bleeding of the gums. I would recommend a cleaning of your teeth. But this can only be done on Wednesday mornings. Please go to the nurse to make an appointment，firstly. Then I'll give you a medicinal liquid. You will apply a little of it on the edges of the gums after brushing your teeth in the evening. It is very important that you should pay more attention to the dental hygiene. And the teeth should be brushed twice a day, once in the morning and once in the evening. The upper and lower rows of teeth should be brushed separately, and one after the other. All the crevices must be cleared of remnant food. Besides, I'll give you a kind of Chinese powder. Massage your gums with it twice a day, about three or four minutes each time, after you have brushed your teeth.

我来给你检查一下。嗯,你牙齿上的牙垢有很多,这可能会引起牙龈发炎、出血,所以我建议你做一次洁齿(洗牙)。不过,这只能在每星期三上午做,先到护士那里约个时间。然后,我给你开一种药水,每天晚上刷完牙后在出血牙龈处涂一点。以后,你必须注意牙齿卫生了。最好每天刷两次牙,早晚各一次。上面一排牙和下面一排牙要分开刷,刷完上面再刷下面。仔细认真地把缝隙里的残余食物刷干净。我再给你开一种中药粉,每天刷完两次牙后,用它涂擦按摩牙龈,每次三四分钟。

Patient：Thanks, doctor. Should I come back for another consultation?
谢谢你,医生。我还需要再来复诊吗?

Doctor：It would be better if you come back once more after the teeth-cleaning.
洗完牙后最好再来一次。

2. Extracting a Tooth 拔牙

Patient：Doctor, I have a bad tooth. Should it be filled?
医生,我的一颗牙齿坏了,你看还能补吗?

Doctor：Oh, my god. This tooth is too bad to be filled any more. It has to be pulled. Do you agree to have it extracted?
噢,这牙坏得太厉害了,已经不能补了。需要拔掉了,你同意吗?

Patient：It's up to you to decide what to do, doctor.
医生,你看着决定吧。

Doctor：OK. But at first, I want to know if you have ever had an injection of procaine. Have you ever been allergic to anything?

好的,不过首先我想了解一下,你以前是否注射过普鲁卡因?另外,你有没有对什么东西过敏过?

Patient：No.

没有。

Doctor：That's fine. Now I'll give you an injection. Please open your mouth as wide as you can. But relax. It won't hurt much. Now you've gotten the injection. Please wash your mouth and spit out the water into the spittoon. If you feel your heart palpitate a little, it doesn't matter. That's the effect of the procaine, and it'll soon be over. Now, do you feel numb? Do you have a sensation of swelling on the lips and the tongue? This tooth is in very bad condition. It needs a careful operation, which may last a little longer than usual. Now, the tooth is out. Please bite and hold the cotton ball tightly in place. Don't spit it out until half an hour from now. You may eat in two hours. But don't rinse your mouth today because it may cause bleeding. Please go to make the payment and get the medicines.

那好。我现在给你打麻药。请尽量把嘴张大,放松。不会太疼的。好的,针打完了。请漱一下口,水就吐在痰盂里吧。如果你觉得有点心慌,那是普鲁卡因的正常反应,没什么关系,一会儿就过去了。现在你感觉嘴麻了吗?你的嘴唇和舌头有肿胀的感觉吗?你这牙的确很糟糕,要想彻底拔掉,可能会多用点时间。好,出来了。现在在拔出牙的地方咬紧一个棉球,过半小时以后再吐出来。记着两小时后才可以吃东西。今天别漱口,以防出血。现在你去交费,取药吧。

3. For False Teeth 镶牙

Patient：Doctor, I want to have fixed false teeth.

医生,我希望做个固定的假牙。

Doctor：No problem. Let me see whether the teeth on either side of the jaw are fixed or not. Then the fixed bridge can be made.

可以,没问题。我得先检查一下缺的牙两旁的基牙是否稳固,然后才可以做固定桥。

Patient：Oh, I see.

噢,我明白了。

Doctor：Tell me what kind of material do you prefer for the fixed bridge? Gold-alloy or stainless steel? Let me show you some samples.

告诉我,你喜欢哪种材料的固定桥? 合金的还是不锈钢的? 我给你看看样品吧。

Patient：I prefer the gold one, doctor.

医生,我喜欢金的。

Doctor：Well, in that case you must bring some gold, for example, gold rings, earings. But they should be 20 or 24 carat. If you haven't get any, you can buy them at the Friendship Store. Or you can order here, but it will be costly.

那么,你可以以自己拿金子来这儿做——金戒指、金耳环都可以用。金子的成分要 20 或 24 开的。如果没有这些,你可以到友谊商店去买,或者干脆直接在这里定制,不过这样花费可能会贵点儿了。

Patient：How much do I need?

需要多少量呢?

Doctor：Eight or nine grams will be enough for one.

八九克就够做一个固定桥了。

Patient：OK. I'll come back later.

好吧,我买完以后再来吧。

Doctor：Let me make an appointment for you. Here is the card. Please try to be punctual.

我给你预约个时间。这是预约卡,请按时前来。

4. An Injury 外伤

Parent：My child has been wounded in a fall, doctor.

医生,我的孩子跌了一跤受伤了。

Doctor：Where did it happen?

在什么地方摔伤的?

Parent：Right at home.

就在家里。

Doctor：His upper lip has been cut. Several teeth have become loose. One of them has to be extracted, and some others need refixing.

他上嘴唇破了,有几颗牙也松动了,其中有一颗需要拔掉,其余几颗需要固定一下。

Parent：How about the lip?

那裂开的嘴唇怎么办呢?

Doctor：Don't worry, madame. I'll give him a shot of anaesthetic and have the lip washed clean and the cut sewn up. Please explain this to your chlid and ask him not to be afraid.

别担心,夫人。我给他打一点麻药,把嘴唇洗净,把裂口缝合上。你跟孩子解释一下,叫他不要害怕。

Parent：Please just go ahead, doctor. Don't worry about him.

医生,这一点你不必担心,该缝就缝吧。

Doctor：The operation is over, madame. Your boy has been very good and cooperative. Please take this slip of paper to the nurse so that she will give him an injection of TAT. Come back in five days to have the stitches taken out. If anything unexpected should develop in the meantime, then don't wait but come back any day for a consultation.

缝合完了,夫人。你孩子表现真棒,配合得很好。拿着这单子到护士那里,她会给他注射一针破伤风抗毒素的。五天以后来拆线。如果五天内有什么异常情况,随时来看门诊。

5. Pulpitis 牙髓炎

Doctor：Sit in the chair please. Lean your head back against the chair now. What's the trouble?

请坐到手椅上。把头往后靠在椅子上。有什么不舒服吗?

Patient：I have an awful toothache, doctor.

医生,我的牙疼得厉害。

Doctor：Which tooth is causing the trouble?

哪颗牙呢?

Patient：I don't know. The right side of my face and head hurts.

我不知道是哪颗牙。右边的脸和头都疼。

Doctor：How long have you had this pain?

疼了多长时间了？

Patient：Two days.

两天了。

Doctor：Does the pain increase at night?

晚上疼得是不是更厉害呢？

Patient：Yes，it hurt so much at night that I couldn't sleep.

对，晚上疼得都睡不着觉。

Doctor：Does the pain increase when you take hot or cold food?

吃冷的或热的东西也疼得更厉害吗？

Patient：Yes. It's particularly painful if I drink something cold.

是的，一喝凉的东西就特别疼。

Doctor：Please open your mouth and let me examine your teeth. One of your back teeth has a big cavity. We'll take an X-ray picture first. The X-ray room is on the third floor. Let's go there now.

请张大嘴，我给你检查一下。你后面的牙有个大洞。我们先去拍张 X 光片吧。X 光室在三楼，我们现在到那儿去吧。

Patient：What's the result?

结果怎样？

Doctor：The pulp is exposed. I'll give you an injection first，then I'll put some medicine in the cavity to kill the nerve.

哦，牙髓已经露在外面了。我先给你注射一支麻药，然后在牙洞里放点药把神经杀死。

Patient：OK.

好。

Doctor：Rinse your mouth and spit into the basin. Now open your mouth wide，please. This injection may hurt a little，but don't move，the pain will soon stop.

漱口，把漱口水吐在盆里。请张大嘴。打麻药时会有点疼，不要动，很快就不疼了。

Patient：Um…

嗯……

Doctor：Does your mouth feel numb now?

现在嘴麻了吗？

Patient：Yes.

麻了。

Doctor：Good, avoid chewing on that tooth today. I'll give you some tablets for the pain. If necessary, take one tablet. Here is your prescription. Come back in two weeks for the permanent filling.

好了，记住今天不要用坏牙那边嚼东西。我给你一点儿止疼药，疼的时候服一片。这是处方。两周后再来做个永久性的填充。

6. Inflammation of the Mucous Membrane（Stomatitis）口腔黏膜炎症（口炎）

Patient：There are several painful spots in my mouth, doctor, salty and sour things make it sting.

医生，我嘴里有几块地方疼，吃咸的和酸的东西都感觉螫着疼。

Doctor：It's caused by an infection. I'll give you some Chinese traditional medicine, it will soon clear up.

这是感染引起的。我给你开点中药，很快就会好的。

Patient：My gum is inflamed and hurts badly, too.

我的牙龈也发炎了，很疼。

Doctor：It's caused by your denture. Don't wear it for a few days until your gum has healed. I'll prescribe some ointment for local use.

这是你的假牙引起的，牙龈没好之前，这几天先不要戴假牙。我给你开一点软膏，是局部涂擦用的。

Patient：I have prickly and burning ulcers in the mucosa. It happens periodically.

我的口腔黏膜上的溃疡有刺疼和烧灼疼，而且还周期发作。

Doctor：Do you think it occurs for any obvious reason, for example, emotional stress or lack of sleep?

你想想看，它的发作有什么明显的原因吗，比如情绪波动或缺少睡眠？

Patient：Yes, sometimes it happens when I have difficulty falling asleep.

有的，我有时候失眠时总会出现这样的情况。

Doctor：What kind of drugs did you take in the past?

你过去吃过什么药吗?

Patient：Vitamins and antibiotics.

维生素和抗生素。

Doctor：I'll give you some tablets to swallow this time, a mouth rinse to gargle with and powder for local use. They are effective hut they do not guarantee the condition won't recur.

这次我给你开一些口服药,漱口药水和局部用的药粉。这些药都有效,但不能保证它不再复发。

Patient：Why do I have a burning and thickening sensation in my mouth, doctor?

医生,为什么我嘴里有种灼热和增厚的感觉呢?

Doctor：How long have you had this trouble?

多长时间了?

Patient：For about half a year.

大约半年了。

Doctor：Have you been to see a doctor before?

过去看过医生吗?

Patient：Two months ago in Hong Kong, I went to see a dentist. He took a specimen from that particular spot of my mouth for culture. Then he told me that my trouble was caused by some bacteria. I had taken too many antibiotic tablets but there was no improvement.

两个月前在香港我看过牙科医生。他取了一个标本做细菌培养。后来他告诉我是细菌引起的。我吃了许多抗生素片,但是没有见好。

Doctor：Did you notice any rash on your body?

你身上出过皮疹吗?

Patient：No.

没有呀。

Doctor：Let me examine you. There are many white spots and plaque-like lesions on the tongue and buccal mucosa. It may be leukoplakia or lichen planus. A biopsy is necessary, I think.

让我检查一下吧。在你的舌头上和口腔黏膜上发现了一些白点和白斑样的病灶。可能是白斑病或扁平苔藓。我想你需要做个活检。

Patient：What is the cause? Is it a cancer, doctor?

是什么原因引起的呢? 会是癌吗,医生?

Doctor：No. don't worry. The cause of it is not clear, but chronic irritation and emotional stress may play an important role in its development.

不是,别顾虑那么多了。这种病的原因虽然现在还不清楚,但是慢性刺激和情绪波动对病情发展可能会起重要作用。

Patient：What do you propose to do?

你打算怎么治疗呢?

Doctor：First, the sharp edges of your teeth should be smoothed. Keep to a soft diet and no irritants. Take it easy. Rinse your mouth after every meal. Come here for a check-up every month. Here is an ointment for local application, use it three times a day.

首先,要把你牙齿的锐利边缘磨光一下,多吃软食和不带刺激性的食物。此外,精神要放松。养成饭后漱口的习惯。以后每个月来检查一次。这是软膏,局部涂抹,一日三次。

Patient：OK, doctor, thank you for your detailed explanation.

医生,谢谢你这么详细的介绍。

Ⅱ. Sentences 替换句型

(1) I'm having my teeth out next week.

下周我要去拔牙。

(2) I must make an appointment with my dentist. I had toothache all night.

我必须同我的牙科医生预约,我整夜牙痛。

(3) You had better have all your teeth out. They are poisoning your system.

你最好拔掉你的全部牙齿,它们正在危害你的身体。

(4) How long ago were your teeth pulled out?

你拔牙多久了?

(5) Since when have you had this condition?

这种情况有多久了？

(6) There's a hole in my back tooth, doctor.

医生,我后面的牙上有个洞。

(7) A filling has fallen out. This tooth can be filled.

补过的牙里的填充物掉出来了。不过这牙还可以补。

(8) A tooth that has been filled in Shanghai has started to hurt.

我在上海补的牙现在又开始疼了。

(9) I'll clean it now. Let me know if it hurts.

我给你冲洗一下,如果感觉疼就告诉我。

(10) It is a deep cavity, we'll have an X-ray taken of that tooth just to make sure about the apex. If it is in good condition, I'll treat it.

是有一个很深的洞,要照一张 X 光片检查一下根尖情况,如果根尖好,就可以治疗。

(11) It has been like this since I tried to bite something hard.

有一次我咬了硬的东西之后就这样了。

(12) Bite please. Now open your mouth again. Do you feel anything abnormal when you clench your teeth? Please come here for polishing after two or three days.

请咬一下。请再张开口。咬紧时有什么不正常的感觉吗？请两三天后来磨光。

(13) I want to have some false teeth. Shall I make an appointment for you?

我是来镶牙的。我跟你预约一个时间好吗？

(14) My tooth is very sensitive to cold, doctor. What's wrong with it?

医生,我的牙齿对冷特别敏感,这是怎么回事呀？

(15) There's quite a bit of erosion. Which way do you brush your teeth?

你的牙齿上有许多腐蚀的地方。你是用什么方法刷牙的呀？

(16) I usually brush them horizontally.

我习惯于横着刷。

(17) Brushing them up and down is much better. The way you are doing it rubs all the natural enamel off, you know.

还是上下刷牙比较好些。像你那种刷牙方法很容易将牙釉质刷掉。

(18) Let me have a look. The wound has not healed yet, you will have to wait for two months and a half to three months, or your false

teeth won't fit properly.

让我看一下。伤口还没长好,得等两个半到三个月,否则安上的假牙会感觉不合适的。

(19) I have two teeth missing here, doctor. What kind of false teeth can I have made?

医生,我这儿缺了两颗牙。你看我能装什么样的假牙呢?

(20) Well, I'll show you some sample models, then you can choose any one you like, either a fixed bridge or a removable partial denture. The fixed bridge costs three hundred yuan, while the removable partial denture costs one hundred and twenty yuan. They are made of different materials and the former is more complicated to construct.

我先给你看看样品模型,从中你可以选择你喜欢的一种。你既可以选固定桥,也可以选活动的假牙。固定桥是 300 元,假牙 120 元。它们制作的材料不同,而且前者的工序复杂些。

(21) All my teeth have been extracted and I want to have false teeth, doctor.

医生,我全口牙都拔掉了,我想镶牙。

(22) I'll see if the wound has healed. If it has, we can take an impression.

让我检查一下拔牙的创口长好没有。若长好了,我们就可以取印模了。

(23) Here are the sample models, you can have a look. A full denture set costs one thousand yuan. You'll have to come five times according to your appointments before the work can be completed. It is quite a complicated process.

这些是样品模型,你可以先看看。全口假牙是 1000 元。需按预约的时间来,先后五次才能做完,相对来说比较麻烦。

(24) My dental crown has been broken and it can't be fixed. What shall I do, doctor?

我的牙冠坏了,已无法再修了。医生,你看还有什么办法吗?

(25) You can have a new crown made from gold or stainless steel.

可以考虑做一个新的牙冠,用金子或不锈钢做都行。

(26) I fell and broke my tooth. The nerve died, so the color has

changed. What should I do, doctor?

医生,我的牙断了、神经死了,牙齿颜色也变了,我该怎么办呢?

(27) Don't worry. I'll make a plastic crown for you. That will look all right.

不用担心,我给你做一个塑料冠。那就好看了。

(28) I'll make a post-crown for you. But first of all, you should have it X-rayed to see the condition of the root. The nerve of the tooth should be removed before we make the crown.

我给你做一个桩冠。先得照一张 X 光片看看牙根情况怎样。在做桩冠之前必须把牙神经抽掉。

(29) The inlay came off when I was chewing a piece of chewing-gum. What should I do, doctor?

医生,我吃口香糖时把嵌体弄掉了,怎么办呀?

(30) I can stick them together with cement.

我可以用黏固剂给你粘上。

(31) My removable denture is broken. Can you repair it for me, doctor?

医生,我的活动假牙折断了,能修理一下吗?

(32) I'll make an impression. Leave your old denture here. It will take two days to repair it.

我给你取一个印模。你把假牙留下,两天后来取好了。

(33) When I open my mouth, doctor, I feel a pain in front of the ear and in the head. There is also a cracking sound.

医生,我一张嘴,就感到耳朵前面和头都很疼,而且还有很大的响声。

(34) Please open your mouth. Close it. Open again. Move the lower jaw left and right. Do you feel sore here when I press this place?

请张开嘴。合上,再张开。将你的下颌向左右移动一下。当我按这个地方的时候你感到疼吗?

(35) It's mandibular arthralgia and it feels quite sore.

你这是下颌关节疼痛,疼起来可真厉害。

(36) There is something wrong with the mandibular joint. It has been overstrained. I'd recommend physiotherapy. Please go with this paper to the physiotherapy department for treatment.

你的下颌关节因为咬东西时用力过大而发生了问题。我建议你做一下理疗。请你拿着这张单子到理疗科去做治疗吧。

（37）Doctor, I've got a gumboil. A bad tooth may have to be pulled.

医生,我牙龈上长了个包,一个坏牙可能需要拔掉。

（38）There is an abscess round that tooth, and it's called alveolar abscess. An incision should be made to drain the pus.

你这牙旁边长了个脓肿,医学上叫作牙槽脓肿,必须开刀把脓放出来。

（39）The tooth is indeed in very bad condition and should be extracted. But not until the inflammation has subsided. Today I'll drill a little hole in the tooth for pus-drainage to stop the pain.

是的,你这牙已经很不好了,需要拔掉,但要等炎症消了以后才能拔。今天先在牙上钻个小洞将脓引流出来,这样就不会太疼了。

（40）First, I'll give you an injection of anaesthetic. Have you had anaesthetics before?

我先给你打一针麻药,你以前注射过麻药吗?

（41）The injection may hurt a little, but it'll prevent your feeling any pain during the operation. Now the pus has been let out. Please rinse your mouth. A drain has been left at the incision. Please come back again tomorrow to have the drain replaced. Here is a prescription for some medicines for the inflammation, for pain-killing and mouth-rinsing.

注射麻药时有点疼,这样手术时就不感觉疼了。现在脓都流出来了。请漱漱口。我在切口的地方放了一个引流条。明天需要再来一次,换一下引流条。这是处方,有消炎药、止痛药和漱口药水。

（42）Here are the instructions for your removable denture, let me explain it to you.

这是使用活动假牙的各项注意事项,让我给你解释一下吧。

① Trying on. 试装。

When trying on the denture, take a certain direction without force or pressure. Press the clasp down with the index finger to remove the upper denture, and push up the clasp with thumb to remove the lower denture. The newly-made denture is of course not as good as your natural teeth, therefore you'd better avoid hard food. It will occasionally give you some discomfort, making talking awkward, increasing saliva, even nausea or vomiting. Don't worry about this. Keep the denture in your mouth constantly and you will soon get used to it after a few days.

装假牙时应顺一定方向装进去,不要强力推压。取出时上颌的假牙应用食指尖钩着卡环向下拉,下颌的假牙应用拇指顶住卡环向上推。新做的假牙的功能当然比天然牙差,因此最好不吃硬东西。刚戴上假牙时,你会有一些不舒服,比如说话不利索,唾液增多,甚至还会感觉恶心呕吐,等等。不过,不必紧张急躁,坚持使用几天就会习惯的。

② About check-up. 关于复查。

If you still have some pain after a period of time, return to the clinic for a check-up. The dentist will examine your mouth. You should not remove the denture for too long. In case your own teeth become slightly displaced, your denture will eventually be of no use.

假牙戴上几天后,如果持续疼痛,请再到门诊复查。牙科医生会检查你的口腔情况。不能因为疼就索性取下假牙不用,时间久了,就会引起邻牙变位,假牙就会变成废品了。

③ Preservation. 养护。

a. You should keep the denture in your mouth all day. After each meal and at bed time, you should clean it with toothpaste or soap (avoid boiling water and chemical drugs), to prevent food residues accumulating on it.

你需要戴一天的假牙。饭后或睡前要用牙膏或肥皂(忌用开水或化学药物)刷洗一下假牙,以免食物残渣堆积在上面。

b. Remove the denture before you go to bed and put it into a cup of clear, cold water. This not only relaxes the mouth tissue but also avoids any possibility of accidentally swallowing it.

睡前取下假牙,放在一个盛着清洁冷水的杯子里。这样不仅可以使口腔组织得到休息,同时也可避免吞下假牙发生意外。

c. If the denture is cracked or broken, please bring the whole denture to the clinic for repair.

如果假牙折断或破裂了,请把整套假牙带到门诊来修补。

d. The denture should be adjusted or a new one made after several years, because the tissue of the mouth or the plastic may have altered. Such changes may harm the natural teeth or the soft tissue of the mouth.

假牙使用几年以后,应进行调整或换新,因为口腔组织或塑料会发生变化。否则会损伤天然牙齿或口腔内的软组织。

Ⅲ. Words and Expressions 单词和短语

artificial tooth 义齿

bitter /'bɪtə/ *adj.* 苦的

cleaning of the teeth 清洁牙齿

cleft palate 腭裂

digestive function 消化功能

disturbance of the salivary secretion
唾液分泌障碍

disturbance or disorder of the sense
of taste 味觉障碍

disturbance or impairment of
utterance 言语障碍

epidemic parotitis；mumps /mʌmps/
n. 流行性腮腺炎

gargle /'gɑːgl/ *n.* 漱口液

gustatory function 味觉功能

hare lip 兔唇

herpes labialis 唇疱疹

mastication /ˌmæstɪ'keɪʃən/ *n.* 咀嚼

oral cavity 口腔

ozostomia /ˌəʊzɒs'təʊmɪə/ *n.* ;
saburra /sə'bʌrə/ *n.* ;
halitosis /ˌhælɪ'təʊsɪs/ *n.* ;
offensive breath 口臭

parotid gland 腮腺

salivary gland 唾液腺

salivary stone 唾液结石

salt /sɔːlt/ *adj.* 咸的

simple stomatitis 单纯性口腔炎

sour /'saʊə/ *adj.* 酸的

sublingual gland 舌下腺

submaxillary gland 颌下腺

sweet /swiːt/ *adj.* 甜的

tongue coat；fur of the tongue 舌苔

Section 10　Dermatology & Sexually Transmitted Diseases

第 10 节　皮肤病/性病科

Ⅰ. Dialogues 情景对话

1. Neurodermatitis 神经性皮炎

Patient：My neck is itching terribly，doctor.

医生,我脖子很痒。

Doctor：Let me examine it. Oh，there are two thick patches on it. You have neurodermatitis.

让我检查一下。噢,你颈部有两片厚的皮损。你得了神经性皮炎了。

Patient：What is it?

这是怎么一回事?

Doctor：It can be induced by psychosomatic factors. You should avoid getting nervous and anxious and try to live a regular life.

这是由精神因素诱发的。你应该避免紧张、忧虑,并尽量过有规律的生活。

Patient：I see.

我懂了。

Doctor：It's a kind of chronic skin disease. It takes quite a long time and constant treatment to cure it.

这是一种慢性皮肤病,需要较长时间,你要坚持治疗才能治愈。

Patient：But what can you do for it?

那你准备怎么治疗呢,医生?

Doctor：I'll prescribe a bottle of lotion for you for external use only. Apply it on the lesions，twice a day. Here are some tablets too. Take one tablet three times a day.

我给你开一瓶药水，只能外用，擦在患处，一日两次。另外还有些药片，一日三次，一次一片。

2．Urticaria 荨麻疹

Patient：I have a rash all over my body, doctor. I think it's hives.

　　医生，我全身都起了疹子，我看是风疹块。

Doctor：How long have you had it?

　　起了多久了？

Patient：Just since this morning.

　　早晨刚有。

Doctor：Have you had any nausea or vomiting?

　　你恶心呕吐了吗？

Patient：No.

　　没有。

Doctor：Have you had any diarrhea?

　　泻肚了吗？

Patient：Yes, three times this morning.

　　是的，我早晨都泻了三次肚了。

Doctor：Did you eat any fish or shrimps before the rash began?

　　起疹子前你吃过鱼或虾吗？

Patient：Yes. I had some shrimps yesterday.

　　是的，昨天我吃了一些虾。

Doctor：Does it get worse when you feel cold or when it is windy?

　　受冷、吹风时你感觉出疹子的情况有加重吗？

Patient：No.

　　没有。

Doctor：Let me have a look. Yes, it's hives. The medical name is urticaria. It's an allergic reaction to something you've eaten.

　　让我看看。噢，是的，它就是风疹块。医学上叫作荨麻疹，一般是由于吃了某种食物过敏而引起的。

Patient：What food should I avoid?

　　我应该忌吃哪些食物呢？

Doctor：Avoid spicy food, wine, fish, shrimps and lobster.

最好不要吃辛辣食品,还有不要饮酒,不要吃鱼、虾和龙虾之类的。

Patient：All right, doctor. I'll remember that.

好吧,医生。我记住了。

Doctor：I'll give you some pills, a lotion and an injection to relieve the itching.

我给你一些药丸和外用药,再打一针脱脱敏、止止痒。

Patient：Thank you very much, doctor.

非常感谢你,医生。

3. Herpes Zoster 带状疱疹

Patient：Doctor, I don't know why there are several blisters on the right side of my chest and back.

医生,不知道怎么回事,我右胸右背上起了几个水疱。

Doctor：How long have you had them?

起这些水疱有多久了?

Patient：Three days.

三天了。

Doctor：Let me examine you. Do they hurt?

让我检查一下。疼吗?

Patient：The pain is awful.

是的,疼得厉害。

Doctor：It's caused by virus. And it will take ten to fifteen days to subside. Don't worry, everything will be OK.

这是病毒引起的。十到十五天就会好的。别着急,一切都会好起来的。

Patient：Can you give me something for the pain?

你有办法解除我的疼痛吗?

Doctor：I'll give you a bottle of lotion. Apply it to the blisters twice a day. Then you should have an injection once a day, and take two kinds of tablets. Don't break the blisters or you'll get a secondary infection. If they do break, apply some gentian violet solution.

我给你开一瓶药水。擦在水疱上面,一日两次。另外,每日打一次针,再口服两种药品。最好不要弄破水疱,以免引起继发感染。如果水疱破了,上点龙胆紫药水就行了。

4. Tinea Pedis (Athlete's Foot) 脚癣

Patient：Doctor, why are my feet so itchy?

医生,为什么我的脚这么痒呢?

Doctor：Let me take a look at them.

让我检查一下你的脚吧。

Patient：OK, let me untie my shoes.

好的,让我解开鞋带。

Doctor：You have a fungus infection on your feet. It usually clears up in the winter, but returns in the summer, isn't it?

你脚上感染了霉菌。它常常是冬天见好,夏天又复发,对吗?

Patient：Yes. Is it because the shoes I wear?

是的。是不是我穿的鞋引起的呢?

Doctor：Kind of. Shoes with poor ventilation and nylon socks which are bad at absorbing water keep the feet hot and sweaty all the time.

有点关系。如果鞋子透风不好,还有像穿尼龙袜这样吸水不好的,都会使脚总是汗热潮湿的。

Patient：What about cotton or linen socks?

穿棉袜或麻纱短袜好吗?

Doctor：They are much better, of course.

当然,肯定要好多了。

Patient：I heard there is no cure for it. But I really want to get rid of it. What's your advice, doctor?

我好像听说这脚病是没法儿治好的。但是我真希望你能治好它。你看我该注意些什么呢,医生?

Doctor：The most important thing is to keep the infected area clean and dry. Change your socks often.

最要紧的是保持患处的清洁和干燥。要勤换袜子。

Patient：All right.

好的。

Doctor：I'll prescribe some fungicides to put on the infected area，twice a day. Even after the itching and redness have disappeared you must keep on using it for a few days.

我给你开些杀霉菌的药，涂抹在患处，一日两次。即使红、痒消退了，也要坚持用药再多巩固几天。

5. Gonorrhea 淋病

Patient：Doctor，I have difficulty and a burning sensation when I pass urine.

医生，我排尿困难而且有烧灼感。

Doctor：Are you passing urine more frequently?

你感觉小便次数比以前多了吗?

Patient：Yes.

是的。

Doctor：Have you had intercourse recently?

你最近有过性生活吗?

Patient：Yes.

是的。

Doctor：All right. We would like a specimen of your pus. Please wait for the result of the examination.

好的，我们先要取些你的脓性分泌物化验一下。请在这儿等待检查结果。

Patient：Thank you, doctor.

好的，医生。

Doctor：The smear shows a lot of gonococci. You have gonorrhea. We would like to give you penicillin injections twice a day. Firstly, we'll do a skin test to see if you are allergic to it. You'll have to wait twenty minutes for the result. If the reaction is negative, then you can buy the penicillin from the pharmacy.

涂片查到许多淋球菌。你得了淋病。我们准备给你每天注射两次青霉素，请你先来做皮试吧，等二十分钟看看结果，若是阴性反应，再去药房买药。

Patient：When shoud I come for the injections?

　　　　我什么时间来打针呢？

Doctor：From nine to ten in the morning and three to four in the afternoon.

　　　　请在早晨九点至十点,下午三点至四点来注射吧。

Patient：All right.

　　　　行。

Doctor：I'll make an appointment for you to come back in three days.

　　　　我给你开一张预约条,三天后再来。

Patient：Thank you, doctor。

　　　　医生,谢谢你。

Ⅱ. Sentences 替换句型

（1）The dermatologist has diagnosed the patient's skin disorder as contact dermatitis.

　　皮肤科医生已经诊断病人的皮肤病为接触性皮炎了。

（2）When did the spots appear?

　　这些斑是什么时候出现的?

（3）Doctor, my baby cries all night especially when I touch her left ear. I don't know if there is something wrong with the skin of her ear.

　　医生,我的孩子通宵啼哭,尤其是我碰到她左耳的时候,是不是她的耳朵皮肤有什么问题了呀?

（4）Your child has an infantile eczema over her external ear. Please apply a thin layer of ointment over her affected ear twice a day. By the way I would suggest that you stop feeding her with cow's milk for a couple of months.

　　你的孩子的外耳部长了婴儿湿疹。请在她患病的耳朵上薄薄地敷些药膏,一天两次。另外,我还建议你连着几个月不要喂她牛奶。

（5）I'll leave a small cotton ball soaked with medicine in her ear canal. Be sure to bring her back to change the dressing in twenty-four hours.

　　我要在她的耳道里放上一个浸了药的棉花球。24 小时之后务必带她回来换药。

(6) I've got some pimples on my face. Perhaps it's just my age, but they are so dreadful, doctor.

医生,我脸上长了一些小疙瘩,也许正是我这种年龄应该长的,但是感觉实在是太糟糕了。

(7) The acne vulgaris doesn't look too bad to me.

这种痤疮看起来还不太厉害。

(8) You're still at school, aren't you? How long have you had the pimples?

你还在念书,是吗? 小疙瘩长多久了?

(9) Since junior high school, but they've gotten worse these past few years.

从我初中时就有了,但最近几年好像又加重了。

(10) Please help me. I've done everything I can, but these pimples won't go away.

请给我治治吧。我想尽了一切办法,但总去不掉这些小疙瘩。

(11) The medical name for them is acne vulgaris.

这些小疙瘩在医学上称作寻常痤疮。

(12) What can I do about them? How can they be prevented?

我能用哪种办法治疗? 怎样才能预防呢?

(13) Firstly, you should wash your face with warm water and soap three times a day. Washing will keep the pores open and prevent them getting clogged with oil. Secondly, don't pick or squeeze the pimples with your fingers. This damages the skin and spreads the bacterial infection. Thirdly, don't eat too much fat or spices such as pepper, curry, chilli, onion or garlic. Fourthly, apply this lotion to your face twice a day. For infected pimples, apply this clear lotion in the small bottle, twice a day.

其一,你应该用温热水和肥皂洗脸,一日三次。擦洗能使汗毛孔打开,这样可以预防油腻物质堵塞汗毛孔。其次,请不要用手挖或挤小疙瘩,因为这样会损伤皮肤,造成细菌感染。其三,尽量少吃肥肉和像胡椒、咖喱、辣椒、洋葱、大蒜这样的调味品。其四,在脸上使用我给你开的这种药水,一日两次。小瓶里的清亮药水用在受感染的疙瘩上,一日两次。

(14) Doctor, I don't know why I'm losing my hair rapidly.

医生,我不知道为什么最近我的头发掉得这么厉害。

(15) How long have you had hair loss (this problem)?

你脱发有多久了?

(16) Were there any small scapes as well?

你是不是也有头皮屑呢?

(17) There are many causes for hair loss, such as mental stress, lack of sleep and shampooing too frequently. Don't worry, lead a regular life and shampoo your hair once a week.

脱发的原因很多,例如精神紧张,睡眠不足,洗头太勤,这些都是重要的因素。不必着急,你应该保持规律的生活,每周洗一次头。

(18) Although there were a few scapes, yet it's a problem. Here are two kinds of tablets. I'm also giving you some hair tonic and a bottle of lotion. Please apply the lotion to the scalp with a dropper twice a day.

尽管你头皮屑不多,可这也是个问题。这里给你开了两种药片。我还会再给你开一些生发剂和一瓶外用药水,请用滴管把药水滴在头皮上,每日两次。

(19) I know you have a rash all over the body. But did you take any medicine before it began?

我知道你全身起满了疹子。问题是你起皮疹前用过什么药吗?

(20) I had pneumonia ten days ago and took penicillin for one week. Is there any relationship with the rash?

我十天前患了肺炎,注射了一周青霉素,可这跟出疹子有关系吗?

(21) Have you had anything like the rash before?

你以前出过像这样的疹子吗?

(22) You are allergic to penicillin. Stop it and drink plenty of fluids to help wash it out.

你对青霉素过敏。请停用青霉素吧,并多喝水加强排泄。

(23) Here are some anti-allergic tablets and a bottle of lotion to apply to the rash.

我给你开些针对疹子的抗过敏药片及一瓶外用药。

(24) Please remember to tell other doctors in future that you are hypersensitive to penicillin, otherwise you'll get the rash again if you take it. It's called dermatitis medicamentosa.

以后看病时,记住告诉医生你对青霉素过敏;要不然,你再用青霉素时,又会全身起疹子了。你这叫药物性皮炎。

(25) Doctor, I got this rash after I used some make-up.

医生,我脸上用了化妆品后就起了皮疹。

(26) It itches a lot. And there are some blisters on my face.

非常痒,而且我脸上出了些水疱。

(27) Avoid using soap to wash your face at the moment.

这时要避免用肥皂洗脸了。

(28) You're allergic to cosmetics. I advise you to stop using them for the time being.

你对化妆品过敏,我劝你暂时停用这种化妆品吧。

(29) Please apply a cold compress and then this paste. For the cold compress, wet five or six pieces of gauze with 3% boric acid solution. Squeeze out some solution from the gauze if it drips. Then spread the wet gauze over the rash and leave it there for five minutes. Then dip the gauze into the solution and apply the compress again. Apply it twice a day, each time for half an hour.

先冷敷,再使用这个药膏。冷敷的做法如下:把五六层纱布浸进3%的硼酸溶液里,取出来挤去一些水,以不滴水为度。然后把湿纱布铺在皮疹上湿敷五分钟。然后再把纱布浸入硼酸溶液,取出再做湿敷。一日两次,每次半小时。

(30) The rash may not respond to treatment for the first day or two, because some traces of the cosmetics are still left on your skin. After these have been removed the rash will disappear rapidly, and it is contact dermatitis.

由于皮肤上仍残留有化妆品,在治疗的头一两天皮疹不会明显见好。等到化妆品都去除掉了,皮疹很快就会消失了,这种皮疹叫接触性皮炎。

Ⅲ. Words and Expressions 单词和短语

dermatology /ˌdɜːməˈtɒlədʒi/ n. 皮肤科学

acne /ˈækni/ n. 痤疮

acquired syphilis 后天性梅毒

alopecia /ˌæləˈpiːʃə/ n. 秃头(发)

aseptic wound 无菌创伤

atheroma /ˌæθəˈrəʊmə/ n. 粉瘤

bedbug /'bedbʌg/ *n*. 臭虫

blister /'blɪstə/; vesicle /'vesɪkl/ *n*. 水疱

blowing wound 开放性(气胸)创伤

burn /bɜːn/ *n*. 灼伤

carbuncle /'kɑːbʌŋkl/ *n*. 痈

carcinoma /ˌkɑːsɪ'nəumə/ *n*. 癌

congelation /ˌkɒndʒɪ'leɪʃən/ *n*.; frost bite; cold injury 冻伤

congenital syphilis 先天性梅毒

contused wound 挫伤

corium /'kɔːriəm/ *n*.; true skin 真皮

cosmetic treatment 美容疗

crust /krʌst/ *n*. 痂皮

cut wound 切伤

cyst /sɪst/ *n*. 囊肿

dermatitis /ˌdɜːmə'taɪtɪs/ *n*. 皮炎

dermatophyte /'dɜːmətəuˌfaɪt/ *n*. 皮肤真菌

dermoid /'dɜːmɔɪd/ *n*. 皮样囊肿

drug eruption 药物疹

eczema /'eksɪmə/ *n*. 湿疹

emphysema /ˌemfɪ'siːmə/ *n*. 气肿

epidermis /ˌepɪ'dɜːmɪs/ *n*. 表皮

erosion /ɪ'rəuʒən/ *n*. 糜烂

erysipelas /ˌerɪ'sɪpɪləs/ *n*. 丹毒

erythematous dose 红斑剂量

erythema /ˌerɪ'θiːmə/ *n*. 红斑

esthetic /iːs'θetɪk/ *adj*. 美容的

fibroma /faɪ'brəumə/ *n*. 纤维瘤

fourth venereal disease 第四性病

furuncle /'fjuərʌŋkəl/ *n*. 疖

gangrene /'gæŋgriːn/ *n*. 坏疽

glycerine /'glɪsə'riːn/ *n*. 甘油

gonorrhea /ˌgɒnə'riə/ *n*. 淋病

hard chancre 硬性下疳

hemal-fibroma 血管纤维瘤

hemangioma /hiːˌmændʒiː'əumə/ *n*. 血管瘤

herpes /'hɜːpiːz/ *n*. 疱疹(热性)

incised wound 刀伤

lacerated wound 撕裂伤

leprosy /'leprəsi/; lepra /'leprə/ *n*. 麻风

lipoma /lɪ'pəumə/ *n*. 脂肪瘤

louse /laus/ *n*. 虱子

lupus /'luːpəs/ *n*. 狼疮

lymphangioma /lɪmˌfændʒɪ'əumə/ *n*. 淋巴管瘤

lymphogranuloma inguinal 腹股沟淋巴肉芽肿

melanoma /ˌmelə'nəumə/ *n*. 黑色素瘤

melanosarcoma /ˌmelənəusɑː'kəumə/ *n*. 黑(色)素肉瘤

neoplasm /'niːəuˌplæzəm/ *n*. 新生物

node /nəud/; nodule /'nɒdjuːl/ *n*. 结节

ointment /'ɔɪntmənt/ *n*. 软膏

open wound 开放性创伤

papillomatosis /ˌpæpəˌləumə'təusɪs/ *n*. 乳头(状)瘤病

papilloma virus 乳头(状)瘤病毒

papula /'pæpjulə/ *n*. 丘疹

paste /peɪst/ *n*. 糊膏

pemphigus /'pemfɪgəs/ *n*. 天疱疮

penetrating wound 刺伤伤口

phlegmon /'flegmən/ *n*. 蜂窝织炎

pigmentation /ˌpɪgmen'teɪʃn/ *n*. 色素沉着

plaster /'plɑːstə/ *n*. 硬膏

poisoned wound 染毒创伤

powder /'paudə/ *n*. 粉剂

primary lesion；primary sore 梅毒初疮
primary lesion 原发疹
psoriasis /səˈraɪəsɪs/ *n.* 牛皮癣
pulmonary emphysema；emphysema
　of lungs 肺气肿
puncture wound 感染性创伤
purpura /ˈpɜːpjʊrə/ *n.* 紫癜
pustule /ˈpʌstjuːl/ *n.* 脓疱
pyoderma /ˌpaɪəʊˈdɜːmə/ *n.* 脓皮病
regulative function 调节作用
sarcoma /sɑːˈkəʊmə/ *n.* 肉瘤
scabies /ˈskeɪbiːz/ *n.* 疥疮
sebaceous gland 皮脂腺
secondary lesion 继发疹
sensation /senˈseɪʃən/ *n.*；sensory

feeling 感觉
sexually transmitted disease（STD）
　性传播疾病
soap /səʊp/ *n.* 肥皂
soft chancre 软性下疳
subcutaneous emphysema 皮下气肿
sweat gland；sudoriferous gland 汗腺
syphilis /ˈsɪfɪlɪs/；lues /ˈluːiːz/ *n.* 梅毒
ulcer /ˈʌlsə/ *n.* 溃疡
ultraviolet lamp；ultraviolet radiator
　紫外线灯
venereal disease 性病
venerology /ˌvenəˈrɒlədʒi/ *n.* 性病学
wheal /(h)wiːl/ *n.* 风疹
wound /wuːnd/ *n.* 伤口；创伤

Section 11　Neurology and Psychiatry
第11节　神经和精神科

I. Dialogues 情景对话

1. Depression 抑郁症

Patient's wife：Doctor, I am sure my husband has become mad. About half an hour ago, I went home with my son. No sooner had we walked into the yard, than I saw a man standing under the biggest tree. Oh! What a dreadful sight! A rope was hanging on that tree. The very man preparing to hang himself was my husband, so we immediately drove him to the hospital. We trust you, doctor, you can save him.

医生,我的先生真的是疯了。半小时以前,我和我儿子一同回家。刚进院子就看到一个人站在那棵最大的树下面。真可怕呀,一根绳子挂在树上。原来那个要上吊的人竟是我的先生。所以我们马上开车送他来医院了。医生,我们相信你能救他的。

Doctor：(Turns to the patient) What's the matter?

(转向病人)你感觉怎么了?

Patient：I am tired of life. I don't get enough sleep. I get extraordinarily irritable. Although nothing seems worth bothering about, I get annoyed at little things and even one word from my superiors makes me feel anxious. Any news upsets me quite a bit. I feel that everything in the world and even my life is senseless to me. I am not only useless but also a heavy load on other human beings. I think that killing myself will benefit other human beings, so I want to commit suicide.

我对生活已感到厌倦了。我睡眠不足,而且特别容易激动。虽然没有什么事可值得烦恼的,但是一点小事就会使我生气,就连上级说的一句话,都会让我觉得急躁不安。任何消息都会使我心烦。我觉得世界上无论什么东西,甚至我的生命对我都已毫无意义了。我活着不仅无用,而且对别人也是沉重的负担。我想自己死了可能对其他人会有好处,所以我就想自杀。

Doctor：(Says in low voice to the patient's wife) His condition is very serious. I would prefer to refer him to a psychiatric hospital. It is a special hospital for treating such patients. A stay in that hospital for a short period of intensive treatment may be necessary. (Turns to the patient) Everyone has something bothering him, but they don't always look at the world through dark-colored glasses, and they can correctly deal with such things. Don't worry too much. I am sure your condition can soon be cured, if you cooperate well with the doctor in charge of you. From now on, you don't have to be upset about trifles.

(对病人的妻子小声说)他的病情很严重,我建议你们将他转到精神病院去。那是治疗这种病人的专门医院。在那样的医院里住一段时间进行积极治疗是很必要的。(转向病人)谁都有伤脑筋的事,但是我们不能总是戴着黑色的眼镜看待世界,我们应该以正确的态度对待我们遇到的一切事情。遇事不要过于焦虑,要是你能和你的医生配合的话,我相信你的情况会很快好起来的。从今以后,你再也不必为一些小事而烦恼了。

2. Mania 躁狂症

Patient's wife：Doctor, can I tell you something about my husband's condition? My son is looking after him now in the waiting room.

医生,我可以给你说一下我先生的情况吗? 我的儿子现在正在候诊室照顾他呢。

Doctor：Certainly, what's your husband's trouble?

当然可以,你先生怎么不舒服了呢?

Patient's wife：My husband may be mad, doctor. At night he sings loudly. During the day, he buys a lot of unnecessary things and behaves strangely, like an actor. Sometimes he lies on his bed, turns around continuously, laughs in a loud voice like a child, and says he is a spaceman in a moving space rocket.

医生,我先生他可能疯了。晚上他大声地唱歌。白天他还去买了好多没用的东西,而且举止奇怪,像个演员似的。他有时躺在床上不断地翻来覆去的,像个孩子似的大声笑,还说他自己是宇宙火箭里的宇宙飞行员。

Doctor：How long has he been like this?

他像这样有多久了?

Patient's wife：Ah, for about one month. But his condition has been getting worse for about two weeks.

啊,差不多一个月了。但是最近两星期好像病情有所加重了。

Doctor：Has he had a similar condition in the past?

他过去有过同样的情况吗?

Patient's wife：Yes, about twelve years ago, he had a similar condition lasting two months or so.

有过,大概在十二年前有过一次同样的情况,差不多持续了两个月才好。

Doctor：Has this happened to anyone else in his family?

　　他们家里还有别的什么人也有过这种情况吗?

Patient's wife：When we got married I was told that his father might have had a similar condition.

　　我们结婚时听说他的父亲好像有过同样的情况。

Doctor：Would you please call him in here?

　　你能把他叫进来吗?

Patient's wife：All right.

　　好吧!

(The patient comes in)

(病人进入诊室)

Doctor：Hello. How do you feel today?

　　你好哇,今天你觉得怎样啊?

Patient：(Euphorically) I feel marvelous.

　　(欣快地)我觉得好极了。

Doctor：What are you?

　　你是做什么工作的呢?

Patient：(Carelessly) I should say I am an engineer but I am a spare-time spaceman and an actor too.（Warmly）Shall I give a performance for you?

　　(不在乎地)照理说我应该是个工程师,但实际上我既是个业余宇航员,又是个演员。(热情地)我给你表演个节目行吗?

Doctor：No, thank you. Now let me examine you.

　　谢谢,不用了。我给你检查检查身体吧。

(After examination)

(检查后)

Patient's wife：（Anxiously）Doctor, is his condition serious? Is it curable?

　　(神情焦虑地)医生,他的情况严重吗? 你看还能治好吗?

Doctor：No, his condition is not too severe. This attack could be overcome, but he may have a relapse.

　　别着急,他的病不太严重,而且能治好,但还可能会复发。

Patient's wife：How long will this attack last and when might he have a relapse?

依你看,他这次病情会持续多久呢? 什么时候还可能会复发呢?

Doctor：It is difficult to tell you exactly, madame, for it varies from individual to individual. Generally speaking，each attack lasts a few months. It may recur several years or even decades later. In a sense，it depends on a great many factors, such as medical treatment，rest，and so on.

夫人,这准确的时间是很难说清楚的,病人的情况因人而异。一般而言,病人每次发病要持续几个月。可能几年或几十年后才复发。我们也可以说,病人的发病是与治疗方法、休息好坏等许多因素有关的。

Patient's wife：What can we do for him? Please give him the best treatment, doctor.

医生,我们应该怎样帮他治疗呢? 请你给他好好地治治吧。

Doctor：Don't worry too much. I'll do my best for him. And I'll give him some medicine to relieve his symptoms and he should have a good rest. Here is his prescription. Pay in the pharmacy and the pharmacist will tell you how to use it.

放心吧。我会尽力而为的。我给他开一些消除症状的药,此外他还需要好好地休息。这是他的处方,请你到药房交款,药剂师会告诉你怎样服用的。

Patient's wife：Is that all, doctor?

这次就这样了吗,医生?

Doctor：That's all. When you run out of medicine, come again.

就这样吧。药用完了请再带他来复诊。

Patient's wife：If his condition gets worse, what shall I do, doctor?

医生,要是他的情况向坏的方面发展我该怎么办呢?

Doctor：You should take him directly to the Psychiatric Department of the Third Affiliated Hospital of Beijing Medical College.

那你就直接带他上北京医学院第三附属医院的精神病科去看吧。

Patient's wife：Thank you so much.

　　　　　多谢了。

Doctor：You are welcome，madame.

　　　　　不必客气，夫人。

3. Psychoneurosis 神经官能症

Patient：Doctor，I've come to you because I think I have a strange disease.

　　　　　医生，我觉得自己得了一种非常奇怪的病，所以我来找你看看。

Doctor：What is it?

　　　　　怎么回事呢?

Patient：I have been suffering from nervousness for two years.

　　　　　近两年来我很神经质。

Doctor：Can you tell me more specifically the symptoms that trouble you?

　　　　　你能明确告诉我你有哪些症状吗?

Patient：Yes. For a little over two years，I have been afraid of noise and strong light. When I am exposed to these，I feel tense and restless.

　　　　　可以。两年多来，我又怕噪声又怕强光，一听到噪声或见到强光，就开始紧张不安。

Doctor：Do you have any other symptoms?

　　　　　还有什么其他症状吗?

Patient：Yes. At times I suffer from palpitations and shortness of breath. I sleep poorly and am troubled almost nightly by frightening dreams. I feel dizzy and weak in the daytime.

　　　　　有。有时我感到心慌气短。也睡不好觉，几乎整夜都在做噩梦，而且一到白天就头晕无力的。

Doctor：What sort of dreams do you have?

　　　　　你都做了哪些梦呢?

Patient：They are different. For instance，once I dreamed that I fell down from a precipice. On another occasion，I was chased by a wolf，and in other dreams I have lost my way in a desert.

　　　　　不同的梦。举例说吧，有一次我梦见自己从悬崖上掉下来了。

还有一次是梦见一只狼在追我,还有一次是梦见自己在荒野中迷了路。

Doctor: Anything else?

还有其他别的症状吗?

Patient: Yes, when I wake up, my heart beats very fast and I am perspiring.

有啊。每当我醒来的时候,我就感觉心跳得非常快,而且还出汗。

Doctor: What do you think all these symptoms mean?

你认为这些症状都说明了什么呢?

Patient: I thought I was having a heart attack.

我想我是得了心脏病了。

Doctor: Oh, no. The physician has clearly told you that you didn't have a heart attack. Your EKG doesn't indicate a heart attack.

哈哈,不是这样的,内科医生已经明确告诉你没有心脏病了。你做的心电图已能证明这一点啊。

Patient: Is that true?

真的吗?

Doctor: The thorough examination didn't reveal anything abnormal in your organs.

根据全面的检查结果,你没有任何器质性的异常。

Patient: Why do I have so many symptoms and feel sick?

那为什么我有那么多症状和不舒服的感觉呢?

Doctor: Your nervousness makes you sick.

你的病是神经质引起的。

Patient: What do you mean?

那是什么意思呢?

Doctor: Generally speaking, the symptoms you mentioned are reflections of your state of mind. You may have an internal conflict that constantly upsets you.

一般说来,你所有的症状都是你思想的反映。你也许有什么令你感到伤脑筋的心事。

Patient: Yes, doctor, you are right. I came to China a little over two years ago. Before I left my country, my mother was in poor shape. She was suffering from heart disease and she would feel faint at the slightest physical exertion. Now my younger sister and brother go to school and my mother has to manage the household. I feel guilty that I cannot share the responsibility with my sick mother who has brought us up so well.

医生,你真的说对了。我来中国两年多了。我离开祖国的时候我母亲的身体状况不怎么好。她有心脏病,稍一做体力活就会晕倒。现在我的弟弟妹妹都在上学,母亲就必须自己操持所有的家务。她那么辛劳地把我们抚养大,而我为不能分担母亲的工作而问心有愧啊。

Doctor: You must have been a good daughter. By the way, how is your mother? Have you received any letters from her?

你肯定是个好女儿。哦,那么,你母亲现在情况怎么样了?你接到过她的信没有?

Patient: Yes, I receive a letter from her every two weeks. She says she is doing fine, and is managing the household duties without discomfort. However, I feel that she may not be telling me the truth.

有,我每两星期接到一封她的信。她说她挺好的,安排家务对她来说,没有任何困难。但是,我想她可能没给我说真话。

Doctor: Have you ever received any letters from your brother and sister? What do you think of your mother's health?

那你曾接到过你弟弟妹妹们的信吗?你想象的你母亲的健康情况会是怎么样的呢?

Patient: They always tell me that mother is doing well, but I think since she suffers from heart disease, she will die sooner or later.

他们也总对我说我母亲的情况很好,但是我想她既然有心脏病,那她早晚是会死的。

Doctor: No. I don't quite agree with you. Under proper treatment and care, a patient with heart disease can live for many years. Is there any reason why your mother, brother and sister might not tell you the truth?

不会的。关于这个问题,我不大同意你的看法。在适当的医疗护理下,心脏病病人可以活很多年。你有什么理由认为母亲、弟弟、妹妹都瞒着你呢？

Patient：Oh，no，doctor.

其实没什么理由的，医生。

Doctor：I think that you will feel reassured when you return home, see, your unnecessary worry makes you feel tense all the time. Your nervousness has caused you to waste a lot of energy. This has produced a series of symptoms, such as a rapid heart beat, shortness of breath, frightening dreams and so forth, that you do not control well. In short, you worry too much and that makes you weary.

我想你如果回到家，你的病情也许会好很多的。想想看，你不必要的忧虑使你总是精神紧紧张张的。其实，你的神经质消耗了你很多的精力，这就产生了一系列你难以控制的症状，比如心跳加快、呼吸困难、做噩梦等等，总之，你的忧虑过度使你终日乏倦。

4. Abdominal Epilepsy 腹型癫痫

Patient's mother：Doctor, my son had a severe pain in his stomach about an hour ago.

医生，我儿子一小时前肚子就开始疼得很厉害了。

Doctor：Oh, I see. What happened?

噢，是吗。怎么回事呢？

Patient's mother：About an hour ago, while my husband and I were chatting about our plan to take a trip to the Great Wall, all of a sudden we heard my son screaming.

大约一小时以前，当我和我先生正在谈去长城游览的计划时，忽然听到我儿子尖声叫起来了。

Doctor：What did you see?

那你看到的情况是什么样的呢？

Patient's mother：When I ran up to him he was suffering from extreme pains. He turned pale and sweated a lot. He was groaning with a stomachache.

我跑到他跟前的时候，看见他疼得非常厉害。他脸色苍白，肚子疼得呻吟着，还大量出汗。

Doctor：Did he feel hot, nauseous, or did he vomit?

　　　　他发烧、恶心或呕吐过吗？

Patient's mother：No, he did not seem to have a fever or feel nauseous.

　　　　　　　　没有，他不像是发烧的样子，而且他也不恶心。

Doctor：Was he mentally clear?

　　　　他神志清醒吗？

Patient's mother：Yes, he was, but he appeared to be fussy, irritable and was hard to please.

　　　　　　　　清醒的，可是他看上去显得很急躁，爱发脾气，而且我们还没办法让他高兴起来。

Doctor：Has he had a similar attack of abdominal pain before?

　　　　他以前有过同样的肚子疼的情况吗？

Patient's mother：Yes, he has had several such episodes.

　　　　　　　　犯过，他犯这样的病已经好几次了。

Doctor：How frequently has he had such attacks?

　　　　像这种发作，每次大概都相隔多久呢？

Patient's mother：About two or three times a year for the past three years, doctor.

　　　　　　　　一年发作两三次，已经有三年了，医生。

Doctor：Has he had symptoms other than abdominal pain?

　　　　除了肚子疼，还有什么其他的症状吗？

Patient's mother：At times he has complained of headaches.

　　　　　　　　有时候他说他头痛。

Doctor：Is that all?

　　　　全部情况就这些了吗？

Patient's mother：Oh, doctor. I forgot to tell you that my son sometimes has fits when his body temperature goes up.

　　　　　　　　噢，医生，我忘记告诉你了，我儿子在体温高的时候还会不省人事。

Doctor：Has he been seen by doctors elsewhere?

　　　　他是否还在别处看过医生呢？

Patient's mother：Yes. He was seen and treated by doctors at home and abroad.

是的,我们国内和国外的医生都给他治疗过。

Doctor：Did he pass worms or blood in his stools?

他的大便里是否有血或是否查过有寄生虫呢?

Patient's mother：The doctors told me that he did not have any worms and there was no evidence of a peptic ulcer or appendicitis. His brain waves were normal.

医生们跟我说过,他大便里没有寄生虫,也没有像胃溃疡或阑尾炎的症状。他的脑电波检查也是正常的。

Doctor：Did medicine help him?

服用药物对他有效吗?

Patient's mother：Yes，his pain would stop immediately after a shot of luminal.

有效,要是它发作时,注射一支鲁米那,疼痛马上就消失了。

Doctor：Does he receive medication regularly，madame?

那他定时服药吗,夫人?

Patient's mother：No. The doctor said it is not necessary because the attacks have not been frequent.

没有。医生说因为他不经常发作,所以没有必要定时服药。

Doctor：Do you consider his birth history and development normal?

你认为他的出生史以及发育都还正常吗?

Patient's mother：Yes，doctor. His birth was uneventful. He is as active and healthy as other children.

是的,医生。他出生时很顺利,而且他和别的孩子一样活泼健康。

Doctor：Has anyone in the family had a similar condition?

家里其他人也有过同样的情况吗?

Patient's mother：No，but his maternal uncles have suffered from migraines for a number of years.

没有,不过他的几个舅舅们得偏头痛有好多年了。

Doctor：(To the patient) What's your name, my little friend?

（对病人）小朋友，你叫什么名字呀？

Patient：My name is John Smith.

我叫约翰·史密斯。

Doctor：How old are you?

你多大了？

Patient：I'll be six years old next month.

到下月我就六岁了。

Doctor：John，can you tell me more about your illness?

约翰，你能再告诉我一些你的病情吗？

Patient：Yes. I would hurt a lot in the middle of my stomach. It is a sort of dull cramp over which I have no control. After a shot it goes away very fast. Then I feel sleepy. When I wake up I feel all right again.

好的。我的肚子当中疼得厉害。是那种止不住的隐隐的拧着的疼。注射一针后就不疼了，然后我就感觉发困。睡醒过来一切就都又好了。

Doctor：Very well. Let me give you a check-up.

很好。我给你检查一下吧。

Patient：Please do it and help me get rid of my nasty stomachache.

好的，你给我检查吧，请你尽快解除我这讨厌的肚子疼好吗？

Doctor：That is all.

检查完了。

Patient's mother：Doctor，what is your opinion of my child's illness?

医生，我这孩子的病，你的看法是怎样的呢？

Doctor：I feel your child is suffering from epileptic equivoke which we call abdominal epilepsy.

我想你孩子得的是双关型的癫痫。我们医学上有时也把它叫作腹型癫痫。

Patient's mother：Yes，you are right. The other doctor also made the same diagnosis.

是的是的，你说对了。别的医生也是这样诊断的。

Doctor：When did he have his last EEG，madame?

夫人,他最后一次脑电图是什么时候做的呢?

Patient's mother：About six months ago. Is there anything else we
should do, doctor?

大约是六个月以前了。医生,我们还要做些什么吗?

Doctor：I think he should have another EEG, and regular doses of
phenobarbital for a period of time.

还需要做一次脑电图,同时他在一段时间内必须定时服用苯巴
比妥。

Patient's mother：OK, no problem, doctor.

好的,医生,没问题。

Doctor：I have read his EEG which strongly supports our diagnosis.
Please have this prescription filled.

我看过他的脑电图了。它支持了我们的诊断。请去取药吧。

Patient's mother：Thank you, doctor.

谢谢你了,医生。

II. Sentences 替换句型

(1) ECT is a form of treatment used to clear up depressive states
quickly.

电休克疗法是用于迅速清除抑郁状态的治疗方法。

(2) Group therapy has been shown to be particularly useful in dealing
with moderate and mild depression.

群体疗法在处理中度和轻度抑郁症中已显示其特别有效的作用。

(3) Many drugs used for the treatment of depression have disadvantages
and dangers which seriously limit their usefulness.

用于治疗抑郁症的许多药物都有缺陷和危险,大大限制了这些药物
的有效性。

(4) By watching the child at play, the psychiatrist found the boy was
seriously disturbed emotionally.

精神病医生通过观察这个男孩玩耍发现他在感情上受过严重创伤。

(5) Doctor, this is the patient, my son. He is having convulsions.

医生,这病人是我儿子。他在不断抽搐。

(6) The trouble is that while we were enjoying our luncheon in the

park，all of a sudden，my child fell down on the ground and threw a fit，which subsided in ten minutes but came back four times that hour. Since his first attack，he has not woken up. The last attack occurred more than half an hour ago.

我们正在公园吃午餐的时候，忽然间我儿子就倒在地下抽起风来了，过十分钟就停了，但是在一小时之内发作了四次，从第一次发作后他就没有清醒过来。最后一次发作是在半个多小时之前。

(7) Is this the first time he has had such episodes?

这是他第一次发作吗？

(8) Let me see. He had his first attack when he was two，without any apparent cause，and since then it's happened once or twice a year.

让我想想。头一次是他两岁的时候，发作时并没有什么明显的原因，此后每年都发作一两次。

(9) Does he receive medication regularly?

他按时接受药物治疗吗？

(10) No，he has been off medication for half a year.

没有，他停药都有半年了。

(11) How is my child? (The child jerks once in a while) Oh，God. Have mercy on him.

我的孩子怎样？（孩子一会儿抽动一下）唉，上帝啊，可怜可怜这孩子吧。

(12) Please be calm. Your son's condition is serious，but we will do our best for him. First of all，we'll give him an injection (a mild tranquilizer).

别着急，你儿子的病情的确很严重，不过我们会尽最大的努力治疗他。首先我们要给他打一针（让他服一些镇静剂）。

(13) His condition may get better in a few hours. Although sudden deterioration of his condition is possible.

几小时后他的病情会有所好转的，但是情况也可能会急剧地恶化。

(14) Nurse，will you please give the patient an intravenous injection of 10 mg of diazepam before he goes to the ward?

护士，你能在这孩子住院之前先给他静脉注射一支 10 毫克的安定吗？

(15) We have heard from the press at home that diazepam is a very

effective treatment for so-called status epilepticus.

在我们国内的报纸上就听说过安定对治疗所谓的持续性癫痫是很有效的。

(16) That is what we are going to give him. I should say that small and regular doses are even more important in the prevention of such mishaps.

那就是我们要给他注射的药。应该说小剂量地定时服用这种药物，对预防发病更为重要。

(17) I think he should stay in the hospital for a few days. Nurse, the patient is ready to go to the ward. After checking up on another patient, I'll be there.

我想他需要在医院住上几天。护士，先把这病人送进病房，等我给另一个病人检查完就过去(那儿)。

(18) Any physical problems haven't been found, madame, all the test results are normal.

夫人，体格检查未能查出你有什么异常的变化，所有检查结果也一切正常。

(19) This should be a kind of reactive depression, and an anti-depressant and some sleeping pills are needed for some time.

这应该是反应性抑郁症了，你需要服用一段时间的抗抑郁和催眠的药物了。

(20) Sir, your problem seems to be connected with psychological factors. Normally speaking, changes in living habits or environmental factors would bring about some mental stress or pressure, and sometimes unexpected surprise or shock would also lead into mental disorder.

先生，你的情况可能与精神因素有关。一般来说，生活习惯的改变、外界环境的变化都会对个体产生极不适应的精神压力和紧张，有时突发的意外也往往会导致精神有异常的表现。

Ⅲ. Words and Expressions 单词和短语

ECT＝electric convulsive therapy 电休克疗法

anesthesia /ˌænəs'θiːziə/ *n.* 感觉缺失；麻醉

anxiety /æŋ'zaɪəti/ *n.* 苦闷

auditory hallucination 听幻觉

behaviour changes or disorders 行为异常

catalepsy /'kætəlepsi/ *n.* 僵硬症

catatonia /ˌkætə'təʊniə/ *n.* 紧张症

chronic alcoholism 慢性酒精中毒

confusion /kən'fjuːʒn/ *n.* 错乱

delirium /dɪ'lɪriəm/ *n.* 谵妄

delusion /dɪ'luːʒn/ *n.* 错觉

dementia paralytica 麻痹性痴呆

dementia praecox 早发痴呆

dementia /dɪ'menʃə/ *n.* 痴呆

depressive state 抑郁状态

difficulty in walk 行走困难

dimness of sight 蒙视症

diplopia /dɪ'pləʊpiə/；double vision 复视

disturbance of gait 行走障碍

disturbance of memory 记忆障碍

disturbance of movement of extremities 四肢运动障碍

disturbance of speech 言语障碍

disturbance of vision 视力障碍

drunkenness /'drʌŋkənɪs/ *n.* 醉酒

ecstasy /'ekstəsi/ *n.* 狂喜

emotion changes 情绪异常

emotional disorder 感情障碍

enuresis /ˌenjʊ'riːsɪs/；bedwetting /'bedˌwetɪŋ/ *n.* 遗尿

epilepsy /'epɪlepsi/ *n.* 癫痫

eyeball pain 眼球痛

fainting /'feɪntɪŋ/ *n.* 失神

feeling of numbness 麻木感

fit of convulsion 癫痫发作

formication /ˌfɔːmɪ'keɪʃən/ *n.* 蚁走感

general paralytica progressive 进行性麻痹性痴呆

general paralytic 全身麻痹

gustatory hallucination 味幻觉

hallucination of hearing 幻听

hallucination of sensibility 感觉性幻觉

hallucination /həˌluːsɪ'neɪʃən/ *n.* 幻觉

hebephrenia /ˌhiːbɪ'friːniə/ *n.* 青春型精神分裂症

hyperesthesia /ˌhaɪpəriːs'θiːziə/ *n.* 感觉过敏

hypoesthesia /haɪpəʊs'θiːziə/ *n.* 感觉减退

hysteria /hɪ'stɪəriə/ *n.* 癔病

idea of flight 想逃

illusion of sight 错视

illusion /ɪ'luːʒn/ *n.* 错觉

indifference /ɪn'dɪfrəns/，apathy /'æpəθi/ *n.* 不关心

lameness /'leɪmnɪs/ *n.* 跛

lame /leɪm/ *adj.* 跛行的

mania state 躁狂状态

manic-depressive psychosis 躁狂抑郁性精神病；躁郁病

mannerism /'mænəˌrɪzəm/ *n.* 习惯

melancholy delusion 抑郁性妄想

mental deficiency 精神衰弱(缺陷)

mental retardation 智力延迟

morbid elation 痛快

mutism /ˈmjuːtɪzəm/ n. 缄默症；哑症

negativism /ˈnegətɪvɪzəm/ n. 拒绝症；
否定态度

neurasthenia /ˈnjuərəsˈθiːniə/ n. 神经
衰弱症

neurosis /njʊəˈrəʊsɪs/ n. 官能症

nervosity /nɜːˈvɒsɪti/ n. 神经质（缺
陷）

nightmare /ˈnaɪtmeə/ n. 噩梦

olfactory hallucination 嗅幻觉

paralysis /pəˈrælɪsɪs/ n. 麻痹

paranoia /ˌpærəˈnɔɪə/ n. 偏执症

paresthesia /ˌpærəsˈθiːʒə/ n. 感觉异常

persecutory delusion 被害妄想

personality changes or disorders 性格异常

psychogenic reaction 精神性反应

psychopathy /saɪˈkɒpəθi/ n. 精神病理

schizophrenia /ˌskɪtsəˈfriːniə/ n. 精神
分裂症

senile dementia 老年性痴呆

senium praecox 早衰

involuntary movement 不随意运动

somnambulism /sɒmˈnæmbjəlɪzəm/
n. 梦游症

stereotypy /ˈsteriətaɪpi/ n. 刻板症

stupor /ˈstjuːpə/ n. 昏迷

swimming of objects before the eyes
飞蚊症

symptomatic epilepsy 症状性癫痫

syncope /ˈsɪŋkəpi/; fainting /ˈfeɪntɪŋ/
n. 昏厥

tactile hallucination; haptic
hallucination 触幻觉

thumb-sucking 吸指

tinnitus /ˈtɪnɪtəs/ n. ;
singing in the ear 耳鸣

traumatic neurosis 外伤性神经官能症

tremor /ˈtremə/; trembling
/ˈtrembləŋ/ n. 颤抖

true epilepsy 真癫痫

vertigo /ˈvɜːtɪgəʊ/; dizziness /ˈdɪzɪnɪs/;
faint /feɪnt/ n. 眩晕

visual hallucination 视幻觉

agony /ˈægəni/ n. 苦恼

Section 12　Clinic of Blood Diseases

第12节　血液科

Ⅰ. Dialogues 情景对话

1. Scarlet Fever 猩红热

Patient：Doctor，my child has a temperature，headache，sore throat and rash，and I don't know how to deal with it.

　　　　医生，我孩子发烧，头痛，嗓子疼，身上还起了疹子，我不知道该怎么办才好。

Doctor：Don't worry，tell me，please，how long has he been ill?

　　　　别着急，请你告诉我，他病了多久了?

Patient：He's had the temperature since yesterday，doctor.

　　　　他是从昨天才开始发烧的，医生。

Doctor：Are there any children around or at school also sick?

　　　　邻居中或者孩子学校里有没有别的小孩儿也病了呢?

Patient：His classmate had a fever and complained of a sore throat five days ago.

　　　　他有个同学在五天前发了烧，也是嗓子疼。

Doctor：Let's have a look at him. Open your mouth，please show me your tongue. His tonsils are swollen and red. His tongue is as red as a strawberry. Now，take off your clothes. En… There is a rash all over his body. Wait a moment，make a blood test for him.

　　　　让我检查一下。张开口，伸出舌头。他的扁桃体又红又肿，舌头红得像草莓一样。脱下衣服，噢，他全身都起了疹子了。等一会儿，给他化验个血。

Patient：Here is the result，doctor. Is it normal?

　　　　这是化验结果，医生。检查结果正常吗?

Doctor：His white blood cell count is high. He is suffering from scarlet fever. It's an infectious disease. You should keep him away from other children as much as possible.

白细胞偏高。他得了猩红热。这是一种传染病。你应该尽可能把他跟其他小孩隔离开。

Patient：What can I do for him?

那我该怎样照顾他呢?

Doctor：He should stay in bed until his fever goes down. Let him eat easily digested food and drink plenty of fluids. I'll prescribe penicillin injections for a few days.

他应该卧床直到体温降至正常。让他吃些易消化的食物,多喝水。我给他注射几天青霉素吧。

Patient：What should I do about his sister?

他妹妹我应该怎么办呢?

Doctor：I'll prescribe something to prevent her catching it.

我给她开一点预防这病的药吧。

Patient：Thank you, doctor.

谢谢你,医生。

2. Abnormal Bleeding 异常出血

Doctor：So you say that you are having problems with bleeding or bruise easily?

你是说你不舒服,经常发生出血和瘀血吗?

Patient：Yes, I am.

是的,医生。

Doctor：Can you tell me what do you mean by that? Do you bleed or bruise easily?

你能说得详细点吗? 是很容易就出血或瘀血了吗?

Patient：Yes. Every time I scrape myself or bump into something I get bruised.

是的,每次一擦伤或者身体稍有碰撞就会瘀血。

Doctor：Have you always had this problem, or is it a recent development?

是经常这样还是最近才出现这种情况呢?

Patient：I noticed that the problems started about the time I started shaving.

我是刮胡子时才发现出血的。

Doctor：Do your gums bleed when you brush your teeth?

刷牙时你牙龈出血吗?

Patient：Yes，quite a bit / lot.

是的，出一点/很多。

Doctor：Do you have any trouble stopping the bleeding?

那你感觉止血困难吗?

Patient：Oh，yes. Even from the most minor cuts.

难，就是很小的伤口也很难止住血。

Doctor：How long does it take to stop the bleeding?

每次止住血大概需要多长时间?

Patient：At least ten or fifteen minutes.

至少十或十五分钟。

Doctor：Are there any other members of your family with bleeding tendencies?

你家人中还有谁有过类似情况吗?

Patient：No，not that I know of.

好像没有。

Doctor：Have you ever needed a blood transfusion，or have you given blood recently?

你曾经输过血或最近献过血吗?

Patient：I don't like needles，so I don't give blood，but I needed a transfusion after a car accident a few years ago，when I was fifteen.

我怕疼，所以从没献过血。可是几年前，我十五岁时，因为遭受车祸曾经输过血。

Doctor：Do you remember how many units of blood you received?

你还记得当时输了多少血吗?

Patient：No，I don't remember，sorry.

抱歉，我记不清了。

Doctor：Do you know what your blood type is?

你知道你是什么血型吗？

Patient：I think it is AB negative，doctor，but I'm not sure.

这一点我可不敢确定,医生,可能是 AB 阴型吧。

Ⅱ. Sentences 替换句型

(1) What seems to be the trouble / problem?

你怎么了？

(2) I am having a lot of trouble with bleeding even from the smallest shaving cut or scratch.

即使有点小的刮伤我也会血流不止。

(3) Are you likely to bleed? And how long does it take to stop the bleeding? Or have you had a blood test before?

常出血吗？ 止血需要的时间长吗？ 你以前查过血吗？

(4) My father and my elder brother had the same troubles，doctor. And they died ten years ago，so I worry about me very much.

我父亲和哥哥就是这样,十年前他们就死了,所以我现在很害怕。

(5) You need a thorough examination. / I'll give you a thorough check-up.

你需要做个全面的检查。

(6) First of all，I would like to have a detailed history，how long have you been like that?

首先说一下你的病史吧,你得这个病多长时间了？

(7) Any other complaints?

你还有其他什么不适吗？

(8) I want you to have a blood test now and I'll wait for the result.

你去验一下血吧,我在这儿等你的检查结果。

(9) According to the blood test，you are suffering from an iron deficiency anaemia.

检查结果显示你得了缺铁性贫血。

(10) I have no idea about my blood type，doctor.

医生,我不知道我的血型。

(11) My blood type is B.

我是 B 型血。

(12) I have had bleeding problems recently. My gums had bleeding before I brushes my teeth, and I had never bruised easily.

医生,我最近遇到了出血问题,刷牙前牙龈总是出血。我以前也没发现有瘀血情况的。

(13) Doctor, it started after an operation five years ago in which I had a blood transfusion.

医生,我在五年前的一次手术中输了血,从那以后开始的。

Ⅲ. Words and Expressions 单词和短语

abdominal purpura 腹部紫癜

abdominal wall reflex 腹壁反射

absent /'æbsənt/ adj. 消失

accentuate /ək'sentʃueɪt/ v. 亢进

achilles jerk 跟腱反射

activated partial thromboplastin time (APTT) 活化部分凝血活酶时间

acute lymphoblastic leukemia 急性淋巴细胞白血病

acute myeloid leukemia 急性髓性白血病

aleucia /ə'ljuːsiə/ n. 无白细胞症

alkylating agent 烷化剂

anal region 肛门区域

anemia /ə'niːmiə/ n. 贫血

angiopathy /ˌændʒɪ'ɒpəθi/ n. 血管病

ankle-clonus 踝阵挛

anuria /ə'njuəriə/ n. 尿闭

ape hand 猴样爪

aplastic anemia 再生障碍性贫血

arteriosclerosis /aːˌtɪəriəusklə'rəusɪs/ n. 动脉硬化

ascites /ə'saɪtiːz/ n. 腹水

atrophy /'ætrəfi/ n. 萎缩

Babinski sign 巴宾斯基征

bending /'bendɪŋ/ n. 弯曲

biceps-reflex 二头肌反射

bleeding time 出血时间

bone marrow aspiration 骨髓抽吸

bone marrow transplantation 骨髓移植

B symptoms B 症状

bulging /'bʌldʒɪŋ/ adj. 膨隆

Burkitt lymphoma 伯基特淋巴瘤

cecum /'siːkəm/ n. 盲肠

central nervous system leukemia 中枢神经系统白血病

cerebellar ataxia 小脑性共济失调

chorea /kə'riə/ n. 舞蹈症

chronic leukemia 慢性白血病

claw-hand 鹅样爪

club foot 足内翻

coagulation time 凝血时间

colon /'kəulən/ n. 结肠

complete remission 完全缓解

contour of intestine 肠形

Coombs test 抗人球蛋白实验

cramp in the calf 腓肌痉挛

cremasteric reflex 提睾反射

cyclophosphamide /ˌsaɪkləu'fɒsfəˌmaɪd/

n. 环磷酰胺

cytarabine /sɪtɑːˈræˈbɪn/ *n*. 阿糖胞苷

daunorubicin /ˌdɔːnəˈruːbɪsɪn/ *n*. 道诺霉素

differentiation therapy 分化治疗

disseminated intravascular coagulation 弥散性血管内凝血

doxorubicin /ˌdɒksəˈruːbəsɪn/ *n*. 阿霉素

duodenum /ˌdjuːəʊˈdiːnəm/ *n*. 十二指肠

end of the bone 骨骺

epigastric region 心窝部

Epstein-Barr virus 爱-巴病毒

erythroblast /ɪˈrɪθrəʊblæst/ *n*. 幼红细胞

erythrocyte /ɪˈrɪθrəsaɪt/ *n*. 红细胞

erythropoiesis /ɪˌrɪθrəʊpɔɪˈiːsɪs/ *n*. 红系造血

erythropoietin /ɪˌrɪθrəʊpɔɪˈiːtɪn/ *n*. 红细胞生成素

essential hypertension 原发性高血压

essential thrombopenic purpura 特发性血小板减少性紫癜

expiratory fixation 呼气固定

extremity /ɪkˈstreməti/ *n*. 四肢

falminant purpura 大片性紫癜

fecal incontinence 大便失禁

fibrin /ˈfaɪbrɪn/ *n*. 纤维蛋白

fibrinolysis /ˌfaɪbrɪˈnɒlɪsɪs/ *n*. 纤溶

finger to nose test 指鼻试验

flat-foot 扁平足

flatus /ˈfleɪtəs/ *n*. 肠胃胀气;屁

frog-belly 蛙腹

genital region 阴部

genu valgum 膝外翻

glossy /ˈglɒsi/ *adj*. 有光泽的

grasping power 握力

ham's test 酸溶血实验

haptoglobin /ˌhæptəˈɡləʊbɪn/ *n*. 珠蛋白

hematocrit /ˈhemətəʊkrɪt/ *n*. 红细胞压积

hematopoietic stem cell transplantation 造血干细胞移植

hemoglobin /ˈhiːməˈɡləʊbɪn/ *n*. 血红蛋白

hemoglobinopathy /ˈhiːməʊɡləʊbɪˈnɒpəθi/ *n*. 血红蛋白病

hemoglobinuria /ˈhiːməʊɡləʊbɪˈnjʊəriə/ *n*. 血红蛋白尿

hemolytic anemia 溶血性贫血

hemophilia /ˌhiːməˈfɪliə/ *n*. 血友病

hereditary hemorrhagic telangiectasis 遗传性出血性毛细血管扩张症

Hodgkin's disease 霍奇金病

idiopathic thrombocytopenic purpura 特发性血小板减少性紫癜

ileum /ˈɪliəm/ *n*. 回肠

inductive chemotherapy 诱导化疗

interferon-2 2-干扰素

intermediate-grade lymphoma 中度淋巴瘤

intestine string 肠系带

involuntary movement 不随意运动

iron deficiency anemia 缺铁性贫血

jejunum /dʒɪˈdʒuːnəm/ *n*. 空肠

Kerning sign 克尼格征

kidney /ˈkɪdni/ *n*. 肾

knee-heel test 跟膝反射试验

knee jerk;knee reflex;patellar reflex 膝反射

knock pain 叩击痛

kyphosis /kaɪˈfəʊsɪs/ *n*. 脊柱后凸

large intestine 大肠

leukemia /luːˈkiːmiə/ n. 白血病

liver /ˈlɪvə/ n. 肝

local projection 龟背

locomotor ataxia 共济运动失调

lordosis /lɔːˈdəʊsɪs/ n. 脊柱前弯

low-grade lymphoma 低度淋巴瘤

lymph node biopsy 淋巴结活检

lymphoma /lɪmˈfəʊmə/ n. 淋巴瘤

lymphogranuloma
/ˌlɪmfəʊˌgrænjʊˈləʊmə/ n. 淋巴肉芽肿

Mc Burney's point 麦氏点

megaloblastic anemia 巨幼细胞性贫血

meteorism /ˈmiːtɪəˌrɪzm/；
tympanites /ˌtɪmpəˈnaɪtiːz/ n. 鼓胀

methotrexate /ˌmeθəʊˈtrekseɪt/ 氨甲蝶呤

morphologic immunologic and cytogenetic classification MIC 分型

multiple drug resistance（MDR）多药耐药

multiple myeloma 多发性骨髓瘤

muscle rigidity 肌肉僵直

muscular daefense 肌性反抗

myelodysplastic syndrome（MDS）骨髓增生异常综合征

myeloproliferative disorder 骨髓增生性疾患

myelo-suppression 骨髓抑制

non-Hodgkin lymphoma 非霍奇金淋巴瘤

pain upon pressure 压痛

palpation /pælˈpeɪʃən/ n. 触诊

paralysis of radial nerve 桡神经麻痹

paroxysmal hemoglobinuria 发作性血尿

paroxysmal nocturnal hemoglobinuria 阵发性睡眠性血红蛋白尿

paroxysmal purpura 发作性紫癜

patellar clonus 膝阵挛

pathologic reflex 病理反射

Pel-Ebstein fever 周期性发热

percussion /pəˈkʌʃən/ n. 叩诊

pernicious anemia 恶性贫血

pes calcaneus 踵足

pes eguinus 尖足

phlebectasis /flɪˈbektəsɪs/ n.；venous dilatation 静脉扩张

plasmin inhibitor 纤溶酶抑制物

plasminogen activator inhibitor 纤溶酶原激活物抑制因子

pointing test 指示试验

polypus /ˈpɒlɪpəs/ n. 息肉

procarbazine /prəʊˈkaːbəziːn/ n. 丙卡巴肼

prostate /ˈprɒsteɪt/ n. 前列腺

protein C 蛋白 C

protein S 蛋白 S

prothrombin time 凝血酶原时间

pseudo-leukemia 假性白血病

Raynaud's disease 雷诺病

rectal examination 肛诊

rectum /ˈrektəm/ n. 直肠

reed-sternberg 里斯细胞

resistance of sphincter 括约肌抵抗

reticulocyte /rɪˈtɪkjʊləˌsaɪt/ n. 网织红细胞

rheumatic purpura 风湿性紫癜

rigidity of the back 背部强直

Romberg sign 昂伯征

scoliosis /ˌskɒliˈəʊsɪs/ n. 脊柱侧凸

shaft of the bone 骨干

small intestine 小肠

smooth /smuːð/ adj. 平滑的

spherocytosis /ˌsfɪərəʊsaɪˈtəʊsɪs/ n. 球形红细胞增生症

spinal ataxia 脊髓性共济失调

splashing sound 泼水音

spleen /spliːn/ n. 脾

spontaneous gangrene 特发性坏疽

static ataxia 静止性共济失调

stomach /ˈstʌmək/ n. 胃

supportive care 支持治疗

surface /ˈsɜːfɪs/ n. 表面

tension of abdominal wall 腹壁紧张

thalassemia /ˌθæləˈsiːmiə/ n. 地中海贫血

the bladder rectum nest 膀胱直肠窝

the human T-cell leukemia virus-1 HTLV-1 病毒

thickening /ˈθɪkənɪŋ/ n. 肿胀部分

thrombin /ˈθrɒmbɪn/ n. 凝血酶

thromboangitis obliterans 栓塞性脉管炎

thrombocytopenic purpura 血小板减

少性紫癜

thromboplastin /ˌθrɒmbəʊˈplæstɪn/ n. 凝血活酶

thrombosis /θrɒmˈbəʊsɪs/ n. 血栓形成

tibial edge 胫骨棱

tissue-type plasminogen activator 组织型纤溶酶元激活物

tonus of sphincter 括约肌紧张

tremor /ˈtremə/ n. 震颤

triceps-reflex 三头肌反射

true polycythemia, essential polycythemia 真性红细胞增多症

tympanitic /ˌtɪmpəˈnɪtɪk/ adj. 鼓的

tympany /ˈtɪmpəni/ n. 鼓音

umbilical cord 脐带

umbilical hernia 脐疝

umbilicus /ʌmˈbɪlɪkəs/ n. 脐

urokinase-type plasminogen activator 尿激酶型纤溶酶元激活物

vascular purpura 血管性紫癜

vincristine /vɪnˈkrɪstiːn/ n. 长春新碱

von willebrand factor 血管性血友病因子

Section 13　Department of Vaccination and Immunization

第 13 节　预防免疫科

Ⅰ. Dialogues 情景对话

1. Well Baby Clinic 健康门诊

Parent：Doctor，my baby is more than three months old. I'd like you to give him a check-up.

医生，我孩子已经三个多月了。你能不能给他检查一下呢？

Doctor：OK，no problem. Let me examine him. His heart and lungs are normal. I'd like to weigh him. What was his birth weight?

好的，我给他检查一下。他的心、肺功能都正常。再来给他称一下体重。他出生时体重多少？

Patient：He weighed 3.8 kilograms at birth，doctor.

出生体重是 3.8 公斤，医生。

Doctor：His weight is 8 kilograms now，that's very good.

现在体重是 8 公斤，发育很好。

Patient：And would you please tell me how I should feed him? He is taking breast milk，milk powder and fruit juice.

医生，你能不能告诉我应该怎样喂养孩子呢？他现在吃我的奶，此外还给他加些奶粉，喂些果汁。

Doctor：You can add egg yolk，vegetable purée and porridge gradually. Remember to start only one new food at a time.

还可以逐渐加一点蛋黄、菜泥和粥之类的。但是记住每次只给孩子加一种新食物。

Patient：Then，what about vaccinations?

那怎样给孩子预防接种呢？

Doctor：Did he have a BCG vaccination soon after his birth?

他出生后种过卡介苗吗？

411

Patient：Yes, he had it when he was three days old. He hasn't had any others.

种过,他是出生后三天接种的卡介苗,还没有接种过其他疫苗。

Doctor：Well, I know. He should be vaccinated against polio and have a triple vaccine when he is four months old. And he should also be vaccinated against measles at his eight months and have smallpox at two years.

哦,出生后四个月应该接种小儿麻痹疫苗和三联疫苗,出生后八个月接种麻疹疫苗,到两岁时可接种牛痘疫苗。

Patient：I see. Thank you very much, doctor.

我知道了,医生,谢谢你。

2. Vaccination 预防接种

Patient：Doctor, my child is healthy. But what vaccinations should he have (take)?

医生,我孩子很健康,他应该怎样接种呢?

Doctor：Don't worry. I'll start him on the triple vaccine today. Altogether three injections you remember. This is the first one.

别担心,今天我给他注射的是三联疫苗,一共是三针。这是第一针。

Patient：Then, when should I bring him back for the second injection?

那我该什么时候再带他来打第二针呢?

Doctor：Four to six weeks from now.

四至六个星期后再来。

Patient：Will there be any reaction after it?

打完针孩子会有什么反应吗?

Doctor：Some children have a little fever one or two days after the injection.

有些孩子打完针一两天后有点发烧。

Patient：Oh. And I have another child who had the triple vaccine last year. And does he need more this year?

好的,我明白了。不过,我还有个孩子,他去年已经打过三联疫苗了,今年还需要打吗?

Doctor：He should have a booster this year. Normally speaking, one injection is enough.

今年他只需要加强一次,只打一针就够了。

Patient：OK, I see, and anything else, doctor?

好的,我知道了。还有别的什么事吗,医生?

Doctor：I'll also give your baby the polio vaccine today, and there are three types. This is a red sugar pill which is type one.

我今天会给你的孩子一些小儿麻痹疫苗,一共三型。这是一型,一粒红色的糖丸。

Patient：When should I give it to him?

我什么时候给他吃?

Doctor：The pill does not keep at room temperature, so you must give it to him as soon as he gets awake. Don't let him take any warm water or food until one hour after taking the pill.

这种糖丸不能室温存放,所以孩子一睡醒就给他吃吧。吃后一小时之内不能喝热水、吃热的东西。

Patient：Will be there any reaction?

会有什么反应吗?

Doctor：Normally, no. There's nothing to worry about. Come back one month from now for the sugar pill type two and type three.

正常情况下没什么反应。不用担心。一个月后请来取二型、三型糖丸。

3. Reaction to Smallpox Vaccination 牛痘反应

Doctor：What's wrong with your child?

你的孩子怎么了?

Parent：He was vaccinated against smallpox a week ago. Yesterday he began to run a fever and he was irritable.

他一个星期前种了牛痘。昨天开始发烧、烦躁。

Doctor：Is there any redness and swelling?

有红肿吗?

Patient：Yes, there is some swelling at the armpit.

有的,腋下肿了。

Doctor：He is having a reaction to the smallpox vaccination. Yet，his axillary lymph gland is swollen.

这是牛痘反应,他的腋下淋巴结肿了。

Patient：When will it get better?

什么时候能好呢?

Doctor：About one week.

一周左右。

Patient：Can I bathe him?

我能给他洗澡吗?

Doctor：Yes，but don't wash the vaccination area.

可以,但是不要洗种痘的地方。

Patient：OK，I see，doctor. Thanks a lot.

噢,我知道了,谢谢你,医生。

Doctor：You are welcome，madame.

不客气,夫人。

Ⅱ. Sentences 替换句型

(1) Have you ever had an injection against tetanus?

你以前打过破伤风预防针吗?

(2) Has she been vaccinated against measles? When was she vaccinated?

她接种过麻疹疫吗? 什么时候接种的?

(3) Does anyone in your family have a heredity allergy?

你们家有家族遗传过敏史吗?

(4) Everything is normal for your baby, remember to take him to the clinic regularly.

你的孩子各项指标都很正常,带他定期来门诊检查就行了。

(5) In case of some symptoms of heat，cough，snuffle，sneeze，nasal mucus，ached belly，vomits，measles，dysentery，headache，being knotted，stupor，haematuria，albuminuria，jaundice，missing to inhale or swollow something，trauma，nose bleed，etc.，parents should be hurry to take your child to receive proper pediatric treatment.

万一你的孩子出现发烧、咳嗽、鼻塞、打喷嚏、流鼻涕、肚疼、呕吐、出疹子、拉痢疾、头痛、抽筋、昏迷、血尿、蛋白尿、黄疸、不明异物的吸入或误服、外伤、鼻出血等情况时，家长一定要带你的孩子到儿科门诊及时就诊。

Ⅲ. Words and Expressions 单词和短语

actinomycosis　/ˌæktɪnəʊmaɪˈkəʊsɪs/ n. 放线菌病

acute articular rheumatism 急性风湿性关节炎

acute infectious diseases 急性传染病

acute polyarthritis 急性多发性关节炎

amoebic dysentery 阿米巴痢疾

anti-epidemic station 防疫站

bacillary dysentery 菌痢

Bacillus Calmette-Guérin（BCG）卡介苗

chickenpox /ˈtʃɪkɪnˌpɒks/；varicella /ˌværɪˈselə/ n. 水痘

cholera /ˈkɒlərə/ n. 霍乱

cholera vaccine 霍乱菌苗

chronic infectious diseases 慢性传染病

chronic rheumatic arthritis 慢性风湿性关节炎

chronic villous polyarthritis 慢性多关节滑膜炎

common cold 感冒

cowpox vaccine 牛痘

diphtheria /dɪfˈθɪəriə/ n. 白喉

environmental hygiene 环境卫生

epidemic parotits mumps 流行性腮腺炎

fly swatter 苍蝇拍

free medical service 公费医疗

garbage wagon 垃圾车

German measles；rubella /ruːˈbelə/ n. 风疹

health service 保健事业

heatstroke prevention 防暑

hemorrhagic fever 出血热

hydrophobia /ˌhaɪdrəˈfəʊbiə/ n. 恐水病

hygiene /ˈhaɪdʒiːn/ n. 卫生

immune /ɪˈmjuːn/ adj. 免疫

industrial hygiene 工业卫生

infectious diseases 传染病

influenza /ˌɪnfluˈenzə/ n. 流感

inoculation /ɪˌnɒkjʊˈleɪʃn/ n. 防疫注射

kala-azar；black sickness 黑热病

leptospiral jaundice 出血性黄疸

measles /ˈmiːzlz/ n. 麻疹

medical kit 卫生箱

mental hygiene 心理卫生

muscular rheumatism 肌肉风湿

network of health protection 保健（健康）网络

paratyphoid fever 副伤寒

patriotic health and sanitation movement 爱国卫生运动

period of recuperation 疗养期

personal hygiene 个人卫生

pest plague 鼠疫

physical checkup 体格检查

prevention /prɪˈvenʃn/ n. 预防

public health 公共卫生

quarantine /ˈkwɒrəntiːn/ *n.* 检疫

quarantine office 检疫所(站)

rabies /ˈreɪbiːz/；lyssa /ˈlɪsə/；
hydrophobia /ˌhaɪdrəˈfəʊbiə/ *n.* 狂犬病

rat-bite disease(fever) 鼠咬病

relapsing fever 回归热

rheumatic fever 风湿热

scarlet fever 猩红热

sepsis /ˈsepsɪs/ *n.* 败血症

small pox；variola /vəˈraɪələ/ *n.* 天花

sterilization station 消毒站(点)

syphilis /ˈsɪfɪlɪs/ *n.* 梅毒

TAB＝typhoid-paratyphoid A and B
（vaccine）伤寒、副伤寒甲、乙三联
菌苗

tetanus /ˈtetnəs/ *n.* 破伤风

thorough cleaning 大扫除

typhus /ˈtaɪfəs/ *n.* 斑疹伤寒

to gain weight 增加体重

to get rid of four pests(mosquitoes，
flies，rats and bedbugs)"除四害"
（蚊子、苍蝇、老鼠和臭虫）

to lead a regular life 过有规律的生活

to lose weight 减肥

to recuperate 疗养

tsutsugamushi disease；Japanese
river fever 恙虫病

tuberculosis /tjuːˌbɜːkjuˈləʊsɪs/ *n.* 结核

typhoid fever 伤寒热

vaccination /ˌvæksɪˈneɪʃən/ *n.* 接种

vaccine /ˈvæksiːn/ *n.* 菌苗

whooping cough；pertussis /pəˈtʌsɪs/
n. 百日咳

Chapter 4　Tests and Diagnoses

第4章　检查与诊断

Section 1　Routine Tests and Examination of Blood and Urine

第1节　血尿常规检查

Ⅰ. Dialogues 情景对话

1. Chronic Hepatitis 慢性肝炎

Patient：I feel very tired and worn out all the time.

我总是觉得身体虚弱无力,非常疲倦。

Doctor：How is your appetite recently?

你最近食欲怎样?

Patient：Not good. I force myself to eat, but everytime I look at food and feel sick.

不太好。不过我还是强迫自己吃点东西,可我一看见饭,就想吐。

Doctor：Have you lost any weight?

你是否也有体重下降的现象呢?

Patient：Yes, quite a bit.

是的,我觉得瘦多了。

Doctor：When did you begin to feel unwell?

你是什么时候感觉不舒服的?

Patient：I don't know, doctor. But recently I've felt really bad.

我没有注意,医生,只是觉得最近病情加重了。

Doctor：Any other symptoms?

还有其他什么不适吗？

Patient：Yes. I can always feel a kind of pressure around the right side of my stomach.

有。我总是觉得肚子右边有一种压迫感。

Doctor：Do you drink a lot of alcohol?

你喝酒多吗？

Patient：Yes, I drink some everyday.

多,我每天都喝酒。

Doctor：How long have you been drinking?

你喝酒有多少年了？

Patient：About eight years.

大概八年了吧。

Doctor：Have you ever had any trouble with your liver?

你的肝脏以前出过毛病吗？

Patient：Yes, two years ago in a check-up, the doctor told me that my liver was enlarged and my liver function tested abnormal.

是的,两年前在一次常规体检时,医生说我是肝肿大,肝功能也有点不正常。

Doctor：Really? You'd better have another liver function test. And would you please come to the clinic tomorrow morning before breakfast with an empty stomach to have a blood test? Remember, don't eat or drink anything. Nor even coffee or tea.

哦,是吗？那你最好再做一次肝功能检查。明早记着不要吃早饭空腹来抽个血,不能喝水,就连茶和咖啡也不要喝,好吗？

Patient：Yes. But can you tell me, doctor, what's wrong with me?

好,不过我得了什么病了,医生？

Doctor：Your liver is enlarged and tender to the touch. It seems to be chronic hepatitis. You'll need absolute rest and avoid strenuous physical exertion. You can't drink alcohol anymore, and you should take the medicine regularly which I prescribe for you. There is no special treatment. It will take you some time to recover, so you have to be patient.

你的肝的确肿大,还有压痛感。看起来像慢性肝炎。你需要卧床休息,避免重体力劳动。另外你要按时吃药,不能再喝酒了,因为这病没有什么特效疗法,所以你必须要有耐心慢慢恢复。

2. At the Waiting Room 等待化验检查

Doctor：There are three more patients before you. Please wait a minute. Please put the thermometer under your arm now.

你前面还有三个病人等着化验,请你稍等一会儿。请把体温计夹在腋下。

Patient：That's OK, thank you, doctor.

好的,谢谢你,医生。

Doctor：We would like to have your stool examined. Will you please give us a specimen?

我们还要检查一下你的大便,你能留点大便标本吗?

Patient：Yes, I'll have a try, doctor.

可以,让我待会儿试试吧。

Doctor：You need to have your blood pressure checked. While, you also need to have a fluoroscopy done.

你需要量量血压,还要做个透视检查。

Patient：Yes, no problem.

好的,我知道了。

Doctor：Have you had your lungs X-rayed this year?

今年你做过胸透吗?

Patient：No. By the way, when can I get the result, doctor?

没有。医生,我的结果什么时候能出来呢?

Doctor：You can have all the results next Monday when you come to see the doctor. Now I'll take some blood from your arm, please take off your coat and roll up your sleeve. Wait, your veins don't stand out very clearly. I'll try to do it carefully, be patient and clench your fist please. OK, now please open your hand and press it with this bit of cotton wool for a while.

下周一你来看病时就能看到结果了。来,脱了上衣,挽起袖子,我来采点血。噢,你的静脉血管不太好找,我小心点,请你耐心等待,握紧拳头。好了,松开手吧,用棉球压一会儿啊。

Patient：Yes, I will, doctor.

好的,医生。

Doctor：More importantly, I'll do a skin test to see if you have any sensitivity.

重要的是,你还要做个皮试看看你是否过敏。

Patient：OK, but I discover a lump on my buttock yesterday. What shall I do, doctor?

好的。医生,昨天我发现臀部有个硬块,你看该怎么处理?

Doctor：Let me have a look. Better put a hot towel on it at home, twice a day and fifteen minutes for each time. Physiotherapy at hospital is needed if it doesn't get better anymore.

让我看看。最好回家用热毛巾热敷一下,一天两次,每次十五分钟。如果效果不好,可来医院做做理疗。

Ⅱ. Sentences 替换句型

(1) Please give some urine for a routine examination. Remember to collect the urine in the middle of urination.

请留点尿做个常规检查,记住最好接中段的尿。

(2) If there is no urine today, you can come tomorrow, but remember to fill about two thirds of this container with urine.

如果今天没尿,明天也行,记住尿液一定要接够杯子三分之二的量。

(3) Drink a lot of water before your collecting/making enough urine.

采尿前最好多喝点水。

(4) Your urine albumin is positive with two plus. You should omit salt from your diet.

尿蛋白两个加号,你应该忌盐了。

(5) It's 200/120 mmHg(26.7/16.0 kPa). That's moderately high. I would like you to do a urinalysis, blood urea nitrogen test, chest X-ray and electrocardiogram examination.

200/120 毫米汞柱(26.7/16.0 千帕),你的血压有点偏高,你最好做个尿常规化验、血尿素氮化验、X 线胸片和心电图检查。

(6) You may have an acute pyelonephritis, a kind of urinary tract infection. And I want a routine urine and a mid-stream clear catch

urinalysis. I'll also send a urine specimen for culture and sensitivity.

你可能得的是急性肾盂肾炎,这是一种尿路感染。你要先去取个中段尿液,做个尿常规检查。再送个尿标本做培养和敏感试验。

(7) There is no doubt that you have acute pyelonephritis, a kind of urinary tract infection.

毫无疑问你患的是肾盂肾炎,一种泌尿系统的感染。

(8) Take this sheet back to the urology clinic and tell your doctor that you could not urinate this morning.

请把这张化验单拿回泌尿科,给你的医生说你今天上午排不出小便。

(9) Let's take a white blood count and a blood amylase test, a kind of test for acute pancreatitis.

给你做个白细胞计数和淀粉酶试验吧,这是一种专门筛查急性胰腺炎的试验。

(10) By the way, I would like to take a drop of blood from his ear for a blood test.

另外,我要从他耳朵上取滴血做个试验。

(11) I'm afraid I have to prick your finger and take a drop of blood.

恐怕我得扎一下你的手指,取一滴血。

(12) Let me prick your ear to check how long it takes for your blood's coagulation. Don't worry, it just hurts a little.

我从耳部采血,给你做个血凝时间的检查。别担心,只稍微有一点点疼。

(13) It doesn't matter. (It's quite all right. / Never mind.)

没什么关系。(那没事。/没有关系。)

(14) Never mind. Bring a specimen in tomorrow, will you?

没关系,明天你再带标本来,行吗?

(15) Now I'm going to take a little blood from your arm. We need some laboratory findings to help us in making the diagnosis and get the type and a cross match for three units of whole blood to hold.

我要从你的胳膊上抽点血,做一些化验来帮助我们建立诊断和进行血型鉴定。做一个交叉配对的实验需要准备三个单位的全血待用。

Ⅲ. Words and Expressions 单词和短语

acid reaction 酸性反应

alkaline reaction 碱性反应

ammoniacal /ˌæməˈnaɪəkl/ *adj*. 氨的

amount of hemoglobin 血红蛋白量

anemic /əˈniːmɪk/ *adj*. 贫血的

aromatic /ˌærəˈmætɪk/ *adj*. 芳香的

ascites /əˈsaɪtiːz/ *n*. 腹水

bacillus /bəˈsɪləs/（pl.，bacilli
   /bəˈsɪlaɪ/）*n*. 杆菌

bacillus tetani 破伤风菌

bad smelling 恶臭

bleeding time 出血时间

blood coagulation rate 血凝率

blood count 血球计数

blood grouping 血型鉴定

blood in sputum 痰带血

blood platelet；thrombocyte
   /ˈθrɒmbəˌsaɪt/ *n*. 血小板

blood pressure 血压

blood test 验血

blood transfusion 输血

bloody urine 血尿

cerebrospinal fluid； cerebrospinal
   liquor 脑脊液

cholesterol /kəˈlestərɒl/ *n*. 胆固醇

clear /klɪə；transparent
   /trænsˈpærənt/ *adj*. 透明的

cloudy urine 浊尿

coagulation time 凝血时间

coccus /ˈkɒkəs/ *n*. 球菌

colon bacillus 大肠杆菌

color index 血色指数

crystal /ˈkrɪstl/ *adj*. 结晶的

deposit /dɪˈpɒzɪt/ *v*. & *n*. 沉淀

epithelial cell 上皮细胞

expectoration /ɪkˌspektəˈreɪʃn/ *n*. 痰；
   咳出物

exudate /ˈeksjʊˌdeɪt/ *n*. 渗出物

fat drops 脂肪滴

fecal /ˈfiːkl/ *adj*. 粪样的

filterable virus 滤过性病毒

fragrance /ˈfreɪɡrəns/；scent /sent/ *n*.
   香味

fruity /ˈfruːti/ *adj*. 果味的

germ /dʒɜːm/；bacteria /bækˈtɪəriə/
   n. 细菌

gonorrhea fiber 淋丝

hyperchromic /haɪpəˈkrəʊmɪk/ *adj*.
   高血色的

hypertension /ˌhaɪpəˈtənʃn/ *n*. 高血压

hypochromic /haɪpəʊˈkrəʊmɪk/ *adj*.
   低血色的

hypoproteinemia /haɪpɒprəʊtiːˈniːmiə/
   n. 低蛋白血症

hypotension /ˌhaɪpəʊˈtenʃən/ *n*. 低血压

leucocyte /ˈluːkəsaɪt/ *n*.；white cells；
   white blood corpuscle 白细胞

lumbar puncture 腰穿

mould /məʊld/ *n*. 霉菌；霉

neat and acid test 煮沸酸试验

number of leukocyte 白细胞数

number of red cells 红细胞数

pathogenic bacteria 病原菌

pathogeny /pəˈθɒdʒɪni/ *n.* 病原

pathological fluid 病理液

pericardial fluid 心包液

peritoneal fluid 腹腔液

plasma protein 血浆蛋白

polycythemia /ˌpɒlɪsaɪˈθiːmiə/ *n.* 红细胞增多症

precipitate /prɪˈsɪpɪteɪt/ *n.* 沉淀物

pressure of fluid 液压

red blood corpuscle；erythrocyte /ɪˈrɪθrəʊˌsaɪt/ *n.*；red cells 红细胞

sedimentation /ˌsedɪmenˈteɪʃn/ *n.* 血沉

serum protein 血清蛋白

specific gravity 比重

spinal /ˈspaɪnl/ *adj.* 脊柱的

sputum /ˈspjuːtəm/；phlegm /flem/ *n.* 痰

staphylococcus /ˌstæfɪləˈkɒkəs/ *n.* 葡萄球菌

suboccipital puncture 枕下穿刺

thrombocytopenia 血小板减少

thrombocytosis 血小板增多

transudate /ˈtrænsjʊˌdeɪt/ *n.* 漏出液；渗出液

turbid /ˈtɜːbɪd/ *adj.* 浑浊

Tyndall phenomenon 丁铎尔现象

unclear like milk 奶样的

urinary cast cylinder 管型尿圆柱

urinary stone 尿石

urine analysis 尿分析

urine /ˈjʊərɪn/ *n.* 尿

virus /ˈvaɪrəs/ *n.* 病毒

vomitus /ˈvɒmɪtəs/ *n.* 呕吐物

white cell count 白血球计数

xanthochromia 黄褐色

Section 2　Tests and Examination of Stool

第2节　粪便检查

Ⅰ. Dialogues 情景对话

1. Bacillary Dysentery 细菌性痢疾

Patient：Doctor, I have had a terrible diarrhea for two days.

医生,我严重腹泻已经两天了。

Doctor：What are your stools like? Watery or soft? Is there blood or mucus in the stool?

你的粪便是什么样的？水泻还是软便？有没有血和黏液？

Patient：Watery with blood and mucus.

水泻带有血和黏液。

Doctor：How frequent are they each day?

你每天大便几次?

Patient：They are very frequent. I don't know how many.

许多次,具体也不知道有多少次。

Doctor：Do you have a temperature?

发烧吗?

Patient：I feel hot and sometimes shivery.

有时觉得发烧,有时又觉得发冷。

Doctor：Have you had any abdominal pain?

肚子疼吗?

Patient：Yes, I have lower abdominal cramps.

疼,感觉是下腹部绞痛。

Doctor：Give a stool specimen to the laboratory please. And I'll wait for the results… Look, the stool shows blood, mucus and pus as well as some ascaris eggs. It's bacillary dysentery.

去化验室送一个粪便标本,我在这里等化验结果……看,化验单结果表明粪便里有血、黏液和脓,还有蛔虫卵。这是细菌性痢疾。

Patient：Doctor, is it serious?

医生,严重吗?

Doctor：It isn't serious. I'll give you some antibiotics. You should have a complete rest and drink large amounts of fluids, otherwise you will be dehydrated. If you like, you should have a liquid or semi-liquid diet that is easily digestible. Eat small quantities frequently. Avoid spicy, fibrous residue or greasy foods for a few days. By the way, it's an infectious disease, you should wash your hands thoroughly after going to the toilet.

不严重。我给你开点抗生素。不过你需要卧床休息、多喝水,不然的话,你会脱水的。吃些流质或半流质而且易于消化的食物。你还应该少吃多餐。最近几天,忌食辛辣、高纤维和油腻食物。由于这是传染病,便后一定要把手洗干净,以防再度传染。

Patient：Thank you, I will follow your advice.

谢谢,我会照办的。

2. Collecting the Sample 标本采集

Doctor：Mr. Smith，here is a glass and a paper box. Please collect your first urine in the glass and some of your stool in the box tomorrow morning.

史密斯先生,给你一个杯子和纸袋,明天你的第一次晨尿接在这个杯子里,纸袋用于装大便。

Patient：OK. Where shall I put them?

好的,这些东西明天我放在哪儿呢?

Doctor：Please put them in the basket at the corner of the nurses' office or you can directly send them to the laboratory. By the way, which doctor is in charge of your case?

你可以放在护士办拐角的筐里,也可以直接送到化验室。还有,谁是你的主治医生呀?

Patient：I think Dr. Wang is.

可能是王医生吧。

Doctor：Oh，I know. Mr. Smith，you look so tired. Please lie down and have a rest. I'll come to see you later and thank you for your cooperation.

知道了。史密斯先生,你看上去很累,躺下好好歇息吧。我待会儿再来看你,谢谢你的配合。

Patient：Doctor，what shall I do since I'm afraid I will not have any bowel movements tomorrow morning.

医生,我明早要是没有大便该怎么办?

Doctor：Never mind，Mr. Smith，you may collect it the day after tomorrow.

没关系,史密斯先生,后天有大便再化验也行。

Ⅱ. Sentences 替换句型

(1) It looks like bacillary dysentery，I'd like to send a stool specimen for culture.

看起来像是细菌性痢疾。我要送个粪便标本做培养。

（2）Infectious gastroenteritis is an infection of the digestive tract, causing vomiting and diarrhea. And a wide variety of bacteria can cause gastroenteritis. Some bacteria cause symptoms by producing toxins, while others grow on the intestinal wall.

感染性肠胃炎是消化道的一种感染症状,可以引起呕吐和腹泻。引起肠胃炎的细菌很多。有些细菌通过产生毒素引起症状,而有些则直接生长在肠壁上。

（3）To diagnose the cause, a doctor will normally consider whether the patient has been exposed to source of infection, such as particular food, an animal or an ill person.

为了能准确诊断出病因,医生一般都会考虑病人是否接触到了比如某些食物、动物或病人等传染源。

（4）Other infants and otherwise healthy children are given antibiotics only for certain bacteria and parasites, such as those that cause bloody diarrhea or cholera.

对于稍大一些的婴儿和其他方面健康的儿童,只是在抑制某些细菌和寄生虫,比如导致血性腹泻和霍乱的细菌和寄生虫的时候,才会考虑使用抗生素。

（5）A client's pertinent assessment data should include decreased dietary fiber and limited fluid intake, no bowel movement for three days, decreased bowel sounds, distention of lower abdomen, hard fecal material extracted during digital rectal examination, and a guaiac-negative stool specimen.

有关病人的评估资料包括膳食纤维的减少和液体摄入的不足,三天不排便,肠鸣音减少,下腹部胀气,直肠指检时有坚硬的粪便,粪便标本检查愈创木脂阴性。

Ⅲ. Words and Expressions 单词和短语

abnormal ingredient 异常的成分

acidity /əˈsɪdəti/ n. 酸性

ameba /əˈmiːbə/ n. 阿米巴

ancylostomas duodenal hook worms 十二指肠虫

ascaris eggs 蛔虫卵

ascaris teambricoides round worms 蛔虫

bile /baɪl/ n. 胆汁

bilious /ˈbɪliəs/; choleric /ˈkɒlərɪk/ adj. 胆汁状的

bladder worm；cysticercus /ˌsɪstɪˈsɜːkəs/ *n.* 囊虫

bright-yellow *adj.* 浅黄色的

brown /braʊn/ *adj.* 褐色的

coffee-ground like 咖啡样的

consistance /kənˈsɪstəns/ *n.* 硬度

dark brown 深褐色

distome hepatic 肝吸虫

distome salmonella 裂钩绦虫

dry (hard) stool 干粪

duodenal juice 十二指肠液

duodenal tube 十二指肠管

echinococcus /ɪˌkaɪnəˈkɒkəs/ *n.* 包虫

eggs of worm 虫卵

fart /faːt/ *n.* 屁

fecaloid /fɪkæˈlɔɪd/ *adj.* 粪样的

fibrous /ˈfaɪbrəs/ *adj.* 纤维的

filaria /fɪˈleərɪə/ *n.* 丝虫

flagellate /ˈflædʒəˌleɪt/ *n.* 鞭毛虫

form /fɔːm/ *n.* 形状

gallstone /ˈɡɔːlˌstəʊn/；cholelith /ˈkɒlɪˌlɪθ/ *n.* 胆石

gastric juice 胃液

granular /ˈɡrænjʊlə/；granulated /ˈɡrænjʊleɪtɪd/ *adj.* 颗粒状的

greenish /ˈɡriːnɪʃ/ *adj.* 绿色的

HCL-deficit 胃酸缺度

hematemesis /ˌhiːməˈtemɪsɪs/ *n.* 吐血

hemorrhagic /ˌheməˈrædʒɪk/ *adj.* 大出血的

hemoptysis /hiːˈmɒptɪsɪs/ *n.* 咯血

intestinal parasites 肠内寄生虫

itch mite 疥螨

lactic acid 乳酸

light brown 浅褐色

loose (soft) stool 稀粪

lung flukes 肺吸虫

mucous /ˈmjuːkəs/ *adj.* 黏液的

not easily digestible 不易消化的

organic acid 有机酸

pallor /ˈpælə/ *n.* （尤指因疾病、恐惧所导致的脸色）苍白

parasite /ˈpærəsaɪt/ *n.* 寄生虫

pinworm /ˈpɪnˌwɜːm/ *n.* 蛲虫

plasmodium /plæzˈməʊdɪəm/ *n.* 疟原虫

pneumococcus /ˌnjuːməˈkɒkəs/ *n.* 肺炎双球菌

purulent /ˈpjʊərələnt/ *adj.* 化脓的

pyoid /ˈpaɪɔɪd/ *adj.*；purulent /ˈpjʊərʊlənt/ *adj.*；pus-containing 脓样的

quantity /ˈkwɒntəti/ *n.* 量

round worms 蛔虫

rusty /ˈrʌsti/ *adj.* 铁锈的

schistosome /ˈʃɪstəˌsəʊm/ *n.* 血吸虫

soap-like (shaped) 肥皂状

soft /sɒft/；loose /luːs/ *adj.* 软的

stool /stuːl/；feces /ˈfiːsiːz/ *n.* 粪

tapeworm /ˈteɪpwɜːm/；cestode /ˈsestəʊd/；taenia /ˈtiːnɪə/ *n.* 绦虫

test meal 餐试

thematoda flukes 吸虫

total acidity 总酸度

trichomonad /ˌtrɪkəʊˈmɒnæd/ *n.* 毛滴虫

tubercle bacilli 结核杆菌

uncinariasis /ˌʌnsɪnəˈraɪəsɪs/ *n.* 钩虫病

visible /ˈvɪzəbl/ *adj.* 有形的

water fluid 水样的

watery stool 水样便

whipworm /ˈwɪpˌwɜːm/ *n.* 鞭虫

yellowish /ˈjeləʊɪʃ/ *adj.* 黄色的

Section 3　Bultrasonic Examination
第3节　B超检查

Ⅰ. Dialogues 情景对话

1. Peptic Ulcer 消化性溃疡

Patient：I have a pain in my stomach，doctor.
医生,我胃疼。

Doctor：How long have you had it?
疼多久了?

Patient：I have had it off and on for the past three years. It has been really bad these past two weeks.
断断续续已经疼了三年,近两周来疼得很厉害。

Doctor：Do you feel it when your stomach is empty?
肚子空的时候觉得疼吗?

Patient：Yes. After I eat，it goes away for a while.
疼。吃了东西以后疼痛缓解一会儿。

Doctor：When do you get it?
什么时候才疼呢?

Patient：Usually when I get very nervous. Sometimes it wakes me up in the middle of the night.
通常是我一紧张就疼,不过有时半夜能把我疼醒。

Doctor：What kind of pain do you have?
是怎样一种疼痛呢?

Patient：It gives me a burning sensation.
烧灼疼。

Doctor：Usually how do you get relief?

平常你是怎么止疼的呢？

Patient：After I take some sodium bicarbonate, the pain goes away temporarily, doctor.

服点小苏打可暂时缓解疼痛，医生。

Doctor：Have you had any nausea or vomiting?

你感觉恶心、呕吐吗？

Patient：Yes, occasionally.

是的，有时候有这样的情况。

Doctor：Are your bowels regular?　Have you observed your stools?

你大便正常吗？注意过你的粪便有什么异常吗？

Patient：I usually have to go once every other day. I was very worried because last night I went twice and the stool was black (tarry).

平常我每隔一天大便一次。可是昨天晚上我大便了两次，黑黑的颜色（像柏油似的），我很害怕。

Doctor：Go to the next-door room. Let me take you a test of abdominal ultrasonography. Lie down on your back and lower your underwear to expose the abdomen please.

到隔壁屋子，我给你做个B超检查。请仰面躺下，解开衣服，露出腹部。

Patient：OK, doctor.

好的，医生。

Doctor：Please take a deep breath and hold it… OK, I think, it's a duodenal ulcer, you should have a complete rest and give your stomach as little work as possible. Take only fluids. There is nothing better than boiled tepid milk taken regularly in small quantities. In addition, I will give you some medicine. If the black stools persist or your condition gets worse, come back to the hospital at once.

好，深呼吸，屏住气……看来你得的是十二指肠溃疡。你应该卧床休息，尽量不吃那么饱，少食多餐，只吃流食，比如按时喝点少量煮过的温牛奶。另外，我再给你开点药。如果还拉黑便或感觉病情加重，你再马上来看。

Patient：Thank you very much, doctor. And I'll follow your advice.

谢谢你，医生。我会照你说的做的。

2. Regular Ultrasonic Check-up 常规超声检查

Patient：Is there any discomfort in ultrasonic check-up, doctor?

医生,做超声波检查会有什么不舒服吗?

Doctor：No, none at all. Just do what I tell you. Take a deep breath. Extend your belly. Hold your breath for a few seconds.

不会有什么不舒服的。你照我说的去做就行了。好,深呼吸,鼓起肚子。屏住呼吸,持续几秒钟。

Patient：Enn.

嗯。

Doctor：OK! Breathe as usual.

好啦! 可以呼吸了。

Doctor：Have you ever had hepatitis?

你以前得过肝炎吗?

Patient：No, never. (Yes, about three years ago.)

没有,从没得过。(得过,是在三年以前。)

Doctor：Any pain around the liver region?

你肝区疼过吗?

Patient：Yes, I always have pain there.

是的,那里总是很疼的。

Doctor：Has your liver (spleen) ever been enlarged?

你的肝(脾)增大过吗?

Patient：No, my liver (spleen) has never been enlarged. Because I have never been examined, doctor.

没有,我的肝(脾)从来没增大过,因为我从来都没检查过,医生。

3. Pregnancy Ultrasonic Check-up 怀孕超声检查

Doctor：When was your last monthly period?

你末次月经是什么时候?

Patient：The fifteenth of May.

5月15日。

Doctor：How long have you been pregnant?

你怀孕多久了？

Patient：Nearly three months now.

　　　　差不多三个月了。

Doctor：Any complaints?

　　　　有什么不舒服吗？

Patient：I have a little bleeding. Occasionally I have abdominal pains. Is the baby in a good condition?

　　　　我有一点出血。偶尔有腹疼。胎儿的情况好吗，医生？

Doctor：Yes, its heart and movements are all normal.

　　　　是的，很好，胎心和胎动都很正常。

Patient：Will I have one baby, or twins?

　　　　是一个孩子还是一对双胞胎呢？

Doctor：It's twins. (Only one baby.)

　　　　是双胞胎。（是单胎。）

Ⅱ. Sentences 替换句型

(1) What should I do before the ultrasonic examination, doctor?

医生，做超声检查之前应该注意些什么呢？

(2) This test is not painful at all, just lie down on your back and relax.

这个检查一点都不疼，仰面躺下，放松。

(3) Please lift your coat up and lower your underwears to expose your abdomen, then take a deep breath and hold it. Good, now lie down on your right side.

请掀起上衣，解开内衣露出腹部，深呼吸，屏住气。好，换右侧位。

(4) The thyroid scanning reveals that the nodule of thyroid is a "cold" nodule, which means nonfunctional, you just have a goiter.

甲状腺扫描发现你的甲状腺结节是"冷"结节，也就是无功能，你得的是甲状腺囊肿。

(5) Doctor, I suffer from a chest pain and shortness of breath. I wonder whether a watermelon seed has dropped into my windpipe.

医生，我胸痛气促。不知道是不是西瓜子掉进我气管里去了。

(6) Fluoroscopy shows that your right lung is partially collapsed, while the breathing sound is diminishing markedly through auscultation. I

think there is a strong possibility of the presence of a foreign body in your right main bronchus.

透视发现你的右肺有一部分萎陷了,同时听诊时发现,你的呼吸音也明显地减弱了。我想很可能在你的右侧支气管里有一个异物。

(7) I have detected a floating sound in her windpipe. I have a strong suspicion that there is a foreign body in her trachea.

我发现她气管里有游动的响声。我很怀疑在她的气管里有异物。

(8) The foreign body should be removed through the intubation of a bronchoscope. This operation involves some risk for the patient. For safety's sake, we are going to have a consultation with the chest surgeon to discuss the best plan for the treatment.

异物要通过插入的气管镜摘除,这个手术对病人具有一定的危险性。为安全起见,我们正请胸外科医生会诊商讨最好的治疗方案。

(9) Be sure not to let your children talk or cry when they eat. Any solid food should be prohibited before the child's teeth have erupted completely.

切记不要让你的孩子在进食时说话或哭叫。在孩子的牙齿出齐之前禁食固体食物。

(10) Doctor, my daughter fell down from her chair while she was having her dinner. This was followed by a violent fit of coughing and difficulty in breathing, so I bring her to the hospital immediately.

医生,我女儿在吃饭的时候从椅子上摔了下来,接着就是一阵阵厉害的咳嗽,我发现她呼吸困难,就赶快带她到医院来了。

(11) Doctor, my child has had a succession of choking fits for three days. I have also detected a peculiar noise in her throat when she cries.

医生,我的孩子一阵阵憋气已有三天了。我还觉察到她哭的时候嗓子里有一种奇怪的响声。

(12) Please drink more water, but don't urinate before the examination. With urine in your bladder, the image will be clearer.

请多喝些水,但在检查之前不要排尿。膀胱里存着尿,检查时仪器上就可以显示得更清楚些。

Ⅲ. Words and Expressions 单词和短语

acute appendicitis 急性阑尾炎

acute diffuse peritonitis 急性弥漫性腹膜炎

acute enteritis 急性肠炎

acute gastritis 急性胃炎

acute local peritonitis 急性局部腹膜炎

acute pancreatitis 急性胰腺炎

acute yellow atrophy of the liver 肝急性黄萎缩症

anal fissure 肛裂

anal fistula 肛瘘

anal prolapse；prolapsus of anus 脱肛

aorta /eɪˈɔːtə/ n. 主动脉

aortic aneurysm 主动脉瘤

aortic valves 主动脉瓣

apex of lung 肺尖

asthenia /æsˈθiːniə/；atony /ˈætəni/ n. 无力

asthenic /æsˈθenɪk/；atonic /eɪˈtɒnɪk/ adj. 无力的

atony of the stomach 胃无力症

atrophic cirrhosis of liver 萎缩肝硬化

autointoxication /ˈɔːtəʊɪnˌtɒksɪˈkeɪʃən/ n. 自中毒

biliary jaundice；jaundice due to biliary stasis 胆汁性黄疸

calcification /ˌkælsɪfɪˈkeɪʃn/ n. 钙化

cancer of liver；hepatic carcinoma 肝癌

cancer of the intestine 肠癌

cancer of the stomach, gastric cancer 胃癌

cancer of the tongue 舌癌

carcinoma of peritoneum（peritonaeum）腹膜癌

cardia /ˈkaːdiə/ n.；cardiac muscle 心肌

catarrhal appendicitis 卡他性阑尾炎

catarrhal jaundice 卡他性黄疸

cecitis /sɪˈsaɪtɪs/ n. 盲肠炎

cholecystitis /ˌkɒlɪsɪsˈtaɪtɪs/ n. 胆囊炎

cholelithiasis /ˌkɒləlɪˈθaɪəsɪs/ n. 胆石症

chronic peritonitis 慢性腹膜炎

colic of the intestine 肠绞痛

colon cancer 结肠癌

congestion of liver 肝充血

cyst formation 囊肿形成

diaphragm /ˈdaɪəˌfræm/ n. 膈肌

dilatation of oesophagus 食道扩张

dilatation of the stomach；gastrectasia /gæstrekˈteɪziə/ n. 胃扩张

disease of digestive system 消化道疾病

diseases of liver and bile duct 肝胆疾病

diseases of oral cavity 口腔疾病

diseases of peritonization 腹膜病

diseases of the intestine 肠病

diseases of the oesophagus 食管疾病

diseases of the stomach 胃病

distoma hepaticum 胆吸虫

diverticulum of the duodenum 十二指肠憩室

duodenal ampulla 十二指肠壶腹

duodenal bulb 十二指肠球部

duodenal ulcer 十二指肠溃疡

dyspepsia /dɪsˈpepsiə/ n. 消化不良

dystrophy /'dɪstrəfi/; dystrophia /dɪ'strəʊfɪə/ n. 营养不良

early infiltration 早期浸润

echinococcus of liver; liver fluke 肝吸虫

enteritis /ˌentə'raɪtɪs/ n. 肠炎

enteromycosis/actinomycosis of intestine 肠真菌病

enterorrhagia /entərəʊ'reɪdʒɪə/ n.; intestinal bleeding 肠出血

extermal hemorrhoid 外痔

exudative /ɪɡ'zjuːdətɪv/ adj. 渗出性的

fatty liver 脂肪肝

foreign bodies in the oesophagus 食道异物

gangrenous stomatitis 坏疽口腔炎

gastric ulcer 胃溃疡

gastroptosis /gæstrɒp'təʊsɪs/ n. 胃下垂

greater curvature 大弯

hemorrhage from the stomach 胃出血

hepatic abscess 肝脓肿

hilar shadow 肺门阴影

hyperacidity /ˌhaɪpərə'sɪdɪti/ n. 胃酸过多

hypertrophic cirrhosis of liver 肥大性肝硬化

internal hemorrhoid 内痔

intestinal obstruction 肠梗阻

intestinal perforation 肠穿孔

intussusception /ˌɪntəssə'sepʃən/ n.; intestinal invagination 肠套叠

lesser curvature 小弯

lobe of lung 肺叶

lung /lʌŋ/ n. 肺

lung markings 肺纹

miliary tuberculosis 栗粒性肺结核

mitral valves 二尖瓣

niche /niːʃ/ n. 壁龛

noma /'nəʊmə/ 坏疽性口炎

oesophageal doverticulum 食道憩室

oppilation /ˌɒpɪ'leɪʃən/; constipation /ˌkɒnstɪ'peɪʃən/ n. 便秘

pancreas cyst 胰囊肿

pancreas /'pæŋkriəs/ n. 胰腺

pancreatic cancer 胰癌

pancreatic necrosis 胰腺坏死

parotitis /ˌpærə'taɪtɪs/ n. 腮腺炎

perforation of the stomach 胃穿孔

peritonitis /ˌperɪtə'naɪtɪs/ n. 腹膜炎

phlegmonous appendicitis 蜂窝织性阑尾炎

pleural cavity 胸腔

pleura /'plʊərə/ n. 肋膜

portal thrombosis 门静脉血栓症

primary focus 原发症

prolapsus of rectum 直肠脱出

proliferative /prə'lɪfərətɪv/ adj. 增殖的

ptosis /'təʊsɪs/ n. 下垂

ptotic /'tɒtɪk/ adj. 下垂的

pulmonary hilus 肺门

pylorus /paɪ'lɔːrəs/ n. 幽门

rectal cancer 直肠癌

recurrent (recidivistic) appendicitis 再发阑尾炎

region of lung 肺野

schistosoma japonicum 日本血吸虫病

spasm of oesophagus 食道痉挛

stenosis of oesophagus 食管狭窄

stenosis of the pylorus; pyloric stenosis 幽门狭窄

subpancreatic abscess 胰下脓肿

syphilis of liver 肝梅毒

thrush /θrʌʃ/ *n*. 鹅口疮

tuberculous peritonitis 结核性腹膜炎

ulmonary cavity 肺空洞

volvulus /ˈvɒlvjuləs/ *n*. 肠扭转

Section 4　Electrocardiogram and Brain-Wave Examination

第4节　心、脑电图检查

Ⅰ. Dialogues 情景对话

1. Heart Failure 心力衰竭

Doctor：What is troubling you?

你觉得怎么不舒服？

Patient：I have great difficulty in catching my breath. My heart is beating very fast.

我呼吸很困难，心跳得很快。

Doctor：When did you begin to notice these symptoms?

你是什么时候发现不舒服的？

Patient：Well，five years ago in a routine check-up，my school doctor told me that I had heart trouble. But it didn't bother me and I could carry on as usual. About the last two years，I have noticed when I climb stairs my heart beats faster and I have to stop and catch my breath.

五年前的一次常规体格检查时，校医说我心脏有问题。当时我没有任何不适感，照常活动。可是最近两年我发现上楼梯时心跳得很快，而且有时不得不停下来喘气。

Doctor：How many pillows do you use when you sleep?

你睡觉时用几个枕头？

Patient：Two. I used to need only one，but since last year I had to add another.

两个。一般情况下一个枕头，可从去年起，我必须加垫一个才舒服。

Doctor：Do you ever have to sit up to catch your breath at night?

你是不是夜里需要坐起来喘气呢？

Patient：Yes. This has been happening in the past two or three days.

是的。最近两三天更厉害了。

Doctor：Did you ever notice any swelling in your ankles?

你的脚面浮肿吗？

Patient：Yes, recently it occurred in the afternoon and disappeared the next morning.

肿，最近是每天下午浮肿，第二天早晨就消失了。

Doctor：Lie on the bed please. I'll examine you. Wait a moment, I'll give you an EKG and a chest X-ray.

你躺在床上，我给你检查一下。待会儿你还要做一个心电图和X线胸部检查。

Patient：Is it that bad?

有那么严重吗？

Doctor：It seems you had better be hospitalized. (No, it is not very serious, but I don't want to take any risks. You'll be all right soon.)

看来你最好还是住院了。（不，情况不很严重，可是，还是小心点好。你很快就会好的。）

2. Syncope 晕厥

Patient：Doctor, I have been suffering from "fits" for many years. I hope you will help me to calm them down.

医生，很多年来我常会"突然发作"。我希望你帮我把它治好。

Doctor：What do you mean by "fits"?

你所说的"突然发作"是什么意思？

Patient：I mean I suddenly lose consciousness and fall on the floor.

我的意思是我会一下子突然倒在地上，然后就什么都不知道了。

Doctor：Since when?

从什么时候开始的呢？

Patient：Since I was a girl.

从我是个小女孩儿的时候就开始了。

Doctor：For how many years?

　　　　有多少年了？

Patient：About ten years.

　　　　大概十年了吧。

Doctor：How long does each attack last?

　　　　每次大概会持续多久呢？

Patient：Less than a minute.

　　　　不到一分钟吧。

Doctor：How long is the interval between two successive attacks?

　　　　每次发作相隔多久？

Patient：It varies from half a month to a year. Could it be related to circumstances?

　　　　从半个月到一年不等。你说这可能与周围环境有关系吗？

Doctor：What kind of circumstances usually provokes your attacks?

　　　　说说看，通常什么样的环境容易引起你发病呢？

Patient：It is difficult to say exactly. Once when I was crossing the street, a swiftly moving car suddenly drove by and I became very nervous, and I couldn't control myself. I screamed and blacked out.

　　　　很难说。有一次我穿过马路的时候，忽然一辆轿车飞快地开过来了，我马上紧张起来，一下子就控制不住自己了。我尖叫了一声就什么也不知道了。

Doctor：Were you hurt by the car?

　　　　车撞伤你了吗？

Patient：No, the car stopped with a squeal. I came to my senses quickly, then I walked home.

　　　　没有，车子吱的一声停了下来。我也很快醒过来就回家了。

Doctor：Any other attacks?

　　　　你还有其他发作情况吗？

Patient：On another occasion, no sooner had a nurse drawn blood from a patient than I felt perspiration and weakness followed by loss of conscionsness.

　　　　另一次是，我一看到一位护士在给别的病人抽血，我就开始冒汗，腿脚发软，然后就失去知觉晕过去了。

Doctor：Did you have other manifestations during the attack?

在发病的时候还有什么其他的表现吗?

Patient：I was told by eye-witnesses that I became pale and sweated excessively during the attack, but I had no convulsions, incontinence or anything else.

据目击者说,我发病的时候面色苍白,大量出汗,但是没有抽搐、大小便失禁或其他的什么情况了。

Doctor：Have you had any special examinations, such as an electrocardiogram, an electroencephalogram, or a skull X-ray?

你做过什么特殊检查没有,比如心电图、脑电图或头颅 X 光片?

Patient：A doctor working in a local hospital told me that my physical examination, electrocardiogram, and chest and skull X-ray examination results were normal. I've had no other special examinations.

我们当地医院的医生告诉我说,我的体格检查、心电图以及胸部和头颅的 X 光检查都正常,其他的特殊检查就没做过了。

Doctor：Let me give you a thorough physical and neurological examination. (After exams) Some further examinations should be done, including an electroencephalogram and a brain scan. Also the electrocardiogram should be repeated. Here are your referral sheets. After you have had all these examinations, please come back for another check-up.

我给你做一个内科和神经科的全面检查吧。(检查完毕)你还需要做些进一步的检查,包括脑电图和脑扫描检查。还需要重做一次心电图。这是各项检查的单子。把所有的检查做完以后你再来门诊找我看病吧。

(Several days later)

(几天后)

Patient：Doctor, I have had all the examinations you ordered. Are all the results back yet?

医生,你让我做的检查我都做完了。结果出来了吗?

Doctor：Yes, and all the results are normal.

出来了,结果都是正常的。

Patient：Then what is the cause of my "fits"?

那我的"突然发作"是怎么回事啊？

Doctor：The normal results of physical and neurological examinations and other special examinations suggest neither organic heart or brain diseases nor epilepsy. The symptoms and signs which occur during an attack，such as palpitations，paleness and excessive sweating coincide with an imbalance of the autonomic nervous system function. Dysfunction of the autonomic nervous system can lead to a decrease in the cardiac output，cerebral anemia，suppression of brain function，and finally to a loss of consciousness. Such an attack is termed syncope.

根据内科、神经科以及一些其他特殊检查来看，你既不是器质性的心脏病或颅脑病，也不是癫痫。你突然晕倒时的症状和体征，如心跳、苍白和过多的出汗等等，跟你自主神经系统功能失调是相符的。自主神经系统的功能失调能引起心搏出量的减少、脑贫血以及大脑功能抑制，最后导致失去知觉，像这样的病医学上的名称叫晕厥。

Patient：Can you give me some medicine to calm the syncope down?

你有什么药能治我这晕厥病吗？

Doctor：You should pay attention to regulating your life such as getting up and going to bed regularly and not drinking or smoking too much. I'll give you some medicine to regulate the functioning of your autonomic nervous system. If you follow my advice，I am sure your condition will get better soon. Sometimes your symptoms may recur，this is a natural phenomenon. Don't worry，such recurrences don't mean regression. During the struggle against disease，you must feel confident that you can overcome it，then the medicine which I'll give you will help you to defeat the syncope. Medicine is one way，and confidence is another. The latter is more important than the former.

你需要注意的是，生活要有规律，定时起床、睡觉，不要过度地饮酒和吸烟。我给你开点调节你的自主神经功能的药物。假如你能听从我的劝告，我相信你一定会很快好起来的。一些症状有时可能会有反复，这是自然现象。不必着急，症状有反复并不说明病情恶化。你必须树立克服、战胜疾病的信心，加上我给你开的药,会帮助你消除晕厥的。药物治疗仅仅是一个方面,信心却是比药物治疗更为重要的另一个方面呀。

Patient：Thanks a lot, doctor. I'll follow your advice.

谢谢你,医生。我一定听从你的劝告。

3. Test for Blood Circulation 血流变检查

Patient：Is there a tumor, doctor?

有瘤吗,医生?

Doctor：No, there isn't. Have you a headache? Exactly where?

没有。你头痛吗? 在哪一边?

Patient：I have pain all over my head. (On the left side.)

我整个头都痛。(我头的左边痛。)

Doctor：Did you bang your head recently?

最近头部磕碰过吗?

Patient：I knocked my head against a wall a week ago.

一个星期以前我的头碰在墙上了。

Doctor：I'll do a test for your blood circulation.

我要给你做一个血流图的检查。

Patient：Does it hurt?

疼吗?

Doctor：Not at all, just like doing an electrocardiogram. Is your blood pressure high?

一点也不疼,就像做心电图一样。你的血压高吗?

Patient：My blood pressure is usually normal. (My blood pressure is a bit higher than normal.)

我的血压一般是正常的。(我的血压比正常的高一些。)

Doctor：How much? (How high is it?)

多少? (多高呢?)

Patient：Around 140/90 mmHg (18. 7/12. 0 kPa).

在 140/90 毫米汞柱(18. 7/12. 0 千帕)左右。

Doctor：Have you a headache or any dizziness?

你有头痛或头晕的症状吗?

Patient：Not usually, but they've been more frequent recently.

不常有，但最近发作得多些。

Doctor：Don't blink. Breathe gently. Now stop your breath for a few seconds. OK! Breathe as usual. Put this pill under your tongue, and just let it melt in your mouth.

不要眨眼，平稳地呼吸就行了。现在屏住呼吸几秒钟。好，检查完了，你可以正常呼吸了。把这个药丸放在舌头下面，让它慢慢在嘴里溶化。

Ⅱ. Sentences 替换句型

(1) You need an electrocardiogram，sir.

先生，你需要做个心电图的检查。

(2) We take a brain-wave scan (eletroencephalogram) now for you.

我们现在给你做个脑电图检查。

(3) Take off your shoes and undress till the chest. Lie down on your back and relax，let me know if you get ready.

脱掉鞋子，解开衣服，放松平躺在床上，准备好了，咱们就开始做检查了。

(4) Take it easy please and your hair should be cleaned firstly.

放松，检查前先把你的头洗一洗。

(5) The light will take flashes over your eyes，just take it for relexation. If you feel sick please let us know immediately.

检查时会有光在你眼睛上的，别担心，感觉有什么不舒服立即告诉我们。

(6) Open your mouth slightly and relax. Then listen to me，take a deep breath and keep it continuously for three minutes.

轻轻地放松，张嘴。好，现在听我的指令，深呼吸，屏气，我数三分钟。

(7) It doesn't hurt you any more，please close your eyes slightly during the test，so you may sleep if you want.

检查一点都不疼，你只需轻轻闭上眼睛，检查过程中想睡的话睡一觉也行。

(8) OK，that's all for today's examination. The nurse will take you to have a rest，better keep an upright position for a while.

今天的检查到此为止。护士会带你去休息一会儿，最好保持一个半坐位的姿势。

Ⅲ. Words and Expressions 单词和短语

acquired hydrocephalus 后天性脑积水

acute anterior poliomyelitis 急性脊髓灰质炎

amyotrophic lateral sclerosis 肌萎缩性侧索硬化症

apoplexy /ˈæpəpleksi/ n. 中风

aseptic meningitis 无菌性脑膜炎

brain abscess；cerebral abscess 脑脓肿

cerebral anemia 脑贫血

cerebral embolism 脑栓塞

cerebral syphilis；brain lues 脑梅毒

cerebral thrombosis 脑血栓

cerebral tumor；brain tumor 脑肿瘤

chronic spasm of diaphragm 性膈肌痉挛

compression myelitis 压迫性脊髓炎

congenital hydrocephalus 先天性脑积水

cramp in the calf 腓肠肌痉挛

craniotabes /kreɪniˌəʊˈteɪbiːz/ n. 颅结核

diseases of brain 脑病

diseases of meninges 脑膜病

diseases of peripheral nerves 末梢神经疾病

diseases of the external pyramidal system 锥体外系疾病

encephalomalacia /enˌsefələʊməˈleɪʃiə/；softening of the brain 脑软化症

epidemic cerebrospinal meningitis 流行性脑脊髓膜炎

epidemic encephalitis 流脑

facial paralysis 面神经麻痹

facial spasm 面痉挛

hemicrania /ˌhemɪˈkreɪniə/；migraine /ˈmiːɡreɪn/；megrim /ˈmiːɡrɪm/ n. 偏头痛

hemorrhage into spinal cord 脊髓出血

hereditary spinal ataxia 遗传性脊髓性共济失调

hydrocephalus /ˌhaɪdrəʊˈsefələs/ n. 脑积水

hyperaemia of the brain 脑充血

infantile cerebral paralysis 脑性小儿麻痹

lethargic encephalitis 嗜睡性脑炎

meningeal hemorrhage 脑膜出血

mogigraphia /məˌdʒɪɡˈræflə/ n.；writer's cramp 书写性痉挛

multiple cerebrospinal sclerosis 多发性脑脊髓硬化

myelanalosis /maɪlənəˈləʊsɪs/ n.；tabes dorsalis 脊髓结核

myelitis /ˌmaɪəˈlaɪtɪs/ n. 脊髓炎

myotonia congenital 先天性肌强直症

neuritis /njʊˈraɪtɪs/ n. 神经炎

paralysis agitans 震颤性麻痹

paralysis of the median nerve 正中神经麻痹

paralysis of the muscles of the eyes 眼肌麻痹

paralysis of the radial nerve 桡神经麻痹

paralytic dementia 麻痹性痴呆

progressive bulbar paralysis 进行性

球麻痹

progressive muscle atrophy 进行性肌萎缩症

progressive paralysis 进行性麻痹

purulent meningitis 化脓性脑膜炎

sciatica /saɪˈætɪkə/ *n.*； neuralgia sciatica 坐骨神经痛

sea sickness 晕船

serous meningitis 浆液性脑膜炎

sinus thrombosis 窦血栓

spastic spinal paralysis 痉挛性脊髓麻痹

spinal infantile paralysis 脊髓性小儿麻痹

subarachnoidal hemorrhage 蛛网膜下出血

syringomyelia /sɪˌrɪŋɡəʊmaɪˈiːliə/ *n.* 脊髓空洞症

trigeminal neuralgia；prosopalgia /prɒsəˈpældʒə/ *n.* 三叉神经痛

trismus /ˈtrɪzməs/ *n.* 嚼肌痉挛

tuberculous meningitis 结核性脑膜炎

tumor of the spinal cord 脊髓肿瘤

Section 5 X-Ray Examination

第5节 X光检查

Ⅰ. Dialogue 情景对话

Arthritis 关节炎

Patient：Doctor, I have a pain and swelling in my knee.

医生，我的膝关节又肿又疼。

Doctor：When did you first notice it?

什么时候开始觉得疼的？

Patient：About two years ago. At first, the pain occurred only in the mornings right after I woke up, then it gradually eased. But now the pain has become worse and more constant. Sometimes it disturbs my sleep.

大约两年前。起先只有起床时疼，然后慢慢就缓解了，但是现在疼得越来越重，疼的时间也越来越长，有时还影响睡眠。

Doctor：What kind of pain is it?

怎么个疼法？

Patient：Just a dull ache.

隐隐约约地疼。

Doctor：Have you ever had any swelling or pain in your other small joints such as your wrist, fingers, or toes?

其他小关节如腕、指趾关节也疼，也肿吗？

Patient：No.

没有。

Doctor：Is the pain worse when you start to move after resting for a long time?

休息一段时间后，开始活动时疼痛加重吗？

Patient：Yes.

是的。

Doctor：Is it worse when the weather changes?

天气变化时疼得厉害吗？

Patient：Yes. It's worse in cloudy or wet weather.

是的，阴天或潮湿的时候会疼得厉害些。

Doctor：How do you relieve the pain?

你是怎么减轻疼痛的呢？

Patient：If I massage it or put it in hot water, the pain seems to be lessened slightly.

按摩或把关节泡在热水里，疼得就轻些。

Doctor：Did you run any temperature?

你发过烧吗？

Patient：No, never.

没有。

Doctor：Have you lost weight lately?

最近你体重减轻了吗？

Patient：No. Is it serious, doctor?

没有，医生，我的病严重吗？

Doctor：I can't say. We need to make further examinations. The sedimentation rate is normal, the rheumatoid factor is negative, and there is no anemia. The X-ray of your knees shows that the joint space is diminished. Beneath the cartilage there is sclerosis and cysts and the lipping of the margin of the joint. I think you have osteoarthritis.

得做进一步的检查,现在还很难说。你的血沉正常,类风湿因子阴性,没有贫血,X光片显示关节间隙变窄,关节软骨下有硬化和囊性变、膝关节边缘有唇样变,我想你得了骨关节炎。

Patient：What can you do?

那怎么办呢?

Doctor：I'll give you some Chinese traditional medicine pills. Apply a hot water pad over the knees. You can also have short-wave diathermy.

我给你开一点中药丸。你可以在膝关节上做热敷,还可以同时用超短波透热疗法。

Patient：While, my friend suggested I have an operation.

我的朋友建议我做手术。

Doctor：If you do, you would lose the movement of the knee. Total knee replacement has been used recently. If the pain is mild, then the treatment should be conservative. If it gets severe, then we will consider surgery.

如果动手术,你的膝关节就活动不成了。近年来已使用全膝关节置换术了。如果中等程度的疼痛,还是以保守疗法为宜。要是疼痛厉害了,咱们再考虑动手术吧。

Ⅱ. Sentences 替换句型

(1) Come this way to make an X-ray of your chest please. Just like this, press your chest tightly against this board.

做胸透的请这边来。检查时,像这样把胸部紧紧贴在这个板子上。

(2) Take all your jewelries off and undress your coat, bare to your waist please.

请把身上的首饰取下,解开上衣,光着膀子。

(3) Please put this protective cloth on and put your chin on here, just keep relaxed.

穿上防护服,下巴抵住这儿,放松。

(4) Hold your breath please and don't move. OK, now take another breath and move your body as you are told. Lift your right arm.

屏住呼吸,不要动。好的,再吸一口气,按我的指令移动身体。举起右臂。

(5) It doesn't take long. Relax your muscles and keep still. That's it, lower your arms please.

检查很快就完了。放松肌肉,一动都不要动。好的,请放下胳膊吧。

(6) It sounds like a duodenal ulcer, but we have to do some tests, and take an X-ray first before we can be certain.

目前看起来像十二指肠溃疡,不过还需要做一些化验和拍张 X 光片才能确诊。

(7) The chest X-ray suggests the likelihood of tuberculosis.

胸部 X 光片提示可能是肺结核。

(8) Your X-ray and raised blood uric acid level show you have gout.

X 光片和血尿酸浓度升高都证明你得的是痛风。

(9) The X-ray shows a fracture of your left femur.

X 光片显示你左股骨骨折。

(10) Since this is an urgent examination, please take the X-ray film ten minutes later.

因为这是急诊检查,请十分钟后来取 X 光片。

Ⅲ. Words and Expressions 单词和短语

acute endocarditis 急性心内膜炎
aortic insufficiency 主动脉闭合不全
aortic stenosis 主动脉瓣狭窄
chronic endocarditis 慢性心内膜炎
congenital cardiac malformation 先天性心脏病
deep X-ray therapy 深 X 线疗法
dextrocardia /ˌdekstrəʊˈkɑːdiə/ n. 右心病
diseases(troubles) of heart 心脏疾病
dislocation fracture of the spine 脊椎移位骨折
dislocation of the ankle 踝关节脱臼
dislocation of the knee 膝关节脱臼
dorsoventral supine position 仰卧位

endocarditis lenta 迁延性心内膜炎
fibula /ˈfɪbjələ/ n. 腓骨
fluoroscopy /ˌflʊəˈrɒskəpi/ n. 透视
fracture antebrachie 前臂骨折
fracture claviculae 锁骨骨折
fracture /ˈfræktʃə/ n. 骨折
fracture humeri 肱骨骨折
fracture of base of the skull 颅骨骨折
fracture of radius 桡骨骨折
fracture of scapulae 肩胛骨骨折
fracture of the femur 股骨骨折
fracture of the forearm 前臂骨折
fracture of the hand bone 腕骨骨折
fracture of the patella 膝盖骨骨折

fracture of the pelvis 骨盆骨折

fracture of the tibia 胫骨骨折

fracture of the underleg 小腿骨折

fracture of ulna 尺骨骨折

lower limb 下肢

lumbarization /lʌmbəraɪˈzeɪʃən/;
　lumbalization /lʌmbəlaɪˈzeɪʃn/ n.
腰椎化

lumbar vertebra 腰椎

luxation coxae congenital 先天性髋关
节脱臼

luxation /lʌkˈseɪʃən/; dislocation
　/ˌdɪsləˈkeɪʃən/ n. 脱臼

luxation of the coxae 髋关节脱臼

luxation of the elbow 肘关节脱臼

luxation of the finger joint 指关节脱臼

luxation of the hand joint 腕关节脱臼

luxation of the shoulder joint 肩关节脱臼

luxation vertebral; vertebral
dislocation 脊椎脱臼

mitral stenosis 二尖瓣狭窄

myocarditis /ˌmaɪəʊkɑːˈdaɪtɪs/ n. 心肌炎

radiographic appearance X 光像

transillumination /trænziˌluːmɪˈneɪʃən/ n.
　透照试验

ulna /ˈʌlnə/ n. 尺骨

upper limb 上肢

urinary incontinence 小便失禁

valvular disease of the heart 心瓣膜病

vertebral colum 脊柱

visible peristalsis; visible intestinal
　peristalsis 肠型

wrist-drop hand 垂腕手(腕下垂)

wrist /rɪst/ n. 腕关节

X-ray apparatus X 线机

X-ray examination X 线检查

X-ray hurt or burn 放射线灼伤

X-ray photograph X 光拍片

X-ray therapy X 线疗法

Section 6　Fluoroscopy of the Stomach
第 6 节　胃部检查

Ⅰ. Dialogue 情景对话

Peptic-Duodenal Ulcer 胃十二指肠溃疡

Patient：Doctor，my stools have been black for the past two days and I
　　feel weak.
　　医生,我这两天大便发黑而且还感到身体有点虚弱。

Doctor：Have they ever been black before?

你以前有大便发黑的情况吗?

Patient：No. This is the first time.

没有。这是第一次。

Doctor：Have you had any pain?

你还感到别的什么地方疼吗?

Patient：Yes, in my stomach.

是的,胃痛。

Doctor：How long have you had it?

痛了多久了?

Patient：I've had it on and off for the past two years, but it was never as bad as this before.

大概有两年了,时好时坏,不过可从来没有像这次这样疼。

Doctor：When do you feel the pain?

大概什么时候觉得疼呢?

Patient：Just after meals my stomach aches. Sometimes I vomit.

一吃完饭就疼,有时还吐。

Doctor：What kind of pain is it, do you think?

你觉得是怎样的疼呢?

Patient：Like heartburn.

疼得烧心。

Doctor：Does spicy food affect it?

吃辛辣食物你感觉疼痛会加重吗?

Patient：Yes, it's often worse after I eat spicy food or onions.

会的,辛辣食物或洋葱都会使疼痛加剧。

Doctor：Do you have less pain after eating?

吃过东西后,你会感觉疼痛缓和些吗?

Patient：Yes, a little.

会的,稍稍缓和一些。

Doctor：Did you vomit sometimes?

你吐过吗?

Patient：Yes, I did.

吐过。

Doctor：What did you vomit, food or blood?

吐出的是食物还是血呢？

Patient：Food with a little blood.

食物中带有一点血。

Doctor：What was the color of the blood，red or black?

吐的血是鲜红的，还是发黑的？

Patient：Like coffee.

咖啡色的。

Doctor：I'll examine your abdomen. Lie down on your back and loosen your clothes. Please bend your knees. I think we'd better take an X-ray film of your gastrointestinal tract. I think you've got a peptic ulcer (duodenal ulcer). And I'll give you some medicine. Have a good rest at home.

我先给你查一下腹部吧。躺下、解开衣服、屈膝。我想你最好再拍个胃肠 X 光片。你得的像是胃（十二指肠）溃疡。我这就给你开一些药。回家一定好好休息。

Patient：Is there anything else I should do?

还要注意些什么吗？

Doctor：If possible avoid all alcohol. Whenever you have any bleeding，come immediately to the hospital.

如果可能的话，应戒酒。若再有出血，马上到医院来。

Patient：OK，I know，and thank you very much，doctor.

谢谢你，医生，我知道了。

Ⅱ. Sentences 替换句型

(1) It will take twenty minutes to make such an examination. Take all your clothes off and put on the designed colth please. Then change your position as you are told.

检查大概需要二十分钟，请脱下你的衣服换上检查服，然后按照指令变换体位。

(2) Try to take the white liquid. Then we'll give you an injection to stop the movement of your stomach and ease tension during the test.

喝下这种白液体。待会儿我们给你注射一针镇吐剂，检查时你就不会感到难受了。

(3) OK, move slowly and easily, and try every effort not to burp during the examination. It's done soon.

现在轻轻转动身体,尽量不要打嗝。检查马上就完了。

(4) Mmm. Well, it sounds as if she's too ill to have her barium enema performed. We'll leave it for one or two days.

嗯！听起来她的病很重,今天不能进行钡灌肠了,我们再等一两天吧。

(5) On the day of the test, just rinse your mouth. Do remember not to take any food, liquid or medicine. Nor the smoke, either.

检查当天,刷牙漱口、空腹、禁药禁烟。

(6) Before the test, take the medicine when getting on the table. After the test, laxative is given to you immediately. And when you can eat and drink, remember to try to drink plenty of water.

检查前,在检查床上服下钡剂。检查后,立刻服下泻药。等你能进食时,尽量多喝水。

Ⅲ. Words and Expressions 单词和短语

abdominal enlargement；swelling of abdomen 腹胀

abdominal pain；stomachache /'stʌmək‚eɪk/ n. 腹痛

appetite /'æpɪtaɪt/ n. 食欲

bloody stool 血便

boring pain 穿刺痛；钻心状痛

calcareous pancreatitis 结石性胰腺炎

calculus colic 结石绞痛

cancer of the cardia 贲门癌

cancer of the esophagus 食管癌

cancer of the tongue 舌癌

capricious /kə'prɪʃəs/ adj. 多变的；反覆无常的；任性的

carcinoma mamma；carcinoma of the breast 乳腺癌

cardiospasm /'kɑːdɪəʊ‚spæzəm/ n. 贲门痉挛

constipation /‚kɒnstɪ'peɪʃn/ n. 便秘

contrast media 造影剂

crapulent /'kræpjʊlənt/ adj. 暴饮暴食

creatorrhea /‚kriːətə'riːə/ n. 肉质下泻

diarrhea /‚daɪə'rɪə/ n. 腹泻

difficulty in swallowing 吞咽困难

diffuse /dɪ'fjuːs/ adj. 弥漫的

diminished /dɪ'mɪnɪʃt/ adj. 减退；减少

discharge /dɪs'tʃɑːdʒ/ v. & n. 排出

discharge of pus 排脓

drainage gauze 引流线条

drainage tube 引流管

duodenal tube 十二指肠导管

enlargement of liver 肝肿大

epigastric pain 上腹痛

eructation /ˌɪrʌkˈteɪʃən/ *n*. 嗳气

esophagus and stomach 食管及胃

excessive /ɪkˈsesɪv/ *adj*. 亢进

excrement /ˈekskrɪmənt/ *n*. 排泄物

fibrogastroscope *n*. 纤维胃镜

gastric probe 胃探子

gastroscope /ˈɡæstrəskəʊp/ *n*. 胃镜

girdle sensation；zonular pain 带状痛

glycosuria /ˌɡlaɪkəʊˈsjʊərɪə/ *n*. 糖尿

gurgling /ɡɜːˈɡlɪŋ/ *adj*. 咕噜

habitual constipation 习惯性便秘

heartburn /ˈhɑːtˌbɜːn/；pyrosis
   /paɪˈrəʊsɪs/ *n*. 胃灼热；烧心

hunger pain 饥饿痛

intermittent pain 间歇痛

intestine /ɪnˈtestɪn/ *n*. 肠

itch of skin 皮肤痒

jaundice /ˈdʒɔːndɪs/；icterus /ˈɪktərəs/
   n. 黄疸

knock pain 扣痛

lancinating /lightning/ stroke pain 电
   击痛

liver /ˈlɪvə/ *n*. 肝

local /ˈləʊkl/ *adj*. 局部的

loss of appetite 食欲不振

morbid appetite 异味症

mouth pain 口痛

nausea /ˈnɔːsɪə/ *n*. 恶心

neuralgic pain 神经样痛

pain extended to the left arm 绞痛向
   左臂放射

pain in left iliac region 左髂窝痛

pain in region of liver 肝区痛

pain in the ileocecal region 回盲部痛

pain in the right（left） hypochondrium
   右（左）季肋痛

pain upon pressure 压痛

pancreas /ˈpæŋkrɪəs/ *n*. 胰

persistent pain 持续痛

piles /paɪlz/；hemorrhoids
   /ˈheməˌrɔɪdz/ *n*. 痔

polydipsia /ˌpɒlɪˈdɪpsɪə/；excessive
   sense of thirst 烦渴

polyphagia /ˌpɒlɪˈfeɪdʒə/ *n*. 贪食症

pressing feeling 压迫感

proctoscope /ˈprɒktəˌskəʊp/ *n*. 直肠镜

proctoscopy /prɒkˈtɒskəpi/ *n*. 直肠
   镜检查

pus basin 脓盘

retractor /rɪˈtræktə/ *n*. 拉钩；钩子

rumination /ˌruːmɪˈneɪʃən/ *n*. 反刍

salivation /ˌsælɪˈveɪʃn/ *n*. 流涎

sense of discomfort 不快感

sense of fullness 胀满感

slow and steady pain 隐痛

steatorrhea /ˌstɪətəˈriə/ *n*. 脂肪泻

thirst /θɜːst/ *n*. 口渴

thoothache /ˈtuːθeɪk/ *n*. 牙痛

tingle pain；griping pain 刺痛

tumor and（or）pain in the epigastrium
   心窝部肿瘤和（或）疼痛

tumor /ˈtjuːmə/ *n*. 肿瘤

tumour of liver 肝脏肿瘤

vomiting of blood 呕血

Section 7　Pathology
第7节　病理检查

Ⅰ. Dialogue 情景对话

Bladder Cancer 膀胱癌

Patient：What do you think is the matter, doctor?

医生,你说我是什么病啊?

Doctor：It is difficult to say now. Don't worry, Mrs. Smith. In order to clarify the diagnosis, some special tests are necessary. Cystoscopy is the best way I think to establish the diagnosis. Besides, biopsy should provide the microscopic diagnosis.

现在还不好说。别担心,史密斯夫人。为了明确诊断,还需要做一些特殊的检查。我想你最好做个膀胱镜检查,另外还要取活检做显微镜下诊断呢。

Patient：Whatever you say, doctor.

医生,你怎样安排都可以。

Doctor：I've just read the results of your examinations and discussed your case with the urologist, and the best thing for you to do, perhaps would be to come into the hospital for further treatment, Mrs. Smith.

史密斯夫人,我刚看了你的检查结果,也和泌尿外科医生讨论了你的问题。我看你最好能住院做进一步诊治。

Patient：Well… Have you found anything of significance?

怎么,有什么严重问题吗?

Doctor：I'm so sorry, Mrs. Smith. From the history, clinical findings and results of the examination, I believe that you have a bladder cancer.

抱歉,史密斯夫人。根据病史、临床表现以及检查结果,我认为你得了膀胱癌。

Patient：Oh，my God. Is it serious? And what do you advise, doctor?

　　　　哦，天哪！严重吗？医生，你看怎么治好呢？

Doctor：Take it easy，Mrs. Smith. I think you should come into the hospital and receive surgical treatment as soon as possible.

　　　　别担心，史密斯夫人。我认为你需要尽快住院接受手术治疗。

Patient：What kind of operation，I want to know，are you going to perform?

　　　　我想知道你们准备怎么手术？

Doctor：Since the cancer is a superficial small cancer, partial cystectomy or electrodesiccation may be applicable.

　　　　由于肿瘤表浅而小，因此只需进行部分膀胱切除或电灼切除就可以了。

Patient：I'm somewhat worried，doctor. Will it be cured completely?

　　　　我还是有点担心，医生。手术能治愈吗？

Doctor：Don't worry, Mrs. Smith. We'll do our best to cure you，but to tell the truth, the prognosis of bladder cancer depends on the nature and extent of the cancer itself. Generally speaking，when there is no invasion of muscles, the five-year survival rate is 80%. But if with deep invasion of muscles，the chance of five-year survival is much less than ten percent.

　　　　别着急，史密斯夫人。我们会尽最大努力给你治疗的。不过说实话，膀胱癌的预后取决于肿瘤本身的性质和发展程度。如果肿瘤没有浸润到肌肉层，一般而言，五年生存率有80%。而当肌肉深部浸润时，那五年生存率则不到10%。

Patient：I know，doctor. Are there any chemical drugs to treat this cancer?

　　　　我知道了，医生。那么有什么化学药物能治这种肿瘤吗？

Doctor：Yes，madame. But in my opinion，there are no systemic chemotherapeutic agent that warrants recommendation at present. We would like to instill certain medicine into the bladder at weekly intervals for a month or so. It may destroy superficial cancer.

　　　　有的，夫人。不过，依我看，目前还没有针对膀胱癌的全身化疗药物值得推荐。每个星期,我们做局部的化疗,一两个月后,癌细胞基本能杀死。

Patient:Oh, I see. Thanks a lot, doctor.

我明白了,谢谢你了,医生。

Doctor:You are welcome, Mrs. Smith.

不客气,史密斯夫人。

Ⅱ. Sentences 替换句型

(1) Since the diagnosis isn't clear, you'd better have a myelographic examination to rule out tumors.

由于诊断还不清楚,我建议你做一个脊髓造影,这样可以看是不是肿瘤。

(2) In order to be more certain what has happened to him, a lumbar puncture is necessary.

为了更进一步确诊,我们需要做一个腰椎穿刺。

(3) The only way to be certain of breast cancer is to do a biopsy. If she has cancer, she ought to have her breast removed. That's called a radical mastectomy.

乳腺癌确诊的唯一手段是做活检。假如是癌的话,那她就可能摘除乳房。这叫乳瘤根除手术。

(4) I would like to take a smear from your nose and examine it under the microscope.

我想从你的鼻子里取一些黏液做个在显微镜下的涂片检查。

(5) Treatment of children cancers is one of the most remarkable success stories of modern medicine. Although the rate of cancer among children has been rising for more than twenty years, the death rate has plunged.

儿童的癌症治疗是现代医学最显著的成就之一。二十多年来儿童癌症的发病率一直在攀升,而死亡率却在陡降。

(6) Growth hormone deficiency is a frequent complication of chemotherapy and radiation to the central nervous system, and other endocrine problems may include early or late puberty, sterility and thyroid dysfunction.

生长激素缺乏是化疗和放疗对中枢神经系统带来的常见并发症，其他的分泌问题可能会包括青春期的提前和推迟、不育和甲状腺功能障碍。

Ⅲ. Words and Expressions 单词和短语

abduction /æb'dʌkʃən/ *n*. 外展

abscess /'æbses/ *n*. 脓肿

absorption /əb'zɔːpʃən/；sorption /'sɔːpʃən/；resorption /ɪ'sɔːpʃən/ *n*. 吸着；吸收

actinomyces /ˌæktɪnəʊ'maɪsiːz/ *n*. 放线菌

adduction /ə'dʌkʃən/ *n*. 内收

adenopathy /ˌædɪ'nɒpəθi/ *n*. 腺肿大

adhesion /əd'hiːʒən/；synechia /sɪ'nekiə/ *n*. 粘连；粘着

asthenia /æs'θiːniə/ *n*. 无力症

aerobic bacterium 需氧菌

aeroembolism /ˌeərə'embəlɪzəm/ *n*. 气栓

agar-agar 琼脂

agglutination /əˌgluːtɪ'neɪʃən/ *n*. 凝集作用

anaerobic bacillus 厌氧杆菌

anaerobic bacterium 厌氧菌

ankylosis /ˌæŋkɪ'ləʊsɪs/；rigidity /rɪ'dʒɪdɪti/ *n*. 硬化；强直

anorexia /ˌænə'reksiə/ *n*. 无食欲

antiboby /'æntɪˌbɒdi/ *n*. 抗体

antigen /'æntɪdʒən/ *n*. 抗原

antitoxin /ˌæntɪ'tɒksɪn/ *n*. 抗毒素

arsenic /'ɑːsnɪk/；arsenicum /'ɑːsenɪkəm/ *n*. 砷

ascending /ə'sendɪŋ/ *adj*. 升的；上升的

asepsis /ə'sepsɪs/ *n*. 无菌

asphyxia /æs'fɪksiə/ *n*. 窒息

asthenia /æs'θiːniə/；weakness /'wiːknɪs/；debility /dɪ'bɪləti/ *n*. 虚弱

atony /'ætəni/ *n*. 无力

atrichia /'ɑːtrɪkiə/；atrichosis /ɑːtrɪkt'ʃəʊsɪs/ *n*. 无毛症

bacillus anthracis；anthrax bacillus 炭疽杆菌

bacillus coli；escherichia coli 大肠杆菌

bacillus oedematis maligni 恶性水肿杆菌

bacillus influenza hemorrhagic 流感性嗜血杆菌

bacillus leprae；mycobacterium leprae 麻风杆菌

bacillus mallei 鼻疽杆菌

bacillus paratyphosus 副伤寒杆菌

bacillus pertussis 百日咳杆菌

bacillus pestis；pasteurella pestis 鼠疫杆菌

bacillus putrifaction 腐败杆菌

bacillus pyocyaneus 绿脓杆菌

bacillus salmonella 沙门杆菌

bacillus saprophyte 寄生菌

bacillus smegmatis 包皮垢杆菌

bacillus tetani；clostridium tetani 破伤风杆菌

bacillus typhosus；typhoid bacillus 伤寒杆菌

bacillus vibre cholerae 霍乱弧杆菌

bacillus /bəˈsɪləs/; germ /dʒɜːm/ n. 杆菌

bacteric toxin 细菌毒素

bismuth /ˈbɪzməθ/ n. 铋

blastomycosis /ˌblæstəʊmaɪˈkəʊsɪs/ n. 芽生菌病

blindness /ˈblaɪndnɪs/ n. 盲

blood forming organs; hematopoietic organ 造血器官

bloody excrement (stool) 血便

bloody sputum; sputum cruentum 血痰

boric acid 硼酸

cachexia /kəˈkeksɪə/ n. 恶病质

carbonic acid gas 碳酸气

calcification /ˌkælsɪfɪˈkeɪʃən/ n. 钙化

calcinosis /ˌkælsɪˈnəʊsɪs/ n. 钙质沉着症

carrier /ˈkærɪə/ n. 带菌者

cause /kɔːz/ n. 原因

cell division 细胞分裂

cell /sel/ n. 细胞

character /ˈkærɪktə/ n. 性格;特征

choleduchus common bile duct 总胆囊

cicatrix /ˈsɪkətrɪks/; scar /skɑː/ n. 瘢痕

cirrhosis /səˈrəʊsɪs/ n. 萎缩硬化

coccus /ˈkɒkəs/ (pl., cocci /ˈkɒksaɪ/) n. 球菌

collapse /kəˈlæps/; fag /fæg/ n. 虚脱

clot of the blood 血块

coma /ˈkəʊmə/ n. 昏迷

comedo /ˈkɒmɪdəʊ/ n. 粉刺

compensation /ˌkɒmpenˈseɪʃn/ n. 代偿

constipation /ˌkɒnstɪˈpeɪʃn/; obstipation /ˌɒbstɪˈpeɪʃən/ n. 便秘

constriction /kənˈstrɪkʃn/ n. 收缩

continuous fever 持续发烧/热

convalescence /ˌkɒnvəˈlesns/ n.; restoration stage 恢复期

convulsion /kənˈvʌlʃn/ n. 抽搐

corpse /kɔːps/; cadaver /kəˈdævə/ n. 尸体

corrosion /kəˈrəʊʒn/ n. 腐蚀

cortex /ˈkɔːteks/ n. 皮壳

crisis /ˈkraɪsɪs/ n. 危症;危险期

critically ill; dangerously ill 危症

culture fluid 培养液

culture medium 培养基

culture /ˈkʌltʃə/ n. 培养

cyanic acid 氰酸

decompensation /diːˌkɒmpenˈseɪʃən/ n. 代偿破坏

defecation /ˌdefəˈkeɪʃən/; dejection /dɪˈdʒekʃən/ n. 排便

dehydration /ˌdiːhaɪˈdreɪʃən/ n. 脱水

depigmentation /diːˌpɪgmənˈteɪʃən/ n. 脱色素;色素脱出

dermoreaction /dɜːməˌrˈɪækʃn/; cutireaction /kjuːtaɪəˈɪækʃn/ n. 皮肤反应

descending /dɪˈsendɪŋ/ adj. 降的;下降的

development /dɪˈveləpmənt/ n. 发育

diphtheria /dɪfˈθɪərɪə/ n. 白喉

diplococcus /ˌdɪpləʊˈkɒkəs/ n. 双球菌

disease /dɪˈziːz/; sickness /ˈsɪknɪs/; illness /ˈɪlnɪs/ n. 疾病

disinfection /ˌdɪsɪnˈfekʃən/ n. 消毒

dissimilation /dɪˌsɪmɪˈleɪʃən/ n. 异化(作用)

distilled water 蒸馏水

disturbance of compensation 代偿障碍

disturbance /dɪ'stɜːbəns/ *n.* 障碍

division /dɪ'vɪʒən/ *n.* 分裂

dropsy /'drɒpsi/；edema /ɪ'diːmə/ *n.* 水肿

dumb /dʌm/ *adj.* 哑

effusion /ɪ'fjuːʒən/；exudate /'eksjʊdeɪt/ *n.* 渗出

electricity /ɪˌlek'trɪsəti/ *n.* 电力

embolus /'embələs/ *n.* 栓子

enamel of the teeth 牙珐琅质

enterococcus /ˌentərəʊ'kɒkəs/ *n.* 肠球菌

environment /ɪn'vaɪrənmənt/；milieu /'miːljɜː/ *n.* 环境

etiology /ˌiːti'ɒlədʒi/ *n.* 病因学

exfoliation /eksˌfəʊlɪ'eɪʃən/ *n.* 脱落

external cause 外因

exudative /ɪg'zjuːdətɪv/ *adj.* 渗出的

favourable /'feɪvərəbl/ *adj.* 良好的

feeble-minded *adj.* 低能的

felon /'felən/；whitlow /'wɪtləʊ/ *n.* 瘭疽

fibrillation /ˌfɪbrɪ'leɪʃən/ *n.* 纤维震颤

fit /fɪt/；seizure /'siːʒə/；attack /ə'tæk/；stroke /strəʊk/；paroxysm /'pærəkˌsɪzəm/；episode /'epɪˌsəʊd/ *n.* 发作

flask /flɑːsk/ *n.* 长颈瓶

foreign body 异物

freezing /'friːzɪŋ/ *adj.* 冻死的

friction /'frɪkʃən/ *n.* 擦

full-positive location 好发部位

gangrene /'gæŋgriːn/ *n.* 坏疽

glomerulus /glɒ'merʊləs/ *n.* 肾小球

glucose /'gluːkəʊs/ *n.* 葡萄糖

gonococcus /ˌgɒnəʊ'kɒkəs/ *n.* 淋病双球菌

granulation tissue 肉芽组织

granule /'grænjuːl/；granulation /ˌgrænjʊ'leɪʃən/ *n.* 肉芽

grey matter 灰质

growth /grəʊθ/ *n.* 生长

hay bacillus；bacillus subtilis 枯草杆菌

hemolysin /hiːmə'laɪsən/ *n.* 溶血素

hemolysis /hiː'mɒlɪsɪs/ *n.* 溶血

hemolytic streptococcus 溶血性链球菌

hemolytic /ˌhiːməʊ'lɪtɪk/ *n.* 溶血的

hemorrhage /'hemərɪdʒ/；bleeding /'bliːdɪŋ/ *n.* 出血

hunger /'hʌŋgə/；starvation /staː'veɪʃən/ *n.* 饥饿

hydrochloric acid；muriatic acid 盐酸

hydrops /'haɪdrɒps/ *n.* 震荡前水肿；积水

hyperemia /ˌhaɪpə'riːmɪə/ *n.* 充血

hyperglycemia /ˌhaɪpəglaɪ'siːmiə/ *n.* 高血糖症

hypertension and hypotension 高和低血压

hypertrophy /haɪ'pɜːtrəfi/ *n.* 肥大

hyphomycetes /haɪfəmɪ'sets/ *n.* 丝状菌类

hypoglycemia /ˌhaɪpəʊglaɪ'siːmiə/ *n.* 低血糖症

hypoplasia /ˌhaɪpəʊ'pleɪziə/ *n.* 发育不全

imbecile /'ɪmbəsiːl/ *n.* 愚痴

implantation /ˌɪmplɑːn'teɪʃən/；transplantation /'trænsplɑːn'teɪʃən/ *n.* 移植

inanition /ˌɪnə'nɪʃən/ *n.* 饥饿衰弱

induration /ˌɪndjʊ'reɪʃən/ *n.* 硬结作用

infarction /ɪn'fɑːkʃən/ *n.* 梗死作用

infarct /ɪn'fɑːkt/ *n.* 梗死（心肌）

infection /ɪnˈfekʃən/ n. 感染

infiltration /ˌɪnfɪlˈtreɪʃən/ n. 浸润

inflammation /ˌɪnfləˈmeɪʃən/ n. 炎症

injury /ˈɪndʒəri/ n. 损劳

inquest /ˈɪnkwest/ n.；postmortem examination 尸检

insomnia /ɪnˈsɒmnɪə/；agrypnia /əˈgrɪpnɪə/；sleeplessness /ˈsliːplɪsnɪs/ n. 失眠

inspiration /ˌɪnspəˈreɪʃən/ n. 吸入

intelligence /ɪnˈtelɪdʒəns/ n. 天才；智力

internal cause 内因

interstitial /ˌɪntəˈstɪʃəl/ adj. 间质性的

interstitium /ɪntəsˈtɪʃəm/ n. 间质

invagination /ɪnˌvædʒɪˈneɪʃən/ n. 重叠

iodine /ˈaɪəˌdiːn/ n. 碘

keloid /ˈkiːlɔɪd/ n. 瘢痕疙瘩

lack of water 失水

latent period；period of incubation 潜伏期

leishmania dounovanic 黑热病原体

lime /laɪm/ n.；calcium oxide 石灰

lipid /ˈlaɪpɪd/；lipoid /ˈlaɪpɔɪd/ n. 脂质

loss of blood 失血

maceration /ˌmæsəˈreɪʃən/ n. 软化

malacia /məˈleɪʃɪə/ n. 软化

mania /ˈmeɪnɪə/ n. 狂躁

membrane /ˈmembreɪn/；tunic /ˈtjuːnɪk/ n. 膜

memory /ˈmeməri/ n. 记忆

meningococcus /meˌnɪŋɡəʊˈkɒkəs/ n. 脑膜炎球菌

mental alienation；alienation /ˌeɪlɪəˈneɪʃən/ n. 精神错乱

mental deficiency 智力缺陷

mental insanity 精神异常

mercuric cyanide 氰化汞

mercury /ˈmɜːkjʊri/；quicksilver /ˈkwɪkˌsɪlvə/ n. 水银

metamorphosis /ˌmetəˈmɔːfəsɪs/ n. 变形

metastasis /mɪˈtæstəsɪs/；transfer /ˈtrænsfɜː/；abevacuation /əbevækjˈʊeɪʃn/ n. 转移

microbe /ˈmaɪkrəʊb/ n. 细菌；微生物

microbian /maɪˈkrəʊbɪən/ n.；microorganism /ˌmaɪkrəʊˈɔːɡəˌnɪzəm/ n.；microbe derivative 微生物

micrococcus catarrhal 气放杆菌

micrococcus tetragenus 四叠球菌

mixed infection 混合感染

mixed swelling 混合肿胀

mongolism /ˈmɒŋɡəˌlɪzəm/ n. 唐氏综合征

morbid /ˈmɔːbɪd/；pathological /ˌpæθəˈlɒdʒɪkəl/ adj. 病的

mortality /mɔːˈtælɪti/ n.；death rate 死亡率

mucous /ˈmjuːkəs/ adj. 黏液的

mycobacterium tuberculosis 结核杆菌

myxomycete /ˌmɪksəʊmaɪˈsiːt/ n. 黏液菌类

name of disease 病名

necrosis /neˈkrəʊsɪs/ n. 坏死

neoplasm /ˈniːəʊplæzəm/ n. 新生物

nocturia /nɒktˈjʊərɪə/ n. 夜尿

nucleus /ˈnjuːklɪəs/ n. 核

obesity /əʊˈbiːsəti/ n. 肥胖

objective finding 他觉所见

objective/subjective symptom 他觉/

自觉症状

occlusion /ə'kluːʒən/；obstruction /əb'strʌkʃən/ n. 堵塞

oil-emersion 镜油（显微镜用）

osmosis /ɒz'məusɪs/ n. 渗透

osmotic pressure 渗透压

overfatigue /'əuvəfə'tiːg/ n. 过度疲劳

paleness /'peɪlnɪs/ n. 苍白

perionyxis /piəriː'əunɪksɪs/ n. 甲周炎

phagocytosis /ˌfægəsaɪ'təusɪs/ n. 吞噬作用

phenol /'fiːnɒl/ n.；carbolic acid；hydroxybenzene /'haɪdrɒksɪbenziːn/ n. 石炭酸；酚

plasmodium /plæz'məudiəm/ n. 疟原虫

pneumococcus /ˌnjuːmə'kɒkəs/ n. 肺炎球菌

poisoning /'pɔɪzənɪŋ/；intoxication /ɪnˌtɒksɪʃɪŋ/ n. 中毒

polyphagia /ˌpɒlɪ'feɪdʒə/；akoria /eɪ'kɔːriə/ n. 贪食

predisposing cause 诱因

primary /'praɪməri/ adj. 初发的

process /'prəuses/；course /kɔːs/ n. 过程

prodrome /'prəudrəum/ n. 前驱症状；先兆

prognosis /prɒg'nəusɪs/ n. 预后

progressive /prə'gresɪv/ adj. 进行性的

ptomaine poisoning n. 尸碱中毒

purulent /'pjuərələnt/；suppurative /'sʌpjuərətɪv/ adj. 脓性的

pus /pʌs/ n. 脓

putrefaction /ˌpjuːtrɪ'fækʃən/ putridity /ˌpjuː'trɪdəti/ n. 腐败

quarantine /'kwɒrənˌtiːn/ n. 检疫

reagent /rɪ'eɪdʒənt/ n. 反应剂；试剂

recovery /rɪ'kʌvəri/ n. 康复

reinfection /ˌriːɪn'fekʃən/ n. 再感染

relapse /rɪ'læps/；recurrence /rɪ'kʌrəns/ n. 复发

relaxation /ˌriːlæk'seɪʃən/ n. 放松

remission /rɪ'mɪʃən/ n. 恢复；缓解

retention of urine 尿潴留

rupture /'rʌptʃə/ v. & n. 破裂

sarcina /saː'siːnə/ n. 八叠球菌

scab /skæb/；slough /slʌf/ n. 痂

scald /skɔːld/ n. 烫伤

scleroma cutis；scleroderma /ˌsklɪərəu'dɜːmə/ n. 硬皮病

sclerosis /sklɪə'rəusɪs/ n. 硬化

secretion /sɪ'kriːʃən/ n. 分泌

secretory /sɪ'kriːtəri/ adj. 分泌的

segmentation /ˌsegmen'teɪʃən/ n. 分节

sensibility /ˌsensə'bɪləti/ n. 敏感性

sequestrum /sɪ'kwestrəm/ n. 死骨片

serous /'sɪərəs/ adj. 浆液性的

Shigella shigae 志贺痢疾杆菌

solution /sə'luːʃən/；liquor /'lɪkə/ n. 溶液

somnambulism /sɒm'næmbjuˌlɪzəm/；sleepwalking /'sliːpˌwɔːkɪŋ/；noctambulation /nɒkˌtæmbju'leɪʃən/ n. 梦游症

spasm /'spæzəm/ n. 痉挛

specificity /ˌspesɪ'fɪsəti/ n. 特异性

spirochaeta icterohemorrhagica；leptospira icterohaemorrhagial 溶血性黄疸螺旋体

spirochaeta morsur muris 鼠咬热螺旋体

spirochaeta pallida 梅毒螺旋体

Borrelia vincenti 奋森氏螺旋体

spirochaeta /ˌspaɪrəʊˈkiːtə/ n. 螺旋体

spontaneous/natural death 自然死亡

staphylococcus /ˌstæfɪləˈkɒkəs/ n. 葡萄球菌

sterilization /ˌsterəlaɪˈzeɪʃən/ n. 杀菌

sterilize /ˈsterəlaɪz/ v. 灭菌

stimulation /ˌstɪmjʊˈleɪʃən/ n. 刺激

strangulation /ˈstræŋɡjʊˈleɪʃən/ n. 绞窄

streptococcus /ˌstreptəˈkɒkəs/ n. 链球菌

stripping /ˈstrɪpɪŋ/；denudation /ˌdenjʊˈdeɪʃən/；ablation /æbˈleɪʃən/；desquamation /ˌdeskwəˈmeɪʃən/ n. 剥脱

stupidity /stjuːˈpɪdəti/ n. 笨蛋；痴钝

sudden death 突然死亡

suppurant /ˈsʌpjʊərənt/ n. 化脓剂

suppurate /ˈsʌpjʊˌreɪt/ v. 化脓

suppuration /ˌsʌpjʊˈreɪʃən/ n. 化脓

surfeit /ˈsɜːfɪt/ n. 伤食

swelling /ˈswelɪŋ/ n. 肿胀

symptom /ˈsɪmptəm/ n. 症状

syncope /ˈsɪŋkəpi/ n. 晕厥

synthesis /ˈsɪnθəsɪs/ n. 合成作用

terminal stadium 终期

test tube 试管

thrombus /ˈθrɒmbəs/ n. 血栓

tinction /ˈtɪŋkʃən/ n. 染色

tincture /ˈtɪŋktʃə/ n. 酊

tinea alba 白癣菌

tissue /ˈtɪʃuː/ n. 组织

tremor /ˈtremə/ n. & v. 震颤；抖

trypanosoma gambiense 冈比亚锥虫

unconsciousness /ʌnˈkɒnʃəsnɪs/ n. 昏迷

unrest /ʌnˈrest/；instability /ˌɪnstəˈbɪləti/ n. 不安；兴奋

urea /jʊˈriːə/ n. 尿素

uric acid 尿酸

vaccination /ˌvæksɪˈneɪʃən/ n. 接种疫苗

vaccine /ˈvæksiːn/ n. 疫苗

valve /vælv/ n. 瓣

vibration /vaɪˈbreɪʃən/ n. 振动

violent/exogenic death 外因死亡

virulence /ˈvɪrjʊləns/；venom /ˈvenəm/ n. 毒性

virus filterableness 病毒滤过性

water solubility n. 水溶性

widal reaction 肥达反应

Chapter 5　Prescriptions and at the Official Remedy

第5章　处方与指导用药

Section 1　Symptoms

第1节　症状

I. Dialogue 情景对话

A Threatening Miscarriage 先兆流产

Patient：Doctor，I have had some vaginal bleeding for two or three days，and I feel some pain in the lower abdomen.

医生，我下腹疼痛并伴有阴道出血已经两三天了。

Doctor：When was your last period?

你末次月经是什么时间?

Patient：I missed three periods. This is my pregnancy test report.

我已经三个月没来月经了。这是我的妊娠化验单。

Doctor：Oh，it's uric positive. Point directly at where the pain is and tell me what it is like.

噢，尿检阳性。让我看看你什么地方疼，怎么个疼法呢?

Patient：The pain occurs in the central part of the lower abdomen. It comes in attacks accompanied with vaginal bleeding while the pain lasts.

下腹正中间，一阵一阵地疼，疼的时候阴道就出血。

Doctor：These are the signs of abortion. You'd better stay in bed except for eating or going to the toilet. And go to the emergency clinic immediately whenever the bleeding becomes more severe than usual.

这是先兆流产的迹象。除去吃饭和上厕所的时间,你最好卧床休息了。如果出血量增多,立即要看急诊了。

Patient：Oh，no，doctor. The bleeding seems much more and more now，and the attacks of pain reoccur further and further.

哎呀,不好,医生。现在出血好像越来越多了,我觉得疼得越来越厉害。

Doctor：Let me make a check-up. I'm so sorry, madame. The cervix is already open about three centimeters，and part of the fetus can be seen in the cervix. We will prepare the blood for you in case a blood transfusion is needed. Inform your husband that you should be admitted to the hospital at once.

那让我给你检查一下吧。不好,夫人,你已经流产了,子宫口已经开了三厘米宽,宫口可见部分胚胎组织。我们要备些血液以备必要时输用,通知你丈夫你需要马上住院接受治疗。

Ⅱ. Sentences 替换句型

（1）I have a buzzing noise in my head.
　　我感到耳鸣,好像头内有一种嗡嗡的声音。

（2）One of the symptoms of duodenal ulcer is the regurgitation of mouthfuls of scalding, very acid fluid when the pain is at its height.
　　十二指肠溃疡的症状之一是当极度疼痛时,就会有反酸(即少量的、烧灼性酸液体反流)。

（3）Seldom are there any diagnostic signs of duodenal ulcer.
　　十二指肠溃疡经常不带有任何诊断体征。

（4）I've felt dizzy for over a week. I'd better have my blood pressure checked.
　　我感到头晕已经一周多了,最好量一下血压。

（5）When did you have your last dizzy spell?
　　你最近的一次眩晕发作是什么时候?

(6) He might collapse.

他可能会虚脱。

(7) I've had a pain in my chest. When I breathed or bent down I got a pain but my doctor said I had sprained the muscle.

我一直感觉胸痛。当呼吸或弯腰时就会感到疼痛，但我的医生说我是扭伤了肌肉。

(8) He is not so feverish as he was an hour ago.

他不像一小时前那样发烧了。

(9) How long has your hair been falling out?

你头发脱落已经多久了？

(10) An individual's temperature, pulse, respiration and blood pressure are called vital signs, which are measured to detect any changes in normal function and can be also used to determine a patient's response to treatment. In reality, life-threatening situation can be easily recognized from the vital predictors.

一个人的体温、脉搏、呼吸和血压叫作生命体征。通过对生命体征的测量，可以检测出人体正常生理功能的变化，也可以依此来判断病人对治疗的反应。实际上，那些危及生命的病情都是从生命体征上表现出来的。

(11) Physical examination on admission. Body temperature 39.8℃. She was found to be slightly dyspneal. The right lower posterior chest showed dullness on percussion with moist rales at the end of inspiration on auscultation. The X-ray films of the chest showed cloudy patches over the right lower lung field in the posterior-anterior view and over the postero-basal segment of the right lower lobe and the right middle lobe in the lateral view. The white blood cell count was 15,000 per cu mm with a 83% of polymorphonuclear neutrophils in the differential count. The clinical diagnosis was acute pneumonia involving the right middle and lower lobes.

入院查体：体温 39.8℃。轻度呼吸困难。右后下胸部叩诊有浊音，听诊有湿性啰音。X 光胸部正位片可见右下肺叶有斑片状模糊阴影，侧位片可见右下叶后基底段和中叶有斑片状模糊阴影。血白细胞计数为 15,000/立方毫米，其中中性分叶核细胞占 83%。临床诊断为右中、下叶急性肺炎。

(12) On admission her body temperature was 38. 4℃, and her blood pressure 100/60 mmHg (13. 3/8. 0 kPa). Physical examination found no special abnormalities. Laboratory exmination showed white blood cell counts varied from 21,000 to 14,000/cu mm with 90% neutrophils. The X-ray film of the chest showed increased lung markings with a patch of hazy shadow in the left lower lung near the heart border. The heart appeared to be of aortic type with a tortuous and prolonged aorta. Culture of the sputum showed growth of streptococcus pneumonia. Routine urinalysis and tests of the liver and kidney functions showed normal findings.

病人入院时体温 38. 4℃,血压 100/60 毫米汞柱(13. 3/8. 0 千帕)。体格检查无特殊异常发现。化验血白细胞 21,000—14,000/立方毫米,中性白细胞 90%。胸部 X 光片显示肺纹理增厚,左下肺心缘亦可见片状模糊阴影。心脏呈主动脉型,主动脉曲屈延长。痰培养肺炎双球菌生长。尿常规,肝功能、肾功能等检查正常。

(13) Mentally clear with distressing facial expression. Blood pressure 140/90 mmHg (18. 7/12. 0 kPa). Pulse rate 84/min. Body temperature 38. 5℃. The sclera was not icteric. The heart and lungs were normal. The abdomen was flat with marked tenderness over the right upper quadrant, where muscular spasm and rebound tenderness were present. The liver was enlarged with its lower edge 2 cm below the right costal margin. The spleen was not felt. The peristaltic sound was normal.

神志清,痛苦病容。血压 140/90 毫米汞柱(18. 7/12. 0 千帕)。脉率每分钟 84 次。体温 38.5℃。巩膜无黄染。心肺正常。腹平坦,右上腹有明显压疼伴有肌紧张及反跳疼。肝下缘在右肋缘下 2 厘米可触及。脾未触及。肠鸣音正常。

(14) Laboratory examination showed that hemoglobin 16. 0 gm%. White blood cell count 10,800/cu mm with a differential count of 82% polymorphonuclear neutrophils, 16% lymphocytes and 2% monocytes. Bleeding time 1 min 30 sec. Coagulation time 30 sec. Routine examination of the urine was normal. Serum amylase 86 unit%. Blood bilirubin 1. 3 mg% with direct portion of 0. 5 mg%.

SGPT, TTT and TFT were all normal. BUN 12.2 mg%. CO_2 combining power 55 vol%. The blood group was AB and Rh factor negative.

实验室检查：血红蛋白 16.0 克%。血白细胞计数 10,800/立方毫米，中性多核白细胞 82%，淋巴细胞 16%，单核细胞 2%。出血时间 1 分 30 秒，凝血时间 30 秒。尿常规检查正常。血清淀粉酶 86 单位%。血胆红素总量 1.3 毫克%，直接 0.5 毫克%。血清谷丙转氨酶、麝香草酚浊度试验及麝香草酚絮状反应皆正常。血尿素氮 12.2 毫克%。血二氧化碳结合力 55 容积%。血型为 AB 型，血 Rh 因子阴性。

(15) The present health condition of the patient appears much better than three years ago. The intervals of remission between asthmatic attacks were getting longer, while the attacks became less severe than before as well. He is developing fairly well both physically and mentally.

目前患者病情较之三年前有明显改善。哮喘发作间歇也比以前有明显延长，发作程度有较大减轻，智力体力水平均表现良好。

Ⅲ. Words and Expressions 单词和短语

accident /ˈæksɪdənt/ n. 意外事故

air sickness 晕飞机

anemia /əˈniːmiə/ n. 贫血

anhidrosis /ˌænhɪˈdrəʊsɪs/ n. 无汗症

aphonia /əˈfəʊnɪə/ n. 失音症

attack of cough 咳嗽发作

barking cough 犬吠样咳

bite and sting 咬伤及刺伤；叮咬

blood /blʌd/ n. 血液

car sickness 晕车

chill /tʃɪl/；rigor /ˈrɪɡə/；chillness /ˈtʃɪlnɪs/ n. 寒战

circulatory system 循环系统

clearing throat 清嗓样咳

clubbing of fingers and toes 鼓槌指和趾

cold sweating 冷汗

cough with congestion 脸红咳或胀咳

cough with whoop 吼咳

cripple /ˈkrɪpl/；deformation /ˌdiːfɔːˈmeɪʃən/ n. 畸形

croupy cough 格鲁布咳

cyanosis /ˌsaɪəˈnəʊsɪs/ n. 发绀

deafness /ˈdefnəs/ n. 听不清；聋

difficulty in chewing 咀嚼困难

disturbance of consciousness 意志障碍

disturbance of development 发育障碍

dog bites 犬咬伤

dropsy /ˈdrɒpsi/ n. 积水

drowning /ˈdraʊnɪŋ/ n. 溺死

drug addiction 中毒成瘾;吸毒

dry cough 干咳

dysphonia /dɪsˈfəʊnɪə/ n. 发音困难

dyspnea /dɪspˈniːə/ n. 呼吸困难

earache /ˈɪərˌeɪk/; otalgia /əʊˈtældʒɪə/ n. 耳痛

edema /ɪˈdiːmə/ n. 浮肿

emaciation /ɪˌmeɪsɪˈeɪʃən/ n. 消瘦

epistaxis /ˌepɪˈstæksɪs/; rhinorrhagia /ˌraɪnəʊˈreɪdʒɪə/; nosebleed /ˈnəʊzˌbliːd/ 鼻出血

exanthema /ˌeksænˈθiːmə/; eruption /ɪˈrʌpʃən/ n. 发疹

explosive cough 痉挛咳

fatigue /fəˈtiːg/ n. 倦怠;疲劳

fish bites 鱼类咬伤

flea /fliː/ n. 跳蚤

headache /ˈhedeɪk/ n. 头痛

heat stroke 中暑

hemoptysis /hɪˈmɒptɪsɪs/ n.; blood spitting 咯血

hemorrhagic diathesis 出血性体质

herpes /ˈhɜːpiːz/ n. 疱疹

hoarseness /ˈhɔːsnɪs/ n. 嘶哑

husky /ˈhʌski/ adj. 沙哑的

hyperhidrosis /ˌhaɪpəhɪˈdrəʊsɪs/ n. 多汗症

increased sweating 发汗亢进

insect bites 昆虫咬伤

lethargy /ˈleθədʒi/; somnolence /ˈsɒmnələns/ n. 嗜睡状态

marasmus /məˈræzməs/; debility /dɪˈbɪləti/ n. 衰弱;消瘦

mis-swallowing 误咽

moist cough 湿咳

mosquito /məˈskiːtəʊ/ n. 蚊

motion sickness 晕动病

nasal obstruction 鼻塞

night sweating 盗汗

pain in the chest 胸痛

pain in the extremities 四肢痛

pain in the joint 关节痛

pain in the side 肋间痛

pain in the throat 喉痛

pain upon swallowing 吞咽痛

pallor of face 面色苍白

palpitation /ˌpælpɪˈteɪʃn/ n. 心慌

paralysis /pəˈræləsɪs/ n. 麻痹

paroxysmal cough 阵咳

pericardial oppression 心前区压抑

pericardial pain 心前区痛

poisoning /ˈpɔɪzənɪŋ/ n. 中毒

rapid breathing 气急

rhinolalia /ˌraɪnəʊˈleɪlɪə/ n. 鼻音

rhinorrhoea /ˌraɪnəˈriːə/ n. nasal secretion/discharge 鼻涕

sea sickness 晕船

shivering /ˈʃɪvərɪŋ/ n. 颤抖

singultus /sɪŋˈgʌltəs/; hiccup /ˈhɪkʌp/; hiccough /ˈhɪkʌp/ n. 呃逆;打嗝

sneeze /sniːz/ n. 喷嚏

snore /snɔː/ n. 鼾症

splenic enlargement 脾肿大

sputum /ˈspjuːtəm/ n. 痰

stiffness in the shoulder 肩凝

stridulous /ˈstrɪdjʊləs/ adj. 喘鸣的

sweating /ˈswetɪŋ/; perspiration

/ˌpɜːspəˈreɪʃən/ *n.* 发汗
swelling of cheek 颊部肿胀
swelling of lymph nodes 淋巴结肿大
traumatic injury 外伤

trismus /ˈtrɪzməs/ *n.* ；lock jaw 牙关紧闭
under weight 体重不足
weight loss 体重下降
wheeze /wiːz/ ；stridor /ˈstraɪdɔː/ *n.* 喘鸣

Section 2   Cases
第2节   病例

Ⅰ. Dialogue 情景对话

Allergy Test 过敏试验（皮试）

Doctor：Mr. Smith, you've got pneumonia, and I'll give you some penicillin injections. Firstly, a penicillin allergy test will be done to see if you are allergic to it, so I want to know if you have used penicillin before.
史密斯先生，你得了肺炎，需要注射青霉素，但是必须先做个过敏试验，你以前打过青霉素吗？

Patient：Yes, I have used it before, I'm sure I am not allergic to it, never.
打过，我敢肯定我绝不会过敏的。

Doctor：Oh, don't be so nervous with it. Is there anybody in your family allergic to it or are you allergic to any other drugs?
别紧张，你家人有青霉素过敏的吗？你对其他什么药物过敏吗？

Patient：No, no.
没有。也没什么过敏的。

Doctor：OK, it doesn't hurt anymore, just stretch out your right hand to me. Afterwards, within twenty minutes, if you feel any discomforts, such as dizziness, sweating or chest pain, let me know immediately.
好的。也不怎么疼，把右手伸过来吧。之后，在二十分钟内，如果你感到任何不适,如头晕、出汗或胸痛,请立即告诉我。

Patient：All right. Thank you.

　　那好吧。谢谢。

Doctor：Look，Mr. Smith. There is no red or swelling，which shows you are not allergic to penicillin. Please untie your belt and pull your trousers lower，then I'll give you an injection.

　　看看,史密斯先生,没有红肿,这说明你不过敏。来吧,解开皮带,把裤子拉低一点,准备打针吧。

Patient：Please be somewhat tender.

　　轻点好吗?

Doctor：I'll. Take it easy，Mr. Smith. Bend one of your legs and relax your muscles. Now do you feel any pain where I press?

　　我会的。别紧张,史密斯先生。你一条腿稍微弯曲一下,肌肉放松。好的,我手压着的地方疼吗?

Patient：A little.

　　有一点点疼。

Ⅱ. Sentences 替换句型

(1) Constant clearing of the throat may result in the development of a contact ulcer.

不断清洁咽喉可能引起接触性溃疡。

(2) Chest pain is the commonest warning sign of impending acute myocardial infarction.

胸痛是急性心肌梗死前最常见的先兆体征。

(3) When patients are in bed for any length of time, pressure sores are apt to develop.

当病人长期卧床时,易发生褥疮。

(4) Few doctors are willing to be involved in euthanasia.

没有几个医生愿意卷入安乐死事件中。

(5) The smear did not show any bacteria.

涂片没有检出任何细菌。

(6) He has suffered from arthritis for years. Can you give me some advice, please?

他已经患关节炎多年了。请你给我一些建议吧？

（7）Sometimes I have diarrhea and sometimes I'm constipated and I'm tired of all this trouble.

我有时候腹泻，有时候又便秘，我很讨厌这些毛病。

（8）The patient underwent closed mitral valvotomy last year.

病人去年做了闭式二尖瓣瓣膜切开术。

（9）The patient started to have a headache and earache, associated with some vomiting.

病人开始头痛、耳痛，并伴有呕吐。

（10）Over the past two weeks he had begun to vomit but on no occasion had he brought up any blood.

两周前他就已经开始呕吐，但是从没有呕血。

（11）Never had I seen such appalling bedsores.

我从来没有见过这么严重的褥疮。

（12）Not only does the community care too little about these elderly patients, even their relations pay little attention to them.

对于这些老年病人，不仅社会关心太少，甚至他们的家属也很少在意。

（13）The obese man lost weight by dieting and exercising.

这个肥胖的男士通过节食和锻炼来减肥。

（14）Her pulse was very rapid, she was feverish and when I asked her to go to the bathroom, she was too weak to stand up.

她的脉搏很快而且发烧，我喊她去盥洗室的时候，她太虚弱了，站不起来。

（15）We are going to place an intravenous catheter in your neck vein to check the blood volume of the heart. Don't worry, there is no danger. Please turn your head to the right, if you get ready we will sterilize the skin with some tincture.

我们准备在你的颈静脉插入一根静脉导管，来查一下你心脏的血容量。别担心，操作不会有危险的。把头侧转向右边，你如果准备好了，我们就开始用碘酒进行皮肤消毒了。

（16）A 32-year-old lady was admitted to this hospital on July 12, 2006 because of fever and cough of three days' duration.

32岁女病人因发热、咳嗽三天于2006年7月12日住进医院。

(17) A 70-year-old lady was hospitalized in this hospital from March 20 to 26, 2006 because of having coughed for four days with rusted sputum on top of chills and fever of one day's duration.

70 岁女病人因咳嗽四天,发冷发烧伴铁锈色痰一天,于 2006 年 3 月 20 日至 26 日住院诊治。

(18) A 42-year-old male patient was admitted on July 20, 2005 through our emergency clinic because of right upper abdominal pain for 18 hours' duration. He started to have the pain on July 19, soon after his supper. The pain was persistent in nature, gradually increased in severity and radiated to the right scapular region. He vomitted once. No fever was noticed. He had had several similar attacks in the past.

42 岁男性患者于 2005 年 7 月 20 日因右上腹疼 18 小时急诊入院。患者于 7 月 19 日晚饭后即感上腹疼,疼呈持续性并逐渐加重,向右肩胛部放射。呕吐一次。不觉发热。以往有数次类似发作。

(19) Patient's ECG was normal. Ultrasonic examination shows that fluid waves of the gall bladder (at the depth of 3.0-4.5 cm) can be seen under the right costal margin along the midclavicular line, indicating enlargement of the gall bladder. Fluoroscopy of the chest showed normal heart and lung. A plain film of the abdomen revealed nothing remarkable.

病人心电图正常。超声波检查显示右肋缘下近锁骨中线可见胆囊内液平面波深约 3.0-4.5 厘米,提示胆囊有增大。胸部透视心肺正常。X 光腹部平片未见异常。

(20) A patient has been suffering from repeated asthmatic attacks for more than five years. He attended our out-patient clinic in June 2004, complaining of paroxysmal cough and asthma for more than two years. His asthmatic episodes were usually accompanied with symptoms of sneezing and running nose with watery discharge. A clinical diagnosis of bronchial asthma and allergic rhinitis was made. He received a series of specific skin tests for allergy in October. 2004. They showed evidence of positive reaction to house dust, linen fibers, palm fibers, silk, straw, mixed animal hair, polyvalent moulds, mixed early spring pollens, mixed late spring

pollens, and pollens of artemisia (a kind of Chinese weed). A series of specific desensitization treatments for six courses were given from October 2004 to May 2005. There was remarkable improvement in the early stage of desensitization, but it failed to improve further in the later courses of treatment. In the past three years, salbutamol spray, sodium cromoglicate and becotide inhalation were given with appropriate choice. Some Chinese traditional medicines were also used on certain occasions. Some temporary relief was obtained with almost all such treatments, and asthmatic attacks still took place oftentimes as a result of catching cold.

患者发作性哮喘五年有余,曾于 2004 年 6 月门诊就医,主诉阵发性咳嗽哮喘并伴有喷嚏、清水鼻涕二年多。临床诊断为支气管哮喘和过敏性鼻炎。2004 年 10 月的特异性皮肤试验发现患者对屋尘、麻、棕、丝、稻草、混合兽毛、多价霉菌、早晚春花粉及中国特有的艾蒿花粉等有阳性反应。从 2004 年 10 月到 2005 年 5 月,患者曾先后做过六个疗程的脱敏治疗,治疗后期病情改善没有初期效果明显。近三年药物先后用过舒喘宁气雾剂、色甘酸钠及丙酸倍氯米松气雾吸入,也接受过中医治疗。几乎所有这些治疗都能暂时缓解病情,目前病情发作常由着凉感冒引起。

Ⅲ. Words and Expressions 单词和短语

abdomen breathing 腹式呼吸

accentuated /æk'sentʃuˌeɪtɪd / *adj*. 亢进

active dorsal back decubitus 活动性背部褥疮

angina pectoris 心绞痛

apex beat 心尖搏动

aphasia /ə'feɪzɪə/ *n*. 失语(症)

aphonia /ə'fəʊnɪə/ *n*. 失音(症)

aphtha on the palate 腭部鹅口疮

ataxic (stamping) gait 失调性步态

barrel shaped thorax 桶状胸

base of the skull 颅底

brachycardia /bræ'kɪkɑːdɪə/ *n*.; slow pulse 脉缓(心率过缓)

buccal mucous 口腔黏膜

build /bɪld/; physique /fi'ziːk/ *n*. 体格

bulla /'bʊlə/ *n*. 大水疱

calf muscle 腓肠肌

canine /'keɪnaɪn/ *n*. 犬齿

cerebellar gait 小脑性步态

cervical lymph gland 颈淋巴结

Cheyne-Stokes breathing 陈-施呼吸

clavicle /ˈklævɪkl/ *n.* 锁骨

clear /klɪə/ *adj.* 清

clear mental state 清醒神志状态

cleft palate 腭裂

clonic spasm 震颤性麻痹

cold-sweating 出冷汗

coma /ˈkəʊmə/ *n.* 昏迷

consciousness /ˈkɒnʃəsnəs/ *n.* 神志；意识

continued fever 持续热

costa /ˈkɒstə/；rib /rɪb/ *n.* 肋骨

costal breathing 胸式呼吸

croup-membrane 假膜(白喉)

decayed tooth；carious tooth；caries of tooth 龋齿(蛀齿)

decompensation /diːˌkɒmpenˈseɪʃən/ *n.* 代偿不全

decubitus /dɪˈkjuːbɪtəs/；bedsore /ˈbedˌsɔː/ *n.* 褥疮

deep /diːp/；absolute /ˈæbsəˌluːt/ *adj.* 深的；绝对的

deep sensation 深感觉

delirious /dɪˈlɪriəs/ *adj.* 精神错乱的

desquamation /ˌdeskwəˈmeɪʃən/ *n.* 脱屑

diastolic murmur 舒张期杂音

diminished /dɪˈmɪnɪʃt/；poor /pɔː/；bad /bæd/ *adj.* 不良

disorder of sense of taste 味觉障碍

disturbance of consciousness 意识障碍

dullness /ˈdʌlnəs/；stupor /ˈstjuːpə/ *n.* 迷糊

dysarthria /dɪsˈɑːθriə/ *n.* 构音障碍

dyslalia /dɪsˈleɪliə/；stuttering /ˈstʌtərɪŋ/ *n.* 口吃

dyspnea /dɪsˈpniːə/ *n.* 呼吸困难

eczema /ˈeksɪmə/ *n.* 湿疹

edge of tongue 舌缘

epigastric pulsation 心窝搏动

erosion /ɪˈrəʊʒən/ *n.* 糜烂

erythema /ˌerɪˈθiːmə/ *n.* 红斑

exanthem /ekˈsænθəm/；eruption /ɪˈrʌpʃən/ *n.* 发疹

excited condition 兴奋状态

excoriation /ɪkˌskɔːrɪˈeɪʃən/ *n.* 擦伤

fauces /ˈfɔːsiːz/；pharynx /ˈfærɪŋks/；throat /θrəʊt/ *n.* 咽

fissure /ˈfɪʃə/；rhagades /ˈræɡəˌdiːz/ *n.* 皲裂

flaccid paralysis 弛缓性麻痹

formication /ˌfɔːmɪˈkeɪʃən/ *n.* 蚁行

frequency /ˈfriːkwənsi/ *n.* 频率

friction sound 摩擦音

fugue /fjuːɡ/ *n.* 朦胧状态

funnel chest 漏斗胸

fur of tongue 舌苔

gait /ɡeɪt/ *n.* 步态

good nutrition 营养良好

granulation tissue 肉芽组织

grinding of teeth 缀齿

gum /ɡʌm/ *n.* 齿龈

halitosis /ˌhælɪˈtəʊsɪs/ *n.*；bad breath；offensive breath 口臭

hare-lip 兔唇

heart murmur 心杂音

heart sound 心音

high fever 高热

humming murmur 嗡嗡音

Hutchinson teeth 胡钦森牙

icteric /ɪkˈterɪk/ *adj.* 黄疸的

incisor /ɪnˈsaɪzə/ n. 切齿

in good humour 性情良好

in ill humour 性情不好

inspiratory retraction 呼吸性凹陷

intermittent fever 间歇热

internal exanthema 黏膜疹

irregular /ɪˈreɡjʊlə/ adj. 不整齐的

Koplik spots 科泼力克斑（麻疹时）

lameness /ˈleɪmnɪs/ n. 跛行

large（small）fontanelle 大（小）囟门

lateral position 侧位

left edge 左边

limit of cardiac dullness; border of dullness heart 心浊音界

local heat 局部热感

lock jaw; trismus /ˈtrɪzməs/ n. 牙关紧闭

lustrous /ˈlʌstrəs/ adj. 富有光泽

macula /ˈmækjʊlə/; spot /spɒt/; stain /steɪn/ n. 斑

mitral murmur 二尖瓣杂音

motor aphasia 运动性失语症

myocardial in breast pain; myocardial infarct 心肌梗死

myocarditis /ˌmaɪəʊkɑːˌdaɪtɪs/ n. 心肌炎

nape /neɪp/ n. 颈背（项）

nasal alar breathing 鼻翼呼吸（煽动）

neck /nek/ n. 颈

neurosis of the heart 心脏官能症

normal /ˈnɔːml/; moderate /ˈmɒdərɪt/ adj. 正常

oral cavity 口腔

orthopnea /ɔːˈθɒpniə/ n. 端坐呼吸

papule /ˈpæpjuːl/ n. 丘疹

paralalia /ˌpærəˈleɪlɪə/ n. 语言错误

paralysis of the soft palate 软腭麻痹

paralysis /pəˈræləsɪs/ n. 麻痹

paresis /ˈpærɪsɪs/ n. 不全麻痹

paresthesia /ˌpærəsˈθiːʒə/ n. 感觉异常

paretic gait 麻痹性步态

passive ventral position 被动性腹位

pericardial /ˌperɪˈkɑːdɪəl/ adj. 心包性

pericarditis /ˌperɪkɑːˈdaɪtɪs/ n. 心包炎

perleche /pəˈleʃ/ n. 口角疮

permanent tooth 恒齿

petechial rash; blood stain 出血斑

pigeon thorax（breast）鸡胸

pigmentation /ˌpɪɡmenˈteɪʃən/ n. 色素沉着

pleural /ˈplʊərəl/ adj. 胸膜的

poor /pɔː/; lean /liːn/ adj. 贫弱的

position /pəˈzɪʃən/ n. 体位

present condition 目前症状

presystolic /prɪsɪsˈtɒlɪk/ adj. 收缩前期的

pseudo membrane 假膜

pulse /pʌls/ n. 脉搏

pustule /ˈpʌstjuːl/ n. 脓疱

recto-vesical perception 膀胱直肠感觉

reddened /ˈrednd/ adj. 发红

redden /ˈredn/ v. 脸红

redness /ˈrednəs/ n. 发红

regular /ˈreɡjələ/ adj. 规则的

remittent fever 弛张热

rhythm /ˈrɪðəm/ n. 律动

rickety /ˈrɪkəti/ adj. 患佝偻病的

right edge 右边

robust /rəʊˈbʌst/ adj. 强健

saliva flow 流涎

scab /skæb/; crust /krʌst/; scurf

/skɜːf/ *n*. 痂皮

scar /skɑː/; cicatrix /'sɪkətrɪks/ *n*. 瘢痕

sclerosis of the coronary arteries 冠状动脉硬化症

sense of equilibrium 平衡感觉

sense of movement 运动觉

sense of position 位置感觉

sense of temperature 温度觉

sense of touch 触觉

sensory aphasia 感觉性失语症

sensory dissociation 知觉分离

skull /skʌl/ *n*. 颅骨

slight fever 低热

somnolence /'sɒmnələns/ *n*. 嗜睡状态

spasm /'spæzəm/; convulsion /kən'vʌlʃən/; cramp /kræmp/ *n*. 痉挛

spastic gait 痉挛性步态

spastic /'spæstɪk/ *adj*. 痉挛性的

stammering /'stæmərɪŋ/ *n*. 口吃;结巴

stereognosis /ˌsterɪɒg'nəʊsɪs/ *n*. 实体觉

sternum /'stɜːnəm/ *n*. 胸骨

strawberry tongue 草莓舌

subcutaneous fatty tissue 皮下脂肪组织

superficial /ˌsuːpə'fɪʃəl/ *adj*. 浅的

superficial sensation 浅部感觉

suture /'suːtʃə/ *n*. 缝线

syncope /'sɪŋkəpi/ *n*. 晕厥

systolic murmur 收缩期杂音

tachycardia /ˌtækɪ'kɑːdiə/ *n*. 心率过频

tachypnea /ˌtækɪp'niə/ *n*.; rapid breathing 呼吸短促

temporal tooth 乳齿

thickly coated with white furs 厚白舌苔

thinly built 瘦削的

thorax /'θɔːræks/ *n*. 胸部

thrill /θrɪl/ *n*. 猫喘

thyroid /'θaɪrɔɪd/ *n*. 甲状腺

tongue /tʌŋ/ *n*. 舌

tonic spasm 强直痉挛

tonsil /'tɒnsl/ *n*. 扁桃体

uncoated tongue 无舌苔

unilateral lesion of the spinal cord 脊髓单侧病损

upper border 上界

vault of the skull 颅顶

vitiligo /ˌvɪtɪ'laɪgəʊ/ *n*. 白斑病

vomiting reflex 呕吐反射

weak /wiːk/ *adj*. 弱

Section 3   Prescriptions

第3节   处方

Ⅰ. Dialogue 情景对话

Aerobic Exercises 有氧运动

Doctor：Mr. Smith, you look so fresh today. You can go home in the afternoon, congratulations!

史密斯先生,你今天气色真不错。恭喜你,下午就可以出院了。

Patient：Thank you, Dr. Huang. I really feel strong and fit. You are so kind and I can never thank you enough.

谢谢你黄医生,我真的感觉身强体壮。你太好了,我实在是感激不尽。

Doctor：Oh, you are welcome, Mr. Smith. It's really our responsibilities. By the way, you need moderate exercises when you are out of hospital.

噢,别这么客气,史密斯先生。都是我们应该做的。你回到家后一定要做适当的体育锻炼。

Patient：While, which exercises should I take, Dr. Huang?

那么,黄医生,我可以做哪些运动呢?

Doctor：Generally speaking, there are three main kinds of exercises — aerobic exercises, calisthenics and anaerobic exercises.

总的来说,分有氧运动、体操和无氧运动这三类。

Patient：Well, what are aerobic exercises, Dr. Huang?

黄医生,哪些运动是有氧运动?

Doctor：They are exercises such as walking, jogging, skipping rope, badminton, ping-pong, rowing, skating, skiing, boxing, martial arts and some other endurance exercises, which can gradually enhance the abilities of muscle to consume oxygen and improve heart and lung fitness.

像散步、慢跑、跳绳、打羽毛球、打乒乓球、划船、溜冰、滑雪、拳击、形体操和其他一些锻炼耐力的运动统统都是有氧运动。有氧运动可以逐渐增强肌肉运输氧气的能力,改善心肺功能。

Patient：Then the exercises doing without oxygen are called anaerobics?

那么运动中不需要氧气的就是无氧运动喽?

Doctor：Yes, that's right. Take weight lifting for example, it requires just brief spurts of intense efforts, which mainly improves the muscle strength or builds up speed.

完全正确。拿举重来说,它需要瞬间的屏气用力,这种运动可以增强肌肉力量,提高运动速度。

Patient：But what is calisthenics for?

那形体操是干什么用的呢?

Doctor：Good question. It's to warm up before and cool down after the aerobic exercises, and it majorly improves joint flexibility and tone of muscles.

好问题。它主要是为了有氧运动前的热身和运动后的放松,它还能有效地提高各关节的柔韧性及肌肉运动的协调性。

Patient：As for me, Dr. Huang, how can I arrange for each exercise's session?

黄医生,对我来说该怎么安排这些运动时间呢?

Doctor：After five to ten minutes of warming up vigorous exercises, then you take three quarters of moderate aerobic exercises until you somewhat sweat and breathe deeply without getting breathless. Afterwards, you need to cool down for only five minutes, which will prevent your dizziness or faints resulting from so suddenly stopping vigorous exercises.

做五到十分钟的热身运动后,做四十五分钟的有氧运动,记着要用力适当,感觉身体微微出汗,呼吸加深而又不至于上气不接下气就行。最后花五分钟的时间做个全身的放松练习,这样可以防止因剧烈运动突然停止而导致的头晕、昏厥。

Patient：I'm sure I'll follow your advice, Dr. Huang. Thank you very much.

谢谢你,黄医生,我一定按你的建议去做。

Ⅱ. Sentences 替换句型

(1) The doctor prescribed him a long rest in bed.

医生吩咐他要长时间卧床休息。

(2) Doctor, what do (will) you prescribe for this illness?

医生,这种病你准备怎么开药(处置)呢?

(3) He's been losing weight for three months. He'd better get to bed early.

他连续三个月体重下降,最好去早点休息。

(4) Alkalis are still the most effective method of relieving the pain of peptic ulcer.

碱性药物仍然是缓解消化性溃疡疼痛最有效的方法。

(5) The lungs are subject to several diseases which are treatable by surgery. All you need is enough sleep and a balanced diet.

肺病是外科能够治疗的几种疾病之一。你所需要的就是充分的睡眠和平衡的膳食。

(6) The doctor should try as far as possible to investigate and protect the social needs of his patients.

医生应尽可能设法调查和保护其病人的社会需要。

(7) If you need any more information, come and see me.

如果还需要知道什么,请过来找我。

(8) You won't feel a thing. Be careful of your diet. Avoid greasy food, but drink more hot water, and don't be exhausted.

你不会有什么感觉的。注意你的饮食,不要吃太油腻的食物,多喝热水,注意不要过度疲劳。

(9) People live longer than they used to.

如今人们的寿命比过去长。

(10) Did the diabetic get used to giving himself his injections?

这个糖尿病患者习惯于给自己注射吗?

(11) When patients are confined to bed for a long time, every effort must be made to prevent pressure sores.

当患者长期被动卧床上,必须尽一切努力防止褥疮。

(12) Nurse, will you attend to Mrs. Blake's pressure sores, please?

护士,请你关注一下布莱克斯夫人的褥疮好吗?

(13) All diabetics must learn to regulate their diet.

所有糖尿病患者都必须学会调整他们的饮食。

(14) Treatment of Parkinson's disease is now in many ways easier than it used to.

巴金森氏病的治疗在很多方面比过去容易多了。

(15) You need a thorough examination. And avoid sexual relations before the results are made. Besides, take more nourishment such as eggs, vegetables, fruit, milk, meat, vitamins and so on.

你需要做个全面的检查,结果出来前禁止性生活。你应该多吃点像鸡蛋、蔬菜、水果、牛奶、肉类和维生素这样的营养品。

(16) After admission the patient was given gentamycin 80,000 units intramuscularly twice a day and penicillin G 800,000 units intramuscularly three times a day. Her body temperature dropped to normal within three days and her lung condition improved markedly. She was discharged on July 18, 2006. After her discharge, she is advised to take ampicillin 0.5 g orally four times a day for three successive days, aminophylline 0.1 g three times a day and bisolvon (bromhexine) 16 mg three times a day. She is also advised to have further examinations and treatment at intervals in a local hospital.

住院后给予患者庆大霉素 8 万单位,一日两次,肌注;青霉素 G 80 万单位,一日三次,肌注。患者体温三天内降至正常,肺部情况明显好转。患者于 2006 年 7 月 18 日出院。建议出院后口服氨苄西林 0.5 克,一日四次,连服三天;氨茶碱 0.1 克,一日三次;溴己新 16 毫克,一日三次。并建议定期在当地医院继续复查处理。

(17) Clinical diagnosis: Pneumonia, left lower lung. After admission she was treated with penicillin G, gentamycin and anti-cough drugs together with expectorants. The body temperature was dropping gradually. Beginning from the third day on, erythromycin and tablet TMP Co. were administered orally instead. The clinical symptoms improved markedly with increase of her body strength. It was agreed that in keeping with her travelling schedule she will be discharged pretty soon. It is advised that after discharge she should

avoid over-fatigue and cold, take the medication as directed by the physician in charge, and have follow-up observation in a hospital.

临床诊断:左下肺肺炎。住院后即予青霉素 G、庆大霉素及止咳祛痰药治疗。体温逐渐下降。入院后三天起改用红霉素、复方三甲氧苄氨嘧啶片口服,临床症状明显好转,体力恢复。根据患者旅行安排,同意近日出院。出院建议:避免劳累、受凉,按医嘱服药,到医院复查。

(18) It has been suggested that the patient should continue to avoid catching cold and promote his general health with proper nutrition and physical exercises. Symptomatic treatment may be carried out under a physician's supervision if necessary.

建议患者注意补充营养,适当进行体育锻炼,增强体质谨防感冒。必要时遵医嘱进行对症治疗。

Ⅲ. Words and Expressions 单词和短语

artificial pneumothorax 人工气胸
artificial respiration 人工呼吸
aural douche 洗耳
cold compress 冷敷
course of treatment 疗程
cupping /ˈkʌpɪŋ/ n. 拔火罐
daily dose 一日剂量
desensitize /ˌdiːˈsensətaɪz/ v. 使脱敏
dietotherapy /daɪətəʊˈθerəpi/ n. 饮食疗法
dosage /ˈdəʊsɪdʒ/ n. 剂量
dose /dəʊs/ n. 一次量
effect /ɪˈfekt/ n. 疗效
electrotherapy /ɪˌlektrəʊˈθerəpi/ n. 电疗
enema /ˈenəmə/; cyster /ˈklɪstə/ n. 灌肠
gastric gavage 胃输食法
hot compress 热敷
hypnotism /ˈhɪpnətɪzəm/; mesmerism /ˈmezmərɪzəm/ n. 催眠术

hypodermic injection 皮下注射
injection /ɪnˈdʒekʃən/ n. 注射
intradermic injection 皮内注射
intravenous injection 静脉注射
intubation n. 插管法
massage /ˈmæsɑːʒ/ n. 按摩
maximum dose 最大剂量
nasal gavage 鼻饲
once a day 一天一次
once three days 三天一次
oxygen respirator (bag) 氧气袋
oxygen therapy 氧气疗法
pharmacopoeia /ˌfɑːməkəˈpiːə/ n. 处方药
physiotherapy /ˌfɪziəʊˈθerəpi/ n. 理疗
potion /ˈpəʊʃən/ n. 水剂一日量(剂量)
prescribe something for 开药方
prescription charges n. 处方收费
prescription /prɪˈskrɪpʃən/ n. 处方药

rachiochysis injection 椎内注射

radiation therapy；radioactive therapy 放射疗法

radium therapy 镭放射疗法

recipe /ˈresəpi/ *n.* 处方药

roentgenogram /ˈrɒntgənəˌgræm/ *n.*；skiagraph /ˈskiːəˌgraːf/ *n.*；X-ray photo X 光照片

set of fracture 正骨

therapy /ˈθerəpi/；treatment /ˈtriːtmənt/ *n.* 治疗

tissue therapy；histotherapy /hɪstəʊˈθerəpi/ *n.* 组织疗法

twice a day 一天两次

ultra-red ray therapy 红外线疗法

ultra-short wave therapy 超短波疗法

ultrasonic therapy 超声波疗法

ultra-violet ray therapy 紫外线疗法

Section 4　At the Cashier's
第4节　划价收费

Ⅰ. Dialogue 情景对话

Balance Accounts 结清账目

Patient：Please give me my account，sir.
先生,请给我结一下账好吗?

Doctor：OK，I'll get your bill at once.
好的,我马上就给你结。

Patient：How much did I owe you? And may I pay it by the cheque?
我该付多少钱? 问一下,能用支票付款吗?

Doctor：Altogether eight hundred and fifty-five yuan. You may pay either in cash or by cheque.
总共 855 元,你付现金或开支票都行。

Ⅱ. Sentences 替换句型

(1) The cashier's is opened from 9：00 a. m. to 5：30 p. m.
收费处上班时间:上午 9:00 到下午 5:30。

(2) Your bill isn't ready, please wait a moment.

你的账单(费用)还没算好,请稍等。

(3) Mrs. Smith, please wait till your name is called.

史密斯夫人,请稍等,一会儿就轮到你了。

(4) The laboratory costs 298 yuan (The cost is/will be 298 yuan for your laboratory works/items).

你的化验费是 298 元。

(5) Your bill makes (includes) the doctor's fees and the costs of three days' supplies of medicine (the cost of a three-day supply of medicine), and it adds up to (comes to) 967 yuan.

你的费用一共是 967 元,其中包括治疗费和三天的药费。

(6) This prescription is excluded, sir. And you can take it to the pharmacy outside by yourself.

先生,你这张处方没有算在内,你可以自己去药房买药。

(7) Madame, now, please take this receipt to the pharmacy to get your medicine.

夫人,你现在可以拿着这张单子(票据、收据)去药房取药了。

(8) Did the doctor say that you would have any medicine? And let me have a look (check). He shouldn't forget writing your prescription.

医生说过要给你开药了吗? 来让我看看,他该不会忘记开处方吧。

(9) Mrs. Smith, you don't have any medicine prescribed, you can go home now.

史密斯夫人,医生没有给你开任何药,你可以回去了。

(10) Mr. Wang, I checked your medical report, but no medicines are prescribed.

王先生,我看了你的病历,医生的确没开什么药。

(11) Let me ask (phone) your doctor, just wait for a while, please.

让我问问你的医生(给你的医生打个电话)吧,请稍等。

(12) Sorry, there is no delayed billing here.

抱歉,这里不能赊账。

(13) Your bill today is 365 yuan, in addition to the balance of 235 yuan for the cost of yesterday (last visit), the total is 600 yuan.

你今天的费用是 365 元,加上昨天的(上次的)235 元,一共要交 600 元。

(14) The bill will be ready before your discharge, please come back at 10:00 a. m. tomorrow morning, Sir.

先生,你出院前我们一定把账算好,请明早 10:00 再来一次,好吧。

(15) Take care (see you).

保重(再见)。

Ⅲ. Words and Expressions 单词和短语

adrenalin /əˈdrenəlɪn/；epinephrine /ˌepɪˈnefrɪn/ *n.* 肾上腺素

albomycin /ˈælbəmiːsɪn/ *n.* 白霉素

alcohol /ˈælkəhɒl/ *n.* 酒精

aminophylline /æmɪˈnɒfɪliːn/ *n.* 氨茶碱

analgin /ˈeɪnldʒɪn/；novalgin /nəʊˈvældʒɪn/ *n.* 安乃近

antrenyl /æntˈrenɪl/ *n.* 安胃灵

antu /ˈæntjuː/ *n.* 安妥

APC；compound of aspirin 复方阿司匹林

ascorbic acid；vitamin C 抗坏血酸

aspirin /ˈæspɪrɪn/ *n.*；acetylsalicylic acid 阿司匹林

atropine /ˈætrəpɪːn/ *n.* 阿托品

aureomycin /ˌɔːrɪəʊˈmaɪsɪn/ *n.* 金霉素

barbital /ˈbɑːbɪtəl/ *n.* 巴比妥

benadryl /ˈbenədrɪl/ *n.* 苯海拉明

benzathine penicillin；tardocillin /taːdəʊˈsɪlɪn/ *n.* 长效青霉素

benzene hexachloride(BHC) 六六六

berberine /ˌbɜːbəriːn/ *n.* 黄连素

biofermin /ˈbiəfəmɪn/ *n.* 表飞明

bleaching powder 漂白粉

boric acid powder 硼酸粉

boric acid solution 硼酸水

brown mixture 复方甘草合剂

butazolidin /ˌbjuːtəˈzɒlɪdɪn/ *n.* 保泰松

calcium lactate 乳酸钙

camphor liniment 樟脑油

castor oil 蓖麻油

charcoal /ˈtʃɑːkəʊl/ *n.* 炭素片

chloromycetin /ˌklɔːrəʊmaɪˈsiːtɪn/ *n.* 氯霉素眼药水

cocaine /kəʊˈkeɪn/ *n.* 可卡因

codeine /ˈkəʊdiːn/ *n.* 可待因

cod-liver oil 鱼肝油

cortisone /ˈkɔːtɪzəʊn/ *n.* 可的松

DDVP 敌敌畏

dibazol /ˈdɪbəzɒl/ *n.* 地巴唑

dicaine /dɪˈkeɪn/ *n.* 地卡因

digitalis /ˌdɪdʒɪˈteɪlɪs/ *n.* 洋地黄

dipterex /ˈdɪptəreks/ *n.* 敌百虫

dramamine /ˈdræməˌmiːn/ *n.* 乘晕宁

ephedrine /ˈefɪdriːn/ *n.* 麻黄素

ether /ˈiːθə/ *n.* 乙醚

extract belladonna 颠茄片

eyrthromycin /ɪˌrɪθrəʊˈmaɪsɪn/ *n.* 红霉素

fluid extract of ergot 麦角流浸膏

folic acid 叶酸

formalin /ˈfɔːməlɪn/ *n.* 甲醛

furazolidone /ˌfjuːrəˈzɒlɪdəʊn/ *n.* 痢特灵

gargle iodine 含碘喉片

gastropin /ˈɡæstrəpɪn/ n. 胃舒平

gentian violet 紫药水(龙胆紫)

glucose /ˈɡluːkəus/；dextrose /ˈdekstrəʊz/ n. 葡萄糖

glycerine /ˈɡlɪsəriːn/ n. 甘油

griseofulvin /ˌɡrɪzɪəʊˈfulvɪn/；fulvicin /ˈfulvɪsɪn/ n. 灰黄霉素

heroin /ˈherəʊɪn/ n. 海洛因

hydrogen peroxide 双氧水

ichthyol /ˈɪkθɪəʊl/ n. 鱼石脂软膏

insulin /ˈɪnsjəlɪn/ n. 胰岛素

isoniazid /ˌaɪsəʊˈnaɪəzɪd/ n. 导烟肼

isoprenaline /ˌaɪsəʊˈprenəliːn/ n. 喘息定

librium /ˈlɪbriəm/ n. 利眠宁

liver extract 肝精片

luminal /ˈljuːmɪnæl/ n. 鲁米那

lysol /ˈlaɪsɒl/ n. 来苏儿

menthol crystal 薄荷脑

meprobamate /məˈprəʊbəˌmeɪt/； miltown /ˈmɪltaʊn/ n. 眠尔通

mercurochrome /məˈkjʊərəˌkrəʊm/ n. 红汞

mixture pepsin 胃蛋白酶合剂

morphine /ˈmɔːfiːn/ n. 吗啡

naphazoline /næfəzəˈliːn/ n. 滴鼻净

narcotic /nɑːˈkɒtɪk/ n. 麻醉药品

neomycin /ˌniːəʊˈmaɪsɪn/ n. 新霉素

nicotin acid；niacin /ˈnaɪəsɪn/ n. 烟草酸

nitroglycerin /ˌnaɪtrəʊˈɡlɪsəriːn/ n. 硝酸甘油

oil penicillin 油剂青霉素

opium /ˈəʊpiəm/ n. 鸦片

papaverine /pəˈpeɪvəˌriːn/ n. 罂粟碱

para amino salicylic acid (PAS) 对位氨基水杨酸

penicillin /ˌpeniˈsɪlɪn/ n. 青霉素

phenergan /ˈfenəɡən/ n. 异丙嗪

phenformin /fenˈfɔːmɪn/ n. 降糖灵

phenol /ˈfiːnɒl/ n. 石炭酸

phenolphthalein /ˌfiːnɒlˈθeɪliːn/ n. 酚酞

piperazine /pɪˈperəziːn/ n. 驱蛔灵

potassium permanganate 过锰酸钾

probanthine /prəʊˈbænθaɪn/ n. 普鲁本辛

progesterone /prəˈdʒestərəʊn/ n. 黄体酮

proheparin /pˈrəʊpərɪn/ n. 肝宁

protease /ˈprəʊtieɪz/ n. 蛋白酶

psoriasin ointment 牛皮癣素软膏

pyridoxine /ˌpɪrɪˈdɒksiːn/ n. 吡哆醇

quinine /kwɪˈniːn/ n. 奎宁

rauwolfia /rɔːˈwʊlfiə/ n. 降压灵(萝芙木)

reserpine /ˈresəpɪn/ n. 利血平

riboflavin /ˌraɪbəʊˈfleɪvɪn/ n.；vitamin B₂ 核黄素(维生素 B₂)

rutin /ˈruːtɪn/ n. 芦丁

santonin /ˈsæntənɪn/ n. 山道年(用作驱蠕虫剂)

silver nitrate 硝酸银

sippys powder 西皮氏粉

sodium bicarbonate solution 苏打水

sodium bicarbonate 小苏打

sodium salicylate 水杨酸钠

streptomycin /ˌstreptəˈmaɪsɪn/ n. 链霉素

sulfadiazine /ˌsʌlfəˈdaɪəziːn/ n. 磺胺嘧啶

sulfaguanidine /ˌsʌlfəˈɡwænɪdiːn/ n. 磺胺脒

sulfamethoxypyridazine /ˌsʌlfəmɪˈθɒksɪpɪrəˈdæziːn/ n. 长效磺胺

sulfathiazole /ˌsʌlfəˈθaɪəzəʊl/ n. 磺胺噻唑

sulfur ointment 硫黄软膏

syntomycin /ˌsɪntəˈmaɪsɪn/ n. 合霉素

terramycin oculentum 土霉素眼膏

terramycin /ˌterəˈmaɪsɪn/ n. 土霉素

tetracycline /ˌtetrəˈsaɪklɪn/ n. 四环素

thiamine /ˈθaɪəˌmiːn/ n. 硫胺素；维生素 B₁

tincture camphor compound 复方樟脑酊

tincture iodine 碘酒

tincture psoraleae 补骨脂

toclase /təkˈlæs/ n. 咳必清

turpentine /ˈtɜːpəntaɪn/ n. 松节油

urea /jʊˈriːə/ n. 尿素

Vaseline /ˈvæsəˌliːn/ n. 凡士林

vitamin B₁₂ 维生素 B₁₂

vitamin /ˈvɪtəmɪn/ n. 维生素

yeast /jiːst/ n. 酵母片

Section 5　Pharmacy
第 5 节　药房

Ⅰ. Dialogue 情景对话

Instructions of Taking Medicines 指导合理服药

Patient：How can I take these medicines，doctor?

我该怎样服这些药呢，医生?

Doctor：One tablet，three times a day.

一天三次，一次一片。

Patient：And how do I use this suppository?

那我该怎样用这个栓剂呢?

Doctor：Insert one into your anus (vegina) every night before getting to bed.

每晚睡觉前往肛门(阴道)里塞一个。

Patient：Besides，is this for internal use too?

请问，这也是内服药吗?

Doctor：Oh, no. This is for gargling only.

噢，不是，这是含漱剂。

Ⅱ. Sentences 替换句型

（1）This is a special adhesive for easing the pain. Apply it to the painful area and change it every two days. Take one tablet of this pain-killer if you feel much pain，but not more than once every four hours.
这是专门止痛用的药膏，贴在痛处，两天一换。如果你疼得厉害，可以服一片止疼片，但是每两次服药的间隔必须要在四小时以上。

（2）Please put one of the sucking lozenges under your tongue，don't swallow it. And as for this syrup，one line，almost one full teaspoonful，three times a day，and shake it well before taking it.
把含片放于舌下，不要吞咽。而这种糖浆，喝之前摇匀，一天三次，每次一格，也就是一满勺的量。

（3）This will loosen your stools. Please squeeze it into your anus every night after cleaning.
这是通便用的，请每晚清洗肛周后往肛门里挤一些。

（4）This is a suppository which can be put into the anus. Please follow the（read these）detailed directions（instructions）.
此类栓剂，用时放入肛门里，详见说明。

（5）Remove suppository as in（follow）the picture. Put it into your anus，pointed end first.
取出栓剂方法如图所示。尖端朝前，塞入肛门。

（6）You may take the prescription to the pharmacy for dispensing the medicine. And you have to get this filled within three days.
拿此药方去药房配药，三日内取药有效。

（7）Hold it in the rectum. It will be easier to be inserted if you use a little water.
栓剂使用前沾些水，既容易放入肛门，又能保证长时间停留在直肠里。

（8）Apply some of the ointment，and rub it into the skin.
涂一些这种药膏并揉搓进皮肤里去。

（9）Paint this lotion to the itching spot with this small brush（cotton swab）.
用小刷子（棉花棒）把洗剂涂在身体瘙痒处。

(10) Please dissolve the tablet(powder) in hot water, then soak your hands (feet) in it for twenty minutes and twice a day.

请用热水把这药片(药粉)溶化,然后再把你的手(脚)泡在里面。每日两次,每次 20 分钟。

(11) Doctor, how can I use these eye-drops and ointment?

医生,我怎样使用这些眼药水和眼药膏呢?

(12) As for eye ointment, pull down your lower eyelid tenderly and apply (take) the ointment gently. Don't let the tube touch your eyes.

用眼药膏时,轻轻翻开下眼皮,往里面挤少许眼膏。记住,不要让瓶嘴儿碰触眼睛。

(13) Put the eye-drops into your right eye four to six times a day, each time one to two drops. And squeeze a bit of the ointment on your eyelid every night.

将这种眼药水滴入右眼,每天四到六次,每次一到两滴。每晚往眼皮里挤一点眼药膏。

(14) And how do I apply (use) the nose drops?

那我怎样使用这滴鼻剂呢?

(15) Nose drops, spray five to six times a day.

滴鼻剂,一日五到六次喷鼻。

(16) Tilt your head back and apply one to two drops in each nostril.

头往后仰,每个鼻孔滴一到两滴。

(17) Bend your head back as far as possible and then put them in.

尽量把头向后仰然后将药滴进去。

(18) In which way, can I apply the ear drops?

怎样使用滴耳剂效果更好呢?

(19) Turn your head to the side, and put one to two drops in your ear. Then press the tragus for a few seconds.

将头歪向一侧,往耳朵里滴一到两滴药水,再把耳屏按几秒即可。

(20) Chew and swallow the small bits with water or put one of these big pills in water to dissolve it. But remember to remove the wax before taking it.

咀嚼并用温水冲服。或者把大药丸溶化在水里,服用前记得去掉外面的腊皮。

Ⅲ. Words and Expressions 单词和短语

action of drugs；medical effect 药效

administration /ədˌmɪnɪˈstreɪʃən/ *n.* 服法

adult dose 成人量

anaphylaxis /ˌænəfɪˈlæksɪs/ *n.* 药物过敏性

capsule /ˈkæpsjuːl/ *n.* 胶囊

compound /ˈkɒmpaʊnd/ *n.* 复方

concentrated /ˈkɒnsəntreɪtɪd/ *adj.* 浓缩的

decoction /dɪˈkɒkʃən/ *n.* 煎剂

diluent /ˈdɪljʊənt/；dilute /daɪˈluːt/ *adj.* 稀释的

disinfectant /ˌdɪsɪnˈfektənt/ *n.* 消毒剂

dose /dəʊs/；dosage /ˈdəʊsɪdʒ/ *n.* 剂量

dragée /ˈdraːʒeɪ/ *n.* 糖衣丸

empirical formula 验方

emulsion /ɪˈmʌlʃən/ *n.* 乳剂

gargle /ˈgaːgl/；mouthwash /ˈmaʊθˌwɒʃ/ *n.* 漱口剂

lotion /ˈləʊʃən/ *n.* 洗液

medicine /ˈmedsn/；medicament /mɪˈdɪkəmənt/；drug /drʌg/ *n.* 药物

medicine dropper 滴管

mixture /ˈmɪkstʃə/ *n.* 合剂

nostrum /ˈnɒstrəm/ *n.* 秘方

ointment /ˈɔɪntmənt/ *n.* 软膏

pain-killer *n.* 止疼片

panacea /ˌpænəˈsiːə/；magisterium /ˌmædʒɪˈstɪəriəm/ *n.* 万应药

pill /pɪl/ *n.* 丸

plaster /ˈplaːstə/ *n.* 硬膏

powder /ˈpaʊdə/；pulvil /ˈpʌlvɪl/ *n.* 粉剂

solution /səˈluːʃən/ *n.* 溶剂

suger-coated 糖衣

syrup /ˈsɪrəp/ *n.* 糖浆剂

tablet /ˈtæblət/ *n.* 药片

throat spray 喷喉药

tincture /ˈtɪŋktʃə/ *n.* 酊剂

Section 6　Types of Medicine
第6节　药物制剂

Ⅰ. Dialogue 情景对话

Instructions of Taking Chinese Medicines 指导如何服用中药

Patient：Would you mind to tell me that if I must boil it before each time I take it?

医生,你能不能告诉我,是不是每次吃前都要把药煮开一遍呢?

Doctor: No, just put it in a glass (bottle) and warm it in a bowl of hot water.

不必,你可以把药倒入一个玻璃杯(瓶)中,然后放入一碗热水中温热喝就行了。

Patient: And how do I take these big balls?

那这些大药丸该怎么服用呢?

Doctor: Chew (break) and swallow the bits with water or you can put them in water to melt them, then remove the wax before taking it.

嚼碎(掰成小块儿),用水冲服,或者把它泡在水里化开后再喝。服药前,把蜡皮去掉。

Patient: I see. Thank you very much.

我知道了,谢谢你。

Doctor: You are welcome.

不客气。

Ⅱ. Sentences 替换句型

(1) Two tablets are at night, please.

晚上服两片。

(2) Two tablets, four times a day.

一天四次,一次两片。

(3) Take one tablet of this pain-killer if you feel pain, but not more than once every four hours.

假如你觉得疼就吃一片止痛片,但每次必须间隔四小时。

(4) Take this medicine when you must (have pain, itching, trouble in sleeping, a temperature over 39℃).

需要(疼、痒、失眠、发热高达 39℃以上时)时服次药。

(5) One line (half line) three times a day. Shake it well before taking it.

每天三次,每次一(半)格,服前先摇匀。

(6) This medicine may upset your stomach.

此药可引起胃部不适。

(7) You may feel drowsy. Please don't take this medicine when driving (working).

此药可引起嗜睡，所以开车(工作)时禁服此药。

(8) Besides, side effects like dryness and swelling of face, vertigo, dizziness or local nervous tic may also occur.

此外,这种药还有引起面部皮肤干燥,肿胀,眩晕,头昏或局部神经抽搐等副作用。

(9) If you develop(have) any unusual symptoms or if this medicine bothers you, please contact us right away.

服药后,如有任何不适,请立即来就诊。

(10) Please put it under your tongue, don't swallow it.

请把药放在舌下含服,记住不要下咽。

(11) Please suck it.

请含服。

(12) Keep this in the refrigerator, please.

请放于冰箱内冷藏。

(13) This medicine can be taken (take this medicine) with the stomach drugs included in the prescription.

此药可与处方胃药一起服用。

(14) This is a concentrated solution. And dilute it in double amount of water before using (taking).

此药为浓缩型,服用时加二倍水稀释。

(15) Please dissolve the pill in water before taking it.

服前请将药丸放在水中溶化。

(16) Dissolve this in hot water and drink one teaspoon (spoonful) of it each time, three times a day.

喝前,用热水溶化,每天三次,每次一茶匙。

(17) This is oral drugs, please press with your fingers and apply to where it hurts.

此类是口腔用药。用时,用手指把药压附在溃疡处。

Ⅲ. Words and Expressions 单词和短语

absorbent /əbˈzɔːbənt/; sorbent　　　　/ˈsɔːbənt/ *n*. 吸着剂

acid /ˈæsɪd/ n. 酸

alterative /ˈɔːltərətɪv/; alterant medicine 变质药

analgesic /ˌænlˈdʒiːzɪk/;
　antalgic /ænˈtældʒɪk/;
　analgetic /ˌænəlˈdʒetɪk/;
　painkiller /ˈpeɪnˌkɪlə/ n. 止疼药；镇痛剂

anal suppository 坐药

androgen /ˈændrədʒən/ n. 男性激素

angiotonics /ˌændʒɪəˈtɒnɪks/ n. 血管强化剂

anhidrotic /ˌænhɪˈdrɒtɪk/ n. 止汗药

antacid /æntˈæsɪd/ n. 抗酸剂

antagonistic action 拮抗作用

antasthmatic /ænˈtæsθmætɪk/ n. 止喘药

antemetic /ˈæntɪmetɪk/ n. 止吐药

anthracene purgative;
　helminthagogue /ˈhelmɪnθəgɒg/ n. 驱虫药

anti-allergic adj. 防过敏的

antianemic /ˌæntiːəˈniːmɪk/;
　hematopoietics /heˌmætəʊpəʊˈɪetɪks/ n. 造血剂；生血剂

antibiotic /ˌæntibaɪˈɒtɪk/ n. 抗生素

antidiarrheal /ˌæntɪˌdaɪəˈrɪəl/; binding medicine n. 止泻剂

antidote /ˈæntɪˌdəʊt/ n. 解毒药

antiflatulent /æntaɪfˈlætjʊlənt/ n. 排气药

antiphlogistic /ˌæntɪfləˈdʒɪstɪk/ n. 消炎药

antipruritic /ˌæntɪprʊəˈrɪtɪk/ n. 止痒药

antipyretic /ˌæntɪpaɪˈretɪk/;
　antithermic /ˌæntɪtˈhɜːmɪk/ n. 解热剂

antiscolic /ˌæntɪsˈkɒlɪk/;
　antihelminthic /ˌæntɪhelˈmɪnθɪk/ n. 驱虫剂

antiseptic /ˌæntɪˈseptɪk/; preservative /prɪˈzɜːvətɪv/ n. 防腐剂

antisyphilitic /ˈæntɪˌsɪfəˈlɪtɪk/ n. 抗梅毒剂

aphrodisiac /ˌæfrəˈdɪzɪæk/ n. 春药

apocrustic astringent 收剑剂

bitters /ˈbɪtəz/ n. 苦味剂

cardiotonic /ˌkɑːdɪəʊˈtɒnɪk/ n.;
　cardiac stimulant 强心剂

choleresis biliation 胆汁分泌

contraceptive /ˌkɒntrəˈseptɪv/ n. 避孕药

cough remedy; antitussive /ˌæntɪˈtʌsɪv/ n.; cough medicine 镇咳药

desensitizer /diːˈsensɪˌtaɪzə/ n. 脱敏药

digestive /daɪˈdʒestɪv/; digestant /daɪˈdʒestənt/ n. 消化剂

digestive ferment 消化酶

disinfectant /ˌdɪsɪnˈfektənt/ n. 消毒剂

diuretic /ˌdaɪjʊəˈretɪk/ n. 利尿剂

emetic /ɪˈmetɪk/ n. 催吐剂

emmenagogue /ɪˈmenəgɒg/ n. 调经药

expectorant /ɪkˈspektərənt/ n. 祛痰药

eyewash /ˈaɪˌwɒʃ/ n. 洗眼药

febrifuge /ˈfebrɪˌfjuːdʒ/; antipyretic /ˌæntɪpaɪˈretɪk/ n. 退烧药

germicide /ˈdʒɜːmɪˌsaɪd/ n. 杀菌药

haematinic /ˌhiːməˈtɪnɪk/ n. 补血药

hemostatic /ˌhiːməʊˈstætɪk/; styptic /ˈstɪptɪk/ n. 止血剂

hepatic protector n. 保肝药

hidrotic /hɪˈdrɒtɪk/; diaphoretic /ˌdaɪəfəˈretɪk/; sudorific

/ˌsjuːdəˈrɪfɪk/ *n.* 发汗药

hormone /ˈhɔːməʊn/ *n.* 激素；荷尔蒙

hypotensor /haɪpəʊˈtensə/ *n.* 降血压药

indication /ˌɪndɪˈkeɪʃən/ *n.* 适应症

inhalant /ɪnˈheɪlənt/ *n.* 吸入剂

insecticide /ɪnˈsektɪsaɪd/ *n.* 杀虫药

laxative /ˈlæksətɪv/ *n.* 轻泻药

lethal dose 致死剂量（或致死量）

lotion /ˈləʊʃən/；washing /ˈwɒʃɪŋ/ *n.* 洗剂

mydriatic /ˌmɪdrɪˈætɪk/ *n.* 扩瞳药

myotic /maɪˈɒtɪk/ *n.* 缩瞳药

narcotic /naːˈkɒtɪk/；anesthetic /ˌænɪsˈθetɪk/ *n.* 麻醉剂

nutrient /ˈnjuːtrɪənt/ *n.* 营养药

obstipantia /ˈɒbstɪpənʃɪə/ *n.* 止泻药

poison /ˈpɔɪzn/ *n.*；poisonous agent；toxicant /ˈtɒksɪkənt/ *n.* 毒药

popular medicine for heat stroke 祛暑药

powerful medicine 剧药

purgative /ˈpɜːgətɪv/；evacuant /ɪˈvækjʊənt/；cathartic /kəˈθaːtɪk/；

eccoprotic /ˌekəʊˈprɒtɪk/ *n.* 泻药

refrigerant /rɪˈfrɪdʒərənt/ *n.* 清凉药

resolutive /ˈrezəluːtɪv/ *n.* 消肿药

sedative /ˈsedətɪv/；calmative /ˈkælmətɪv/ *n.* 镇静剂

sedative /ˈsedətɪv/ *n.* 镇静药

side effect 副作用

sleeping pill/drug；hypnotic /hɪpˈnɒtɪk/ *n.*；soporific /ˌsɒpəˈrɪfɪk/ *n.*；somnifacient /ˌsɒmnɪˈfeɪʃənt/ *n.* 安眠药；催眠剂

stimulant /ˈstɪmjʊlənt/；excitant /ɪkˈsaɪtənt/；analeptic /ˌænəˈleptɪk/ *n.* 兴奋剂

stomachic /stəˈmækɪk/ *n.* 健胃药

styptic /ˈstɪptɪk/；haemostatic /ˌhiːməʊˈstætɪk/；anastaltic /ˌænæsˈtæltɪk/ *n.* 止血药

synergistic action 协同作用

tonic /ˈtɒnɪk/ *n.* 补药；强化剂

vasodilation /ˌveɪzəʊdaɪˈleɪʃən/ *n.* 血管舒张

Section 7   How to Take Medicine
第 7 节   用药

I . Dialogue 情景对话

Bacillary Dysentery 细菌性痢疾

Patient：Doctor, I have had a terrible diarrhea for two days.

医生,我已经腹泻两天了,很厉害。

Doctor：What are your stools like? Watery or soft? Is there blood or mucus in the stool?

你的粪便是什么样的? 水样便还是软便? 大便里带不带血和脓液?

Patient：Watery with blood and mucus.

水样便,带血和脓。

Doctor：How frequent are they each day?

你一天拉几次?

Patient：They are very frequent. I don't know how many.

反正也没数过,很多次的。

Doctor：Do you have a temperature?

你发烧吗?

Patient：I feel hot and sometimes shivery.

有时觉得烧,可有时又发冷。

Doctor：Have you had any abdominal pain?

你肚子疼吗?

Patient：Yes, I have lower abdominal cramps.

疼,下腹部我感觉是那种绞疼。

Doctor：Give a stool specimen to the laboratory please. I'll wait for the results… The stool shows blood, mucus and pus as well as some ascaris eggs. It looks like bacillary dysentery, I'd like to send a stool specimen for culture.

你到化验室去查一个大便吧,我在这儿等你的化验结果……看,你的大便里有血、脓液和蛔虫卵。看起来像是细菌性痢疾。我还想送个你的大便标本去做个培养。

Patient：Is it serious?

严重吗?

Doctor：It isn't serious. I'll give you tetracyline, which is very effective. You should have a complete rest and drink large amounts of liquids, otherwise, you will be dehydrated. Eat small quantities frequently. You should have a liquid or semi-liquid diet that is easily digestible. Avoid spicy, fibrous residue or greasy foods for a few days. It's an infectious disease. You should wash your hands thoroughly after going to the toilet.

不是太严重。我给你开点特效药四环素吧。不过你需要卧床休息,多喝水,不然的话,你会脱水的。你应该少食多餐,多吃些流质、半流质和易于消化的食物。近几天,还要忌食辛辣、油腻和纤维多的食物。细菌性痢疾是传染病,大便后一定要彻底洗手。

Patient：Thank you, I will follow your advice.

　　　　谢谢,我会按照你说的去做的。

Ⅱ. Sentences 替换句型

(1) Take the tablets once a day.

这个药片每天服一次。

(2) Take the medicine three times a day after food.

每天饭后服药三次。

(3) Lock this medicine out of the reach of children.

把药锁在孩子们拿不到的地方。

(4) Don't forget to take the tablets first thing every morning.

每天早上第一件事:不要忘记吃药。

(5) Don't have anything to eat or drink before coming to hospital.

来医院之前不要吃或喝任何东西。

(6) The colour of your urine may change after the medicine, but don't worry (you need not worry about it). Do rest as much as you can.

服药后,小便颜色会有些变化,不必担心,这是正常现象。记住一定尽可能多休息。

(7) Did your doctor prescribe penicillin?

你的医生开青霉素了吗?

(8) I want you to take these tablets to reduce your blood pressure.

我要你吃这些药片来降压。

(9) You must follow the doctor's instructions carefully. And you must have the same amount of insulin every day at the same time.

你必须遵循医生的劝告。必须每天同一时间服用同样剂量的胰岛素。

(10) You must always carry sugar with you and eat it at once if you feel faint.

你必须随身带着糖,一旦感觉头晕,马上吃糖。

(11) The effective dose of this drug for most patients is 60-120 mg per day and side effects can be minimized by beginning with the low dose and gradually increasing medication to the most effective level for that patient.

这种药物对大多数病人的有效剂量是每天 60－120 毫克,开始剂量小,然后逐渐增加到对病人最有效的剂量,这样副作用才能降到最低限度。

(12) You could increase the dose.

你可以增加剂量。

(13) Do the tablets make your mouth dry?

这些药片让你口干吗?

(14) These tablets don't seem to suit you. We'd better try some others.

这些药片似乎不适合你,我们最好试用一些别的药。

(15) Be sure to give the correct dose of the medicine and watch the patient drink it.

给药量一定要准确并看着病人喝下去。

Ⅲ. Words and Expressions 单词和短语

1. General Terms 一般术语

antagonistic action 拮抗作用
daily dose 一日剂量
indication /ˌɪndɪˈkeɪʃən/ 适应证
internal medicine 内服药
lethal dose 致死剂量(或致死量)
maximum dose 最大剂量
medication /ˌmedɪˈkeɪʃən/ n.; administration of medicine 用药
medication/medicament for external application 外用药
medicine bag 药袋
medicine ticket 药笺
once a day 一天一次

once three days 三天一次
potion /ˈpəʊʃən/ n. 饮剂
recipe /ˈresəpi/ n. 处方
six times every four hours a day 四小时一次,一天六次
twice a day 一天两次

2. Abbreviations (服药)缩写语

a. c. (before meals) 饭前
ad lib. (as much as desired) 随意
adst. feb. (when fever is present) 发烧时
ad us. (according to custom) 按习惯
ad us. ext. (for external use) 外用
agit. ante sum (shake before taken) 服用前摇匀

alt. hor. (every other hour) 每隔一小时

b. i. d. (twice a day) 每日两次

c. m. s. （to be taken tomorrow morning）次日晨服用

D；d. in d. (from day to day) 每日

Dieb. Alt (on alternate days) 间日；隔日

Dim. （one half）一半

h. d. (at bed time) 就寝时

h. n. （tonight）当晚

h. s. (at sleeping time) 临睡时

p. a. a. （applied to the affected region）用于患处

p. c. (after meals) 饭后

p. v. (by the vagina) 由阴道送药

q. i. d. (four times a day) 每日四次

t. i. d. (three times a day) 每日三次

Chapter 6 Admission and Discharge

第6章 住院与出院

Section 1 Operation

第1节 手术

I . Dialogues 情景对话

1. Talks Before an Operation 术前谈话

Doctor：We are going to do the operation on you tomorrow morning，I hope you won't worry. If there is anything uncertain，please let me know.

明天早上我们就要给你做手术了,希望你不要紧张。如果还有什么疑问,一定告诉我。

Patient：OK，I will try not to. Ah…but will it hurt?

好的,我尽量做到放松。啊……我还是想问一句,手术是否会很疼呀?

Doctor：We'll give you anaesthesia. If you feel any pain during the operation，just tell us and we will cope with it right away.

手术前我们会给你打麻药的,手术期间你如果感到疼痛,尽管告诉我们,我们会采取措施的。

Patient：I see，thank you，sir.

好的,我明白了,谢谢。

Doctor：And by the way，have you handed in your consent yet?

顺便问一句,你的手术同意书交了吗?

Patient：No, not yet. But how should I write it?

还没呢,我也不知道该怎么填写才好。

Doctor："I (your name here) the undersigned have requested and consented to a certain operation." That's all. Secondly, we need the seal of your embassy and the signature of your ambassador on the consent form.

"我(此处填写你的名字)签名人申请并同意做某某手术。"然后签上名就行了。此外,这张同意书上还需要你们大使的签名以及加盖你们大使馆的印鉴。

2. Preparation for an Operation 术前准备

Doctor：The operation starts tomorrow morning, now I'd like to shave off the hair around the operation area.

明天早上安排你的手术,现在我要给你备备皮(也就是说把你手术区周围的毛剃剃)。

Patient：Doctor, I have never been in the hospital before. So I'm somewhat scared.

医生,我还从来没有住过院,我有点害怕。

Doctor：There is nothing to worry about, madame. The doctor who will operate on you is very experienced and considerate (thoughtful). If you have any discomfort during the operation, please don't hesitate to tell him.

放宽心(不必担心),夫人,给你做手术的医生不仅经验丰富,而且细致耐心。手术过程中如有不适,尽管向他提出来。

Patient：Thank you, I will.

谢谢,我记住了。

Doctor：I'll give you enema tonight. So after that, please don't take any food or water before the operation.

那么,今晚我就准备给你灌肠了。灌肠后,直到手术前,请你不要再吃任何东西和喝水了。

Patient：Does it hurt? And would you please tell me how you do it?

灌肠疼吗? 你能否告诉我你是怎么个做法呢?

Doctor：OK. I'll insert a rubber tube into your anus and let the soap suds solution flow into your rectum. Then, please do let me know if you feel distension. Later, I'll stop the flowing. And you must hold it for several minutes before you expel it, since that may produce a better result.

好的,我先往你的肛门里插根橡皮管,接着就往直肠里灌些肥皂水。当你觉得肚子发胀时就说话,我就不再灌了。不过你排便前,尽量多憋几分钟,这样效果会好些。

Ⅱ. Sentences 替换句型

(1) Her foot was so swollen she couldn't wear her shoes.
她的脚肿胀得已经不能穿鞋了。

(2) I would like to talk about the operation with you. The operation may be the best way to cure you. However, there are certain dangers in operating, such as the hazards of anesthetics, or you may be unable to withstand the stress of operation. Moreover, after the operation, post-operative complications may occur, such as bleeding, infections or even continued intestinal obstruction.
我想和你谈谈手术的问题。手术也许是治疗的最好办法。但是手术也有一定的危险,如麻醉的危害或你的身体本身耐受不住手术,而且可能还会出现如出血、感染、肠梗阻等术后并发症。

(3) A five minutes' scrubbing of hands and forearms with soap and water is the routine for surgeons before operating.
手术前用肥皂和水洗五分钟的手和前臂,对外科医生来说是常规。

(4) Get on the scales and we'll see how much you weigh.
上体重计,我们要看看你体重多少。

(5) Please sign here for consent to the operation.
请在这里签字表示同意手术。

(6) The theatre sister took charge.
手术室护士长负责。

(7) I know you have some housework to do. But you can't receive the treatment in the out-patient clinic anymore, you'd better be admitted in the afternoon.
尽管你有家务事要做,但你不能再耽搁了。最好下午就从门诊转住院吧。

（8）I'll give you an admission slip and have a bed arranged for you. You can go home and prepare yourself. And come back tomorrow morning for admission.

我给你开张住院单先安排个床位,你今天可以回家准备准备,明天一早来住院。

（9）You should be admitted to the hospital for an operation, because it may grow rather rapidly and an ovarian tumor can change quite easily in nature.

因为卵巢肿瘤长得很快,而且极易发生病变,所以你应该马上住院进行手术摘除。

（10）Will you please sign to give permission for an anaesthetic and an operation?

请你签字同意开始麻醉和手术好吗?

（11）These instruments were sterilized.

这些器械消过毒了。

（12）Have we enough plasma?

我们有足够的血浆吗?

（13）In this operation they have to use the heart lung machine.

这次手术中他们不得不使用心肺机。

（14）They had to perform a tracheostomy.

他们只得做了气管造口术。

（15）Pass me that scalpel. Nurse, please. And we'll need some forceps.

护士,请把那个刀片递给我。另外,我们还会需要一些镊子。

（16）We shall be ready to start as soon as you are. And hand me the scissors, please.

你一旦准备好了,我们就开始。请递给我剪刀。

（17）The operation will not produce 100% cures.

手术不会 100%治愈疾病。

（18）A large proportion of the patients with failed renal grafts will return to regular dialysis treatment.

大多数肾移植失败的病人将回来进行定期的透析治疗。

（19）You are going to have a local anaesthetic so you won't feel anything.

做了局部麻醉,你就不会有任何感觉的。

(20) You are going to have a blood transfusion (He needed a blood transfusion at once).

你马上要输血(他需要马上输血)。

(21) Lie still and place your arms by your sides.

安静躺着,把你的双臂放在身体两侧。

(22) Before his operation he used to be in great pain after meals.

手术前他经常在餐后发生剧痛。

(23) The child is lying on the operating table.

这个孩子正躺在手术台上。

(24) Theatre sisters lay the instruments ready for the surgeon.

手术室护士摆好外科医生用的器械。

(25) Patients who sustain severe burns may need a whole series of operations.

受到严重烧伤的病人可能需要一系列的手术。

(26) Prof. Smith, the patient complained of a little numbness and tingling in both hands.

史密斯教授,病人诉说两只手有麻木和刺痛的感觉。

(27) The surgeon is operating on the patient's kidney.

外科医生正在给那个病人做肾脏手术。

(28) The surgeon X-rayed the man's legs and amputated his left leg.

外科医生透视了那个人的腿并截去了他的左腿。

(29) The surgeon found a swelling under his arm and excised the lump immediately.

外科医生在他的臂下发现了一个肿块并迅速将其切除。

(30) The surgeons were fighting to save his life for six hours.

医生们为抢救他的生命奋战了六个小时。

(31) I have fallen in the street and sprained my ankle.

我在街上摔倒了,扭伤了踝关节。

(32) Will you please go to the casualty department?

请你去急救科好吗?

(33) Don't remove the bandages for another day.

过一天才能去掉绷带。

(34) The surgeon repaired the broken arm efficiently.

外科医生有效地修复了这只断臂。

（35）Manual dexterity combined with great personal attributes made him a much-loved surgeon.

灵巧的手加上他个人的高尚品质，使他成为一位备受人们爱戴的外科医生。

Ⅲ. Words and Expressions 单词和短语

abdominal puncture 腹腔穿刺

abdominosacral method 腹骶法

abscess lance 脓肿切开刀

acupuncture anesthesia 针灸麻醉

administration of eye drops 滴眼药

amputation /ˌæmpjʊ'teɪʃən/ n. 截断术（截肢）

amputatis mammanae 乳房切开术

anatomic forceps 解剖钳

annular zone 环带

appendectomy /ˌæpen'dektəmi/ n.；
    appendicectomy /ˌæpendɪ'sektəmi/ n.；ileocecal resection 阑尾切除术

arthrectomy resection of the joint 关节切除术

artificial pneumothorax 人工气胸

artificial pneumoperitoneum 人工气腹

artificial respiration 人工呼吸

artificial sunlight 人工太阳灯

basal anesthesia 基础麻醉

bladder instillation 膀胱注药术

bladder irrigation 膀胱灌洗术

boric acid solution 硼酸水

change of bandage 更换绷带

cholecystectomy /ˌkɒlɪsɪ'stektəmi/ n. 胆囊摘除术

choledochotomy /kəˌledə'kɒtəmi/ n. 胆总管切开术

closure of the intestinal around；enterorrhaphy /entə'rɒrəfi/ n. 肠缝合术

cold anesthesia 冷冻麻醉

cold compress；cold stupe 冷敷

compress /kəm'pres/ n. （压伤口）绷带

contrast /'kɒntrɑːst/ n. 对照剂；造影剂

craniotomy /ˌkreɪnɪ'ɒtəmi/ n. 开颅术

curettement /kjʊə'retmənt/；
    curettage /kjʊə'retɪdʒ/ n. 刮除术

disarticulation /ˌdɪsɑːtɪkjʊ'leɪʃən/；
    exarticulation /'eksɑːtɪkjʊ'leɪʃən/ n. 关节切断术

dorsal (sacral) method 背法（骶法）

drainage of the thoracic cavity 胸腔流术

drainage tube 引流管

drainage /'dreɪnɪdʒ/ n. 引流

drain-gauze 引流纱布

dressing /'dresɪŋ/ n. 敷料

enterectomy /ˌentə'rektəmi/ n. 肠切除术

enterostomy /ˌentə'rɒstəmi/ n. 肠造口术

enucleation of the phrenic nerve 膈神经切断术

excision of hernial sac 疝囊切除术

extirpation /ˌekstə'peɪʃən/；

enucleation /ɪˌnjuːklɪˈeɪʃən/；

　remove /rɪˈmuːv/ n. 摘除

extradural anesthesia 硬膜外麻醉

extrapleural fill 胸膜外补充术

extrapleural pneumolysis 胸膜外肺剥离术

eye irrigation 洗眼

gastric puncure 肠穿刺

gastropexy /ɡæstˈrəʊpeksi/ n. 胃固定术

gastrostomy /ɡæsˈtrɒstəmi/ n. 胃造瘘

gastrotomy /ɡæsˈtrɒtəmi/ n. 胃切开术

general anesthesia 全身麻醉

gypsum /ˈdʒɪpsəm/；plaster /ˈpɑːstə/

　n. 石膏

hand-dynamometer 握力计

hernioplasty /ˈhɜːnɪəplæsti/ n. 疝根治术

herniopuncture /hɜːˈnaɪɒpʌŋktʃə/ n.

　疝穿刺术

herniotomy /ˌhɜːnɪˈɒtəmi/ n. 疝气切开术

hot compress；hot stupe 热敷

hypothermic anesthesia 低温麻醉

incision /ɪnˈsɪʒən/ n. 切口

infiltration anesthesia 浸润麻醉

inhalation anesthesia 吸麻醉

inhalation /ˌɪnhəˈleɪʃən/ n. 吸入

intestinal incision；enterotomy

　/ˌentəˈrɒtəmi/ n. 肠切开术

intramuscular injection 肌肉注射

intravenous anesthesia 静脉麻醉

intravenous injection；drop instillation；

　venous inflow 静脉输入

laminectomy /ˌlæmɪˈnektəmi/ n. 椎板

　切除术

lavage /læˈvɑːʒ/ n. 洗涤

local anesthesia 局部麻醉

lumbar puncture 腰椎穿刺

medicine for stupe 药敷

menthe /ˈmenθi/ n. 薄荷

mouth gag 开口器

mustard /ˈmʌstəd/ n. 芥末

narcosis /nɑːˈkəʊsɪs/；anesthesia

　/ˌænɪsˈθiːziə/ n. 麻醉(全身)

needle holder 持针器

needle /ˈniːdl/ n. 针

neuroexeresis of the phrenic nerve 膈

　神经捻开术

Pean's forceps 环状舌钳

perforation /ˌpɜːfəˈreɪʃən/ n. 穿孔

pleurocentesis /ˌplʊərəʊsenˈtiːsɪs/；

　thoracocentesis /ˌθɔːrəkəʊsenˈtiːsɪs/；

　thoracentesis /ˌθɔːrəsenˈtiːsɪs/ n. 胸

　腔穿刺术

post-operation 术后

post-operative change of bandage

　stretcher 术后换敷料

post-operative rest 术后休息

potential anesthesia 强化麻醉

preparation care 术前准备

preventive gown 预防眼

probe /prəʊb/ n. 擦针

puncture fluid (paracentesis fluid) 穿刺液

puncture /ˈpʌŋktʃə/ n. 穿刺

pyloroplasty /paɪˈlɔːrəˌplæsti/ n. 幽门

　成形术

radical operation of hernia 疝根治切术

rapid spiral bandage 蛇带

rectal anesthesia 直肠麻醉

removal of the spleen；lienectomy

　/laɪəˈnektəmi/ n. 脾切除术

removal of the stomach; gastrectomy /gæs'trektəmi/ *n.* 胃切除术

reposition of the luxation 脱臼复位术

resection of ribs 肋骨切除术

reservation catheter 潴留导管

rivanol solution 雷佛奴尔液

roller bandage 卷带

scale /skeɪl/ *n.* 秤

shaving of field of operation 术野剃毛

silkworm gut 丝线

soap solution 肥皂液

spica bandage 麦穗带

spinal anesthesia 腰椎麻醉

spiral bandage 螺带

spiral reverse bandage 折带

spirometer /spaɪ'rɒmɪtə/ *n.* 肺活量计

sticking plaster bandage 绊创膏带

stomach-intestinal anastomosis 胃肠吻合术

stretcher /'stretʃə/ *n.* 患者运送车

strumectomy /struː'mektəmi/ *n.* 甲状腺切除术

subcutaneous injection; hypodermic injection 皮下注射

superfacial anesthesia 表面麻醉

suture needle 缝合针

suture /'suːtʃə/ *n.* 缝线

testudo bandage 龟甲带

thoracoplasty 胸廓成形术

tissue forceps 组织钳

tongue depressor 压舌板

toothed forceps 有齿钳

tracheostomy /ˌtrækɪ'ɒstəmi/ *n.* 气管造口术

traction bandage 牵引带

transfusion injection 输脉注射

transfusion /træns'fjuːʒən/ *n.* 输液

treatment /'triːtmənt/; therapy /'θerəpi/ *n.* 疗法

triangle bandage 三角带

ultrashort wave 超短波

urethral catheterization 导尿

vagotomy /væ'ɡɒtəmi/ *n.*; gastric neurectomy 迷走神经切断术

X-ray apparatus X 线机

Section 2　Ward Rounds and Nursing

第2节　查房护理

I. Dialogues 情景对话

1. Concerning Admission 有关住院问题

Parent：Doctor, my child is being admitted. Should I stay with him?

医生, 我的孩子已经住院了, 需要我陪他吗?

Doctor：He'll be in a single room. As he's quite small, it's better for you to stay in the hospital and take care of him.

你的孩子住的是单间, 他人又很小, 你最好留在医院照顾他。

Parent：All right. I'll stay in the hospital with him. But I have to go home first to get my clothes. I have two other children. Can they also stay in the hospital?

好吧! 我留下陪他。但是我得先回家取些我的衣服。另外, 我家里还有两个孩子, 我能不能把他们也带来呢?

Doctor：No. Your husband or some of your friends must look after the other children at home. It's better for healthy chlidren not to come to the hospital, madame.

不行, 留在家里的孩子可以由你先生或朋友来照顾。夫人, 健康的孩子最好不要到医院来。

Parent：In that case, all right, I will follow you.

要是这样的话, 那好吧, 我听你的。

Doctor：Before you go home, I would like to ask you some questions about your son's history. Madame, how many children have you? Is he the oldest child? Was he born full time? And what was his birth weight? Did he cry right after birth? And where was he born? In China or in your own country? Were you healthy during the pregnancy? What vaccinations has he received? Has he had any illness in the past, such as measles, chickenpox or pneumonia? Any tuberculosis or hepatitis patient in your family or among your friends? Has he any contact with them?

在你回家以前，夫人，我想就你孩子的病史提几个问题，好吗？你有几个孩子？他是最大的吗？他是足月产的吗？他生下来有多重？他生下来以后马上就哭了吗？他是在哪里出生的？在中国还是在你们国家？你怀他的时候身体健康吗？他做过什么预防接种？他过去得过像麻疹、水痘、肺炎这样的病吗？你们家里人和朋友中有没有谁得肝炎或结核病的？他和这些人接触吗？

Parent：He is my second child. He was delivered by Cesarean section, at my native country. Since then there was no more other child. His birth weight was 3.5 kilograms. The doctor told me he was normal at birth. He received all the vaccinations at the proper time as advised by my family physician. He has occasional fevers and colds, otherwise no important illness. He has always been very healthy. His father got hepatitis three months ago. He's still taking medicine and is much better. I am quite healthy, too. The nursemaid takes care of the chlid.

这是我的第二个孩子。他是在我们国家剖宫产出生的。这以后我就再没生孩子了。他出生时体重是3.5公斤，医生告诉我他出生时很正常。我们都是按家庭医生的嘱咐，按时给他做了各种预防接种。他偶尔发烧感冒，但没得过什么严重的病。他一向都很健康。他的父亲三个月前得了肝炎，现在还在吃药，但是他好多了。我很健康。这孩子由阿姨照顾。

Doctor：That's all I want to know. Thank you, madame. If I have any more questions, I'll ask you later. Now you can go home. Are you going to have your supper here tonight?

我要知道的都问到了，谢谢你，夫人。以后我再有问题的话，再随时问你。你现在可以回家了。你今天晚上在我们这里吃晚饭吗？

Parent：No, thank you, I'll eat at home. And I'll be back in about one hour. Meanwhile, please look after my son. He is very naughty. Thank you very much. Good-bye.

不用了，谢谢，我在家吃。大约一个小时后回来。我的孩子很淘气。谢谢你照顾他,再见。

2. The Nurse's Introduction 主管护士介绍

Nurse：Hi, Mr. Smith. I'm Linda, your chief nurse. Now I'll take you to the ward, this way, please.

你好,史密斯先生。我叫琳达,你的主管护士。现在我带你去病房,请这边走。

Patient：Thank you very much. I'm glad to meet you.

谢谢。很高兴认识你。

Nurse：OK, here is your bed, the call button is here and just push it slightly anytime you want a nurse. This bedside table is only for such things as toilet articles rather than any valuables.

这是你的病床。如果要叫护士帮忙,轻按这个呼叫按钮就行了。这个床头柜是放你的洗漱用品的,不要存放贵重物品。

Patient：Thank you. But where is the washroom?

谢谢。卫生间在哪儿?

Nurse：On the right side of the door. And there is another one at the end of the corridor, and bathroom is there, too.

在门的右边。不过走廊的尽头还有一个公用的,浴室也在那儿。

Patient：I see, thanks.

多谢,我知道了。

Nurse：The sitting room is over there, Mr. Smith. You can have your meals, watch TV and enjoy various recreations there. Inform your relatives to visit you from four to seven in the afternoon everyday and nine to eleven on Sunday mornings.

休息室在那边,史密斯先生。你可以在那儿吃饭、看电视和进行各种娱乐活动。还有,通知你的家人探视时间是在每天下午的四到七点及周日上午的九到十一点。

Patient：OK, thank you for your detailed introduction, Linda.

好的,琳达,谢谢你这么详细的介绍。

Nurse：By the way, Mr. Smith. Whenever you want to leave the ward, please let me know.

史密斯先生,顺便说一句,不管你什么时候离开病房,一定告诉我一声。

Patient：No problem，Linda.

没问题，琳达。

Ⅱ. Sentences 替换句型

（1）How do you do? I'm the nurse in charge of this ward. We hope you will feel at home here. This is nurse Hou，and this is Doctor Smith.

你好，我是主管这间病房的护士长，希望你在这儿过得开心愉快。这位是侯护士，这位是你的主管医生，史密斯。

（2）If you need anything，just press this button. (Press the bell if there is anything you need.)

你有什么需要，请按这个按钮。（如果需要什么，按电铃。）

（3）The doctor has gone out on his rounds.

医生已经出去查房了。

（4）You do your ward round at ten.

你十点钟查房。

（5）They walked round the ward talking to the patients.

他们巡视了病房，并与病人谈话。

（6）When the swelling goes down，you'll be able to get up.

肿胀消退后，你就能起床了。

（7）On the fifth day of admission，on waking，he complained of an upper central abdominal pain，nausea and anorexia.

住院的第五天，他醒来之后说胃脘（即上腹中央）痛、恶心、没食欲。

（8）Your child is very good. You don't have to stay in the hospital unless you want to. The nurses can take care of him.

你的孩子很好，你不必留在医院，除非你自己愿意留下。护士会照顾他的。

（9）If someone stays here with you，she or he has to pay for her or his bed.

如果你需要有人陪护，陪护人是必须要交陪住费的。

（10）We don't think companions are necessary. Your condition isn't so serious.

我们认为你不需要陪护，你的病情没那么严重。

(11) Now, I tell you, patients usually get up at 7:00 a. m. and breakfast starts at 8:00 a. m. The ward rounds and treatment begins at 9:00 a. m. Lunch is at noon. After that, you have a snap or rest. Visiting hours are commonly from 3:30 to 7:00 p. m., and supper is at 6:00 p. m. Bed time is from 9:30 to 10:00 p. m.

好的,我现在就告诉你:病人一般是早上 7 点钟起床,8 点钟早餐。上午的查房和治疗在 9 点钟,12 点钟吃午饭,饭后午休。下午的探视时间是 3:30—7:00。晚饭就餐时间安排在 6 点钟。9:30—10:00 期间是病人准备睡觉的时间。

(12) The patient's temperature fell rapidly (The patient's temperature rose last night).

病人的体温迅速下降了(昨晚病人的体温又升高了)。

(13) You are responding well to the treatment.

你对治疗的反应不错。

(14) Which kind of food do you prefer, Chinese or western? And would you mind telling me if you are a Muslim?

请问,你喜欢吃中餐还是西餐? 另外,你介不介意我问一下,你是穆斯林(回民)吗?

(15) Have you eaten (had) your breakfast (lunch, supper) already? And how is your appetite?

你吃过早饭(午饭、晚饭)了吗? 还有你胃口怎样?

(16) What are your eating habits? And are you allergic to certain foods, such as (like) prawns or shrimps?

你的饮食习惯怎样? 还有你对某些食品过敏吗,比如虾类食品?

(17) Please try to eat a little more, and it will help you recover more quickly.

你尽可能多吃点,这样有助于你早日康复。

(18) She kept up her spirits in spite of her illness. And in fact, sick people need plenty of reassurance.

尽管病了,她仍然能振作精神。其实,患者需要很多的安抚。

(19) You needn't stay in bed any longer. You can get up whenever you feel like it.

你不必躺在床上了,你觉得什么时候想起床,就可以起床。

(20) Mr. Zhang, although you don't eat so much, I'd like you to have a

snack in the late afternoon and before going to bed.

张先生,虽然你吃得不多,但我建议你傍晚和睡觉前吃点东西。

(21) If you like, I'll go and get some cough mixure (a sleep pill, a laxative, a tranquilizer, a pain-killer…).

如果你无异议,我就去给你拿些止咳药(安眠药、泻药、安定药、止疼药……)。

(22) If your wound is still hurting, please do let me know.

如果你的伤口还疼的话,一定要告诉我。

(23) If you still feel uncomfortable, I will turn on (off) the heat (electric fan, light…) or I will adjust the air conditioner.

要是你还感觉不舒服,我把暖气(电风扇、灯……)开开(关上)或者我把空调再调整一下。

(24) Do you want me to give you another pillow (cushion, blanket, dressing gown, clean pajamas…)?

你想再要一个枕头(一个靠垫、一条毯子、一件袍子、一条干净的睡裤……)吗?

(25) Do you want to have a bed-bath (have a shower, have a shave, have your hair washed/cut…)?

要我给你擦个澡(洗个淋浴、刮刮胡子、洗洗头/理理发……)吗?

(26) Mrs. Smith, you are wanted on the phone from your embassy (delegation, a long distance call from Shanghai), and by the way, may I throw those flowers away and put these freshes in the vase?

史密斯太太,有个你们大使馆(代表团)打来的电话(上海来的长途电话),顺便,要不要我把那些不新鲜的花扔了,把这些新鲜的帮你插到花瓶里呢?

(27) Mr. Zhang, Doctor Smith has written a certificate for you. Generally speaking, there are two suggestions. Firstly, try to avoid any mental stress and do have a good rest. And secondly, examinations of blood sugar and an EKG should be done regularly at the hospital.

张先生,史密斯医生已经给你开好了诊断证明。总的来说,给你有两个建议。一是要避免精神紧张,注意好好休息;二是要定期到医院做血糖和心电图的检测。

(28) Altogether two thousand and fifty yuan. You may pay either in

cash or by cheque, Mr. Fox.

福克斯先生,总共是 2050 元,你付现金或开支票都行。

(29) The taxi I call for you is on the way to hospital, and it will be here soon.

我给你叫的出租车正往医院来呢,请稍等,马上就到。

(30) It saves patients much trouble if they are discharged from the ward with enough medicine for a few days.

病人出院时,如果给他们带几天的药,这将减少他们很多麻烦。

(31) You are welcome (Don't mention it). That is our duty (job).

你不必客气,这是我们应该做的(我们的职责)。

Ⅲ. Words and Expressions 单词和短语

1. Doctor's Round of Visit Around the Ward 医生查房

abdominal belt 腹带

abdominal trias 腹部三主征

call on a patient; doctor visit 医生查房

carelessness /ˈkeələsnəs/ n. 忽略;粗心

care of the body 身体护理

corrective /kəˈrektɪv/; orthotic /ɔːˈθɒtɪk/ adj. 矫正的

death /deθ/ n. 死亡

diabetic diet 糖尿病食解

diagnosis /ˌdaɪəgˈnəʊsɪs/ n. 诊断

diet cure 食饵疗法

digital examination 指诊检查

displeasure /dɪsˈpleʒə/ n. 不快

dying hour; last moment 临终

erroneous diagnosis; false diagnosis 误诊

first medical examination 初诊检查

future /ˈfjuːtʃə/ n. 将来

girdle of the chest 胸带(围)

hunger /ˈhʌŋgə/ n. 饥饿

loss of eyesight 视力丧失

medical examination/consultation 内科检查/会诊

nurse /nɜːs/; take charge of; look after(persons who are ill, injured, etc.) 看护;护理

obstetric forceps 产钳

occupation /ˌɒkjuˈpeɪʃn/; career /kəˈrɪə/; job /dʒɒb/ n. 职业

operation /ˌɒpəˈreɪʃən/ n. 手术

overfatigue /ˈəʊvəfəˈtiːg/ n. 疲劳过度

oxygen inhalation 吸氧

physical examination 体格检查

rest /rest/ n. 休息

single /ˈsɪŋgl/ adj. 单身的

suggestion /səˈdʒestʃən/ 暗示;提议

suspicious /səˈspɪʃəs/ adj. 怀疑的

therapeutic action 治疗作用

tinnitus /ˈtɪnɪtəs/ n.; ringing (singing) in the ear 耳鸣

to check blooding 检查血液

unquiet /ʌnˈkwaɪət/ *adj.* 不安

unwell /ʌnˈwel/; uneasy /ʌnˈiːzi/ *adj.* 不舒服

venotomy /vɪˈnɒtəmi/; venesection /ˌveniˈsekʃən/ *n.* 静脉切开

want of sleep 嗜睡；睡眠不足

weight of the body 体重

will /wil/ *n.* 遗言

2. Hospital Instruments 医院用具

abdominal binder 腹带

absorbent cotton ball 棉球

absorbent cotton 药棉；脱脂棉

ambulance /ˈæmbjələns/ *n.* 救护车

bandage /ˈbændɪdʒ/ *n.* 绷带

bed pan 便盆

cardiac catheter 心脏导管

dressing carriage 敷料车

dressing tray 敷料盘

enema can 灌肠筒

esophagoscope /iːˈsɒfəɡəʊˌskəʊp/ *n.* 食管镜

fiberscope /ˈfaɪbəˌskəʊp/ *n.* 纤维镜

first-aid kit 急救箱

fluoroscope /ˈfluərəˌskəʊp/ *n.* 透视仪

forceps /ˈfɔːseps/ *n.* 钳子

gastroscope /ˈɡæstrəˌskəʊp/ *n.* 胃镜

gauze dressing 纱布敷料

haemodynamometer /ˌhiːməˌdaɪnəˈmɒmɪtə/; sphygmomanometer /ˌsfɪɡməʊməˈnɒmɪtə/ *n.* 血压计

hand-spittoon; sputum mug 痰盒

hot-water bag 热水袋

ice bag 冰袋

injection syringe *n.* 注射器

laser beam for surgery 激光手术器

mask /mɑːsk/ *n.* 口罩

mercury manometer 水银柱

nipper /ˈnɪpə/ *n.* 镊子

pacemaker /ˈpeɪsˌmeɪkə/ *n.* 起搏器

plaster /ˈplɑːstə/ *n.*; adhesive tape; strapping /ˈstræpɪŋ/ *n.* 橡皮膏

plaster splints 石膏夹板

radio isotope scanner 同位素扫描仪

rubber air-mattress 橡皮气褥

rubber ball syringe 橡皮灌注器

scissors /ˈsɪzəz/; shears /ʃɪəz/ *n.* 剪子

sickbed /ˈsɪkbed/ *n.* 病床

spittoon /spɪˈtuːn/; cuspidor /ˈkʌspɪˌdɔː/ *n.* 痰盂

stethoscope /ˈsteθəskəʊp/ *n.* 听诊器

stretcher /ˈstretʃə/; litter /ˈlɪtə/ *n.* 担架

suture needle 缝针

suture /ˈsuːtʃə/; stitch /stɪtʃ/ *n.* 缝线

syringe-needle *n.* 针头

thermometer-Celsius（centigrade） *n.* 体温表（摄氏）

thermometer-Fahrenheit *n.* 体温表（华氏）

tongue depressor 压舌板

truss /trʌs/ *n.* 疝带

urinal /jʊˈraɪnl/ *n.* 尿壶

vacuum aspirator 人工流产电吸器

wheel chair 轮椅

wheel stretcher 推床

X-ray apparatus X线机

Section 3　Visiting
第3节　探视

Ⅰ. Dialogue 情景对话

Warm Warns After an Operation 术后温馨提示

Doctor：Congratulations, the operation went very well. Please do remember to turn from side to side every two or three hours.

恭喜恭喜,手术非常顺利。不过,你要记住,每两三个小时要翻一次身。

Patient：Yes, I will, thank you very much. But now I feel a mild pain, and I don't think pain-killer is necessary.

谢谢,我记住了。现在我感到有些微微的疼,不过我想也用不着吃止疼片了。

Doctor：All right, if you can stand it.

好的,如果你能忍受的话,不吃也行。

Patient：Thanks a lot.

多谢你了。

Doctor：Take it easy. Three days later, with others' help, you can try walking around the room or corridor.

放松点。三天后,别人搀扶你,你可以试着在房间、走廊里走动走动了。

Patient：That's perfectly quite right. I'm looking forward to it.

那太好了,我就盼着这天哪。

Ⅱ. Sentences 替换句型

(1) Sorry to bother you all.

不好意思,麻烦你们大家了。

(2) I'm sorry to hear you are not feeling well. How are you right now?

听说你病了我很难过,你现在怎么样了?

(3) How is your cold? Well, I must say you look much better than when I saw you last time.

你的感冒怎么样了? 我看你比我上次来看你时好多了。

(4) Honestly speaking, the intensive care unit is costly.

说实话,特护病房花费太高了。

(5) Is it possible for my sister to stay here with me?

我姐姐可以在这里陪护我吗?

(6) Patients look forward to visiting time.

病人们盼望着探视时间。

(7) The patient tried to raise himself up on his elbows.

病人自己设法用肘支起身子。

(8) Doctor told me to rest as much as possible with my foot up.

医生告诉我抬高脚,尽可能地休息。

(9) What are the hours here for meals?

这儿都是什么时候开饭呢?

(10) Would you please show me where the sitting-room, bathroom and telephone are?

你能告诉我休息室、淋浴间和电话在哪儿吗?

(11) He/she prefers western food.

他/她爱吃西餐。

(12) Doctor, why hasn't she any appetite?

医生,为什么她没胃口呢?

(13) He has no appetite at all.

他一点食欲都没有。

(14) You shouldn't eat so much greasy food, and I suggest you take more vegetables and gruel (porridge, noodles, toast...) than meat.

你不应该吃那么多油腻的食品。我建议你多吃些蔬菜、大米粥(稀饭、面条、烤面包……),少吃些肉类。

(15) Since my teeth are poor, I want to eat some soft sweet food and tender meat.

我的牙不好,所以我想吃些甜软的食品和嫩肉。

(16) I'm hungry (thirsty, constipated…), and I don't sleep well at night.

我饿(渴、便秘……),而且,晚上睡眠不怎么好。

(17) He hasn't had (has had) his breakfast. It seems that his appetite is not so good (just so so).

他还没吃早饭(已经吃过早饭了),不过,他的胃口不怎么好(一般般)。

(18) It's too noisy (hot, cold, draughty) inside (outside).

里面(外面)太吵(太热、太冷、风太大)了。

(19) I brought some flowers for you. Let me put them in that vase over there. Oh, may I close (open) the door (window)?

我带了些花来看你,插在那边的花瓶里吧。噢,我可以关上(打开)门(窗户)吗?

(20) You have been in the hospital for almost two weeks, haven't you?

你已经住院快两个星期了,是吧?

(21) You are going to be discharged the day after tomorrow. Take care of yourself.

你后天就可以出院了,请多保重。

(22) I'll go to the admission office to get your bill at once.

我马上到住院处把你的账给结了。

(23) How much do I owe you? And may I pay it by cheque?

我还欠医院多少钱? 能否用支票结账呢?

(24) I must go now. Would you please call a taxi for me?

我要出院了,请给我叫辆出租车,好吗?

(25) I'm really so grateful to you all. You were all so kind to me.

你们对我都那么好,我非常感谢大家。

(26) My doctor(organization) needs my medical(case) history. May I have it tomorrow before I leave?

我的医生(单位)需要查看我的病历,明天我出院前你们能给我吗?

(27) I hear you've been discharged. And a medical social worker helps patients with personal and domestic difficulties.

我听说你已经出院了。而且,社区的医务工作者帮助病人解决个人和家庭困难。

(28) The hospital that I visited had 700 beds.

我参观的那家医院有 700 张病床。

(29) You should have a good rest. I hope you will be all right soon.

你好好休息吧。祝你早日康复。

(30) I must go now, and I will see you again tomorrow morning and hope to find you better.

我现在得走了。明天上午我再来看你,真的希望你的病会好些。

Ⅲ. Words and Expressions 单词和短语

1. Food and Drinks 饮食

a bit; a bite 一点

a course 一道菜

afternoon tea 午茶

a piece 一块

a portion 一份

appetizer /'æpɪˌtaɪzə/;
　aperitif /əˌperə'tiːf/ *n*. 开胃品

a slice 一片

a strip 一条

barley /'bɑːli/ *n*. 大麦

bar /bɑː/ *n*. 酒吧

bean /biːn/ *n*. 豆类

bean curd 豆腐

bean milk 豆浆

beverage /'bevərɪdʒ/ *n*. 饮料

breakfast /'brekfəst/ *n*. 早饭

buckwheat /'bʌkwiːt/ *n*. 荞麦

café /'kæfeɪ/ *n*. 咖啡馆

carp /kɑːp/; tench /tentʃ/ *n*. 鲤鱼

celery /'seləri/ *n*. 芹菜

cereal /'sɪərɪəl/; grain /greɪn/ *n*. 谷物

cherry /'tʃeri/ *n*. 樱桃

cod-liver oil 鱼肝油

condiment /'kɒndɪmənt/ *n*. 调味品

corn flour 玉米面

crab /kræb/ *n*. 螃蟹

cured meat 腊肉

delicatessen /ˌdelɪkə'tesn/ *n*. 熟食店

diet /'daɪət/ *n*. 规定的饮食

dining hall; commons /'kɒmənz/ *n*. ;
　mess /mes/ *n*. 食堂

dining room 饭厅

dinner /'dɪnə/ *n*. 晚饭;正餐

dried shrimps 海米

edible /'edəbl/; eatables /'iːtəblz/ *n*.
　食用品

eel /iːl/ *n*. 鳗鱼

fat /fæt/ *n*. 脂肪

fillet /'fɪlɪt/ *n*. 里脊

fruit /fruːt/ *n*. 水果

full course 份饭

game /geɪm/ *n*. 野味

good appetite 胃口好

goose egg 鹅蛋

gourmet /'ɡʊəmeɪ/ *n*. 讲究吃的人

grain of rice 米粒

hairtail /'heəˌteɪl/ *n*. 带鱼

ham /hæm/ *n*. 火腿

horse bean 蚕豆

leek /li:k/ n. 韭菜

lettuce /ˈletɪs/ n. 生菜

lime-preserved egg 松花皮蛋

lunch /lʌntʃ/; luncheon /ˈlʌntʃən/;
  tiffin /ˈtɪfɪn/ n. 午饭

malnutrition /ˌmælnjuˈtrɪʃn/ n. 营养不良

meal /miːl/ n. 饭；餐

meat balls 肉丸

meat /miːt/ n. 肉类

menu /ˈmenjuː/ n. 菜单

mineral /ˈmɪnərəl/ n. 矿物质

molecule /ˈmɒlɪkjuːl/ n. 分子

mutton /ˈmʌtn/ n. 羊肉

nourishment /ˈnʌrɪʃmənt/ n. 营养

nurture /ˈnɜːtʃə/; nutriment
  /ˈnjuːtrɪmənt/ n. 营养品

nut /nʌt/ n. 坚果

oatmeal /ˈəʊtmiːl/ n. 麦片

oat /əʊt/ n. 燕麦

on diet 节食；控制体重地吃

parsley /ˈpɑːsli/ n. 香菜

pea /piː/ n. 豌豆

peel /piːl/; pare /peə/ v. 削皮

peptone /ˈpeptəʊn/ n. 蛋白胨

perch /pɜːtʃ/ n. 鲈鱼

pigeon egg 鸽蛋

poor appetite 胃口不好

pork /pɔːk/ n. 猪肉

potato /pəˈteɪtəʊ/ n. 土豆

potato starch 土豆淀粉

poultry /ˈpəʊltri/ n. 禽类

prawn /prɔːn/ n. 大虾

pressing forceps 麦穗钳

protein /ˈprəʊtiːn/ n. 蛋白质

provision /prəˈvɪʒən/ n. 粮食

pump /pʌmp/ n. 汲筒

quail /kweɪl/ n. 鹌鹑

recipe /ˈresəpi/ n.; cook book 食谱

refreshment kiosk 小吃亭

refreshment shop 小吃店

restaurant /ˈrestrɒnt/ n. 饭馆

rib /rɪb/ n. 排骨

salted egg 咸蛋

sausage /ˈsɒsɪdʒ/ n. 香肠

saveloy /ˈsævəlɔɪ/ n. 腊肠

seafood /ˈsiːfuːd/ n. 海鲜

seaweed /ˈsiːˌwiːd/; kelp /kelp/ n. 海带

shell /ʃel/ v. 剥皮

shrimp /ʃrɪmp/ n. 小虾

silver carp; black carp 鲫鱼

simple fare; pot luck 家常便饭

snack /snæk/; fast food 快餐

snack bar 快餐饭店

soft-boiled egg 软熟蛋

spinach /ˈspɪnɪtʃ/ n. 菠菜

staple food 主食

starch /stɑːtʃ/ n. 淀粉

subsidiary food 副食

supper /ˈsʌpə/ n. 晚饭

sweet /swiːt/; candy /ˈkændi/ n. 糖果

veal /viːl/ n. 小牛肉

vegetable /ˈvedʒtəbl/ n. 蔬菜

vegetarian /ˌvedʒəˈteəriən/ n. 素食者

vitamin /ˈvɪtəmɪn/ n. 维生素

walnut /ˈwɔːlnʌt/ n. 核桃

white of egg; egg white;
  albumen /ˈælbjʊmɪn/ n. 蛋白

yellow of egg; egg yolk 蛋黄

2. 人体各组织名称

acoustic organ 听觉器官

circulatory system 循环系统

digestive system 消化系统

endocrine system 内分泌系统

excretory system 排泄系统

hematogenic organ 造血器官

human body 人体

lymphatic system 淋巴系统

muscular system 肌肉系统

nervous system 神经系统

olfactory organ 嗅觉器官

reproductive system 生殖系统

respiratory system 呼吸系统

sense organ 感觉器官

skeletal system 骨骼系统

tissues /ˈtɪʃuː/ *n.* 组织

urinary system 泌尿系统

visual organ 视觉器官

Appendix

附 录

1. 常用国内外知名医学期刊、机构的中英文名称

AAA（Ambulance Association of America）美国救护协会

AAMP（American Academy of Medical Prevention）美国医疗预防学会

AAN（American Academy of Nursing）美国护理学会

AAPM&R（American Academy of Physical Medicine and Rehabilitation）美国物理医学和康复医学学会

AAS（American Academy of Sciences）美国科学院

ABMAC（American Bureau for Medical Aid to China）美国对华医学援助局

ABMS（American Board of Medical Specialties）美国医学专业委员会

ACC（American College of Cardiology）美国心脏病学会

ACGP（American College of General Practitioners）美国全科医师学会

ACLM（American College of Legal Medicine）美国法医学会

ACOG（American College of Obstetricians and Gynecologists）美国妇产科医师学会

ACP（American College of Pharmacists）美国药剂师学会

ACP（American College of Physicians）美国内科医师学会

ACR（American College of Radiology）美国放射学学会

ACS（American College of Surgeons）美国外科医师学会

Acta Pharmacologica Sinica《中国药理学报》

AGA（American Gastroenterological Association）美国胃肠病学协会

AGA（American Genetic Association）美国遗传学协会

AGS（American Geriatrics Society）美国老年病学会

AHA（American Hospital Association）美国医院协会

AHIB（American Health Information Bank）美国卫生信息库

AIBS（American Institute of Biological Sciences）美国生物科学研究所

All-China Association of Traditional Chinese Medicine 中华全国中医学会

AMA（American Medical Association）美国医学会

American Heart Journal《美国心脏杂志》

American Journal of Cardiology《美国心脏学杂志》

American Journal of Clinical Pathology《美国临床病理学杂志》

American Journal of Diseases of Children《美国儿童疾病杂志》

American Journal of Epidemiology《美国流行病学杂志》

American Journal of Human Genetics《美国人类遗传学杂志》

American Journal of Public Health《美国公共卫生杂志》

American Journal of Surgery《美国外科学杂志》

American Journal of the Medical Sciences《美国医学科学杂志》

American Review of Respiratory Diseases《美国呼吸疾病评论》

ANA（American Nurses Association）美国护士协会

ANCD（Australian National Council on Drugs）全国药物委员会（澳）

ARC（American Red Cross）美国红十字会

Archives of Internal Medicine《内科学文献》

Archives of Neurology《神经病学文献》

Archives of Physical Medicine and Rehabilitation《物理医学和康复文献》

Archives of Surgery《外科学文献》

ASA（American Society of Anesthesiologists）美国麻醉学家学会

ASHG（American Society for Human Genetics）美国人类遗传学会

ASII（American Science Information Institute）美国科学信息研究所

Association for the Dissemination of Science and Technology 科技普及协会

BCS（British Cardiac Society）英国心脏学会

Biochemical Journal《生物化学学报》（英）

BMA（British Medical Association）英国医学会

BPA（British Pediatric Association）英国儿科协会

BPC（British Pharmacopoeia Commission）英国药典委员会

British Heart Journal《英国心脏杂志》

British Journal of Cancer《英国癌症杂志》

British Journal of Radiology《英国放射学杂志》

British Medical Journal《英国医学杂志》

British Pharmaceutical Codex《英国药典》

CAHEP（Chinese Association of Health Education and Promotion）中国

健康教育与健康促进协会

CAMS (Chinese Academy of Medical Sciences)中国医学科学院

Cancer Research《癌研究》

CAPM (Chinese Academy of Preventive Medicine)中国预防医学科学院

CATCM (China Academy of Traditional Chinese Medicine)中国中医研究院

CDC (Centers for Disease Control and Pevention)疾病控制和预防中心(美)

Center for Medical Exchange with Foreign Countries 对外医学交流中心

China National Health Education Center 中国健康教育中心

Chinese Association of the Integration of Traditional and Western Medicine 中国中西医结合研究所

Chinese Journal of Cancer Research《中国癌症研究》

Chinese Journal of Integrated Traditional and Western Medicine《中国中西医结合杂志》

Chinese Journal of Traumatology《中华创伤杂志》

Chinese Medical Journal《中华医学杂志》(英文版)

Chinese Medical Sciences Journal《中国医学科学杂志》

Clinical and Experimental Immunology《临床和实验免疫学》

Clinical Science《临床科学》(英)

CMA (Chinese Medical Association)中华医学会

CNA (Chinese Nursing Association)中华护理学会

CPMA (Chinese Preventive Medicine Association)中华预防医学会

Critical Care Medicine《危重医学》(美)

Current Contents《现期文献目录》

CWI (China Welfare Institute)中国福利会

Digestive Diseases and Sciences《消化道疾病与科学》

EDTA (European Dialysis and Transplant Association) 欧洲透析与移植协会

Education Council for Foreign Medical Students 外国医学生教育委员会

Environmental Health Perspectives《环境卫生展望》(美)

FDA (Food and Drug Administration)食品与药物管理局(美)

Genetical Research《遗传研究》(美)

HUGO (Human Genome Organization)人类基因组(国际)组织

IAEA (International Atomic Energy Agency)国际原子能机构

IAPC（International Association for Pollution Control）国际污染控制协会

IAPM（International Academy of Preventive Medicine ）国际预防医学学会

IARC（International Agency for Research on Cancer）国际癌症研究组织

ICN（International Council of Nurses）国际护士理事会

ICRC（International Committee of the Red Cross）国际红十字委员会

ICSU（International Council of Scientific Unions）国际科学联合会理事会

IFCR（International Foundation For Cancer Research）国际癌症研究基金会

IFMBE （ International Federation for Medical and Biological Engineering）国际医学生物工程联合会

IFME（International Federation for Medical Electronics）国际医学电子学联合会

ILSI（International Life Sciences Institute）国际生命科学研究会

IMIC（International Medical Information Center）国际医学信息中心

Index Medicus《医学索引》

Institute of Medical Science Information 医学情报研究所

International Cardiovascular Society 国际心血管学会

International Journal of Cancer《国际癌症杂志》

International Medical Digest《国际医学文摘》

IOS（International Organization for Standardization）国际标准化组织

IPPF（International Planned Parenthood Federation）国际计划生育联合会

IRCD（International Rehabilitation Center for the Disabled）国际残疾人康复中心

ISBN（International Standard Book Number）国际标准图书编号

ISBI（International Society for Burn Injuries）国际烧伤学会

ISC（International Society of Cardiology）国际心脏病学会

ISN（International Society of Nephrology）国际肾脏病学会

ISO（International Standards Organization）国际标准（审定）组织

ISRM（International Society of Reproductive Medicine）国际生殖医学会

ISSN（International Standard Serial Number）国际标准期刊编号

IUPHAR（International Union of Pharmacology）国际药理学联合会

IUPS（International Union of Physiological Sciences）国际生理科学联合会

Journal of American Medicine《美国医学杂志》

Journal of Canadian Medical Association《加拿大医学会杂志》

Journal of Chinese Pharmaceutical Sciences《中国药学》

Journal of Clinical Endocrinology and Metabolism《临床内分泌学和代谢杂志》

Journal of Clinical Pharmacology《临床药理学杂志》

Journal of Clinical Pharmacy《临床药学杂志》

Journal of Immunology《免疫学杂志》

Journal of Medical Education《医学教育杂志》

Journal of Molecular Biology《分子生物学杂志》(英)

Journal of the American Medical Association《美国医学会杂志》

Journal of Thoracic and Cardiovascular Surgery《胸腔和心血管外科杂志》

Journal of Trauma《创伤杂志》

Medical Journal of Australia《澳大利亚医学杂志》

MICA (Maternity and Infant Care Association) 妇婴保健协会

Microvascular Research《微血管研究》

MLA (Medical Library Association)医学图书馆协会

NADUS (National Association of Doctors in the United States)美国全国医师协会

NARS (National Acupuncture Research Society)全国针疗研究会(美)

National Administration of Traditional Chinese Medicine 国家中医药管理局

National Center for Chronic Disease Control 全国慢性病控制中心

National Health Commission of the People's Republic of China 中华人民共和国国家卫生健康委员会

National Medical Journal of China《中华医学杂志》

Nature《自然》(英)

NBME (National Board of Medical Examiners)全国医学考核委员会(美)

NBRF (National Biomedical Research Foundation)全国生物医学研究基金会

NBS (National Bureau of Standards)国家标准局

NCBI (National Center for Biotechnology Information)国家生物技术信息中心(美)

NCLEX-RN (National Council Licensure Examination for Registered Nurses)全国注册护士执照考试委员会

NCMTE (National Council on Medical Technology Education)全国医学

技术教育委员会

New England Journal of Medicine《新英格兰医学杂志》(美)

NFME (National Fund for Medical Education)全国医学教育基金会(美)

NICHD (National Institute of Child Health and Human Development)国家儿童健康与发育研究所(美)

NIEHS (National Institute of Environmental Health Sciences)国家环境卫生科学研究所(美)

NLNE (National League for Nursing Education)全国护理教育联合会(美)

NMAC (National Medical Audiovisual Center)全国医学视听中心(美)

NPHCC (National Patriotic Health Campaign Committee)全国爱国卫生运动委员会

NSF (National Science Foundation)全国科学基金会

PAHO (Pan-American Health Organization)泛美卫生组织

Pediatric Clinics of North America《北美儿科诊所》

Pharmaceutical Abstracts《药学文摘》

Pharmaceutical Archives《药学文献》

Pharmaceutical Bulletin《药学通报》

Pharmacological Reviews《药理学评论》

Pharmacopoeia Galisa《法国药典》

Pharmacopoeia Germanica《德国药典》

Pharmacopoeia Internationalis《国际药典》

Pharmacopoeia Japonica《日本药典》

Plastic and Reconstructive Surgery《整形与再造外科杂志》

Proceedings of the National Academy of Sciences of the United States of America《美国国家科学院院刊》

Progress in Cardiovascular Diseases《心血管疾病进展》

RCS (Royal College of Science)皇家科学院(英)

RCSC (Red Cross Society of China)中国红十字总会

RSM (Royal Society of Medicine)皇家医学会(英)

Science《科学》(美)

Science and Technology Information Center 科技情报中心

Science Citation Index《科学引文索引》

Scientific and Technological Information Research Institution 科技情报研究所

SNM (Society of Nuclear Medicine)核医学学会

Transplantation Proceedings《移植进展》(美)

The Lancet《柳叶刀》(英)

UNICEF (United Nations Children's Fund)联合国儿童基金会

WHO (World Health Organization)世界卫生组织

WMA (World Medical Association)世界医学协会

2. 医学学位、职称、职务常用术语

(1) 医学学位名称。

Bachelor of Medicine 医学学士

Bachelor of Nursing 护理学学士

Bachelor of Pharmacy 药学学士

Bachelor of Science 理学学士

Bachelor of Surgery 外科学士

Doctor of Anesthesiology 麻醉学博士

Doctor of Dental Medicine 牙医学博士

Doctor of Dental Science 牙科学博士

Doctor of Nursing 护理学博士

Doctor of Ophthalmology 眼科学博士

Doctor of Pharmacy 药学博士

Doctor of Philosophy 哲学博士

Doctor of Psychology 心理学博士

Doctor of Public Health 公共卫生博士

Doctor of Radiology 放射学博士

Doctor of Science 理学博士

Doctor of Surgery 外科博士

Master of Anesthesiology 麻醉学硕士

Master of Dental Science 牙科学硕士

Master of Medicine 医学硕士

Master of Nursing 护理学硕士

Master of Pharmacy 药学硕士

Master of Public Health 公共卫生硕士

Master of Radiology 放射学硕士

Master of Science 理学硕士

Master of Surgery 外科硕士

Master of the Art of Obstetrics 产科硕士

Medical Doctor 医学博士

Medicinae Baccalaureus 医学学士

Medicinae Doctor 医学博士

Pharmaciae Baccalaureus 药学学士

Pharmaciae Doctor 药学博士

Pharmaciae Magister 药学硕士

（2）医院内相关职称名称。

professor /prəˈfesə/ *n*. 教授

assistant professor 助理教授（在美国介于副教授和讲师之间）

associate chief surgeon 外科副主任医师

associate chief-physician 副主任医师

associate professor 副教授

associate research fellow 副研究员

attending physician/doctor；visiting physician/doctor 主治医师

chief physician 主任医师

chief surgeon；surgeon-in-chief 外科主任医师

consultant /kənˈsʌltənt/ *n*.（英）顾问医师、专家

consultant cardiologist（英）顾问心脏学家

consultant chest physician（英）顾问胸科医师

consultant obstetrician and gynecologist 顾问妇产科医师

consultant surgeon（英）顾问外科医师

emeritus professor 荣誉退休教授

house officer 住院医师

house physician（英）住院医师

intern /ˈɪntɜːn/；interne /ˈɪntɜːn/ *n*. 实习医师

lecturer /ˈlektʃərə/ *n*. 讲师

registrar /ˌredʒɪˈstrɑː/ *n*.（英）住院医师

research assistant 助理研究员

research fellow；researcher /rɪˈsɜːtʃə/ *n*. 研究员

resident physician/doctor；resident /ˈrezɪdənt/ *n*. 住院医师

senior lecturer 高级讲师

senior research fellow 高级研究员

teaching assistant 助教

visiting professor；guest professor 客座教授

(3) 医院内相关职务名称。

acupuncturist /ˈækjʊpʌŋktʃərɪst/ n. 针灸师

anesthetist /əˈniːsθətɪst/ n. 麻醉科医师

assistant pharmacist 药剂师

cardiac surgeon 心脏科医师

cardiologist /ˌkaːdɪˈɒlədʒɪst/ n. 心脏科医师

chief resident doctor 总住院医师

dentist /ˈdentɪst/ n. 牙科医师

deputy director of the hospital 副院长

dermatologist /ˌdɜːməˈtɒlədʒɪst/ n. 皮肤科医师

dietician /ˌdaɪəˈtɪʃn/ n. 营养医师

director of nursing；head of nursing 护理部主任

director of the hospital 院长

doctor for infectious diseases 传染病科医师

endocrinologist /ˌendəʊkrɪˈnɒlədʒɪst/ n. 内分泌科医师

ENT doctor；ear, nose, and throat specialist 耳鼻喉科医师

eye doctor；oculist /ˈɒkjəlɪst/ n.；ophthalmologist /ˌɒfθælˈmɒlədʒɪst/ n.
眼科医师

gastroenterologist /ˌɡæstrəʊˌentəˈrɒlədʒɪst/ n. 消化科医师

general practitioner 全科医生

gynecologist /ˌɡaɪnɪˈkɒlədʒɪst/ n. 妇科医师

head nurse 护士长

head of…department……科主任

head of the out-patient department 门诊部主任

health doctor 卫生医师

health educator 健康教育工作者

health worker 卫生工作者

inhalation therapist 气雾师

laboratory technician 检验师

massager /ˈmæsaːʒə/ n. 按摩师

matron /ˈmeɪtrən/ n. 总护士长

medical assistant; practitioner with secondary medical school education 医士

medical director 医务部主任

medical man; doctor /ˈdɒktə/ n. 医生

medical officer; military surgeon 军医

medical personnel; medical staff 医务人员

medical student 医学生

medical worker 医务工作者

nephrologist /nɪˈfrɒlədʒɪst/ n. 肾脏科医师

neurologist /njʊəˈrɒlədʒɪst/ n. 神经科医师

neurosurgeon /ˌnjʊərəʊˈsɜːdʒən/ n.; neurosurgical doctor 神经外科医师

nurse /nɜːs/ n. 护士

nursing aide 助理护士

obstetrician /ˌɒbstəˈtrɪʃn/ n. 产科医师

optometrist /ɒpˈtɒmɪtrɪst/ n. 验光师

orderly /ˈɔːdəli/ n. 护理员

orthopedist /ˌɔːθəʊˈpiːdɪst/ n. 矫形外科医师

paramedic /ˌpærəˈmedɪk/ n. 医务辅助人员

pathologist /pəˈθɒlədʒɪst/ n. 病理科医师

pediatrician /ˌpiːdiəˈtrɪʃn/; pediatrist /piːˈdaɪətrɪst/ n. 儿科医师

pharmacist /ˈfɑːməsɪst/; pharmaceutist /ˌfɑːməˈsjuːtɪst/ n. 药剂师

physician /fɪˈzɪʃn/; internist /ɪnˈtɜːnɪst/ n. 内科医师

physician of traditional Chinese medicine 中医师

physiotherapist /ˌfɪziəʊˈθerəpɪst/ n. 理疗科医师

plastic surgeon 整形外科医师

practitioner /prækˈtɪʃənə/ n. 开业医师

psychiatrist /saɪˈkaɪətrɪst/ n.; mental doctor 精神科医师

radiologist /ˌreɪdɪˈɒlədʒɪst/ n. 放射科医师

registered nurse 注册护士

stomatologist /ˌstəʊməˈtɒlədʒɪst/ n. 口腔科医师

student nurse 实习护士

surgeon /ˈsɜːdʒən/ n. 外科医师

technician /tekˈnɪʃn/ n. 技术员

thoracic surgeon; surgeon of thoracic surgery 胸外科医师

urological surgeon 泌尿外科医师

X-ray technician X 线技师

(4) 各级、各类综合及专科医院及相关单位名称。

center for disease prevention and control 疾病预防控制中心

children's hospital 儿童医院

clinic /ˈklɪnɪk/；dispensary /dɪˈspensəri/ *n*. 诊所

community hospital 社区医院

county hospital 县立医院

drugstore /ˈdrʌgstɔː/；chemist's shop；pharmacy /ˈfɑːməsi/ *n*. 药房；药店

epidemic prevention station 防疫站

general hospital 综合医院

hospice /ˈhɒspɪs/ *n*. 临终关怀医院

hospital /ˈhɒspɪtl/ *n*.；health center 卫生院

hospital of oncology 肿瘤医院

hospital of traditional Chinese medicine 中医院

infirmary /ɪnˈfɜːməri/；dispensary /dɪˈspensəri/ *n*. 医务室(所)

in-patient department 住院部

institute for health education 健康教育所

maternity hospital 产科医院

medical station；health center 医疗站

mortuary /ˈmɔːtʃəri/ *n*. 太平间

municipal hospital 市立医院

operating room；operating theater 手术室

out-patient department 门诊部

plastic surgery hospital 整形外科医院

private clinic 私人诊所

private hospital 私立医院

psychiatric hospital；mental home；mental hospital；mental institution 精神病院

public hospital 公立医院

shop（store）of traditional Chinese medicine；Chinese pharmacy；Chinese drugstore 中药店

special hospital 专科医院

stomatological hospital 口腔医院